CONTRIBUTORS ▶

Eleanor K. Flores, M.Ed., B.S.N., R.N. Eleanor is program director for Medical Assisting at Lincoln College of New England in Southington, Connecticut. Eleanor's professional affiliations include membership in the American Association of Medical Assistants and Connecticut Society of Medical Assistant (CSMA), for which she served on the board of directors.

Barbara Marchelletta, B.S. Barbara is program director of Allied Health (including the Medical Assisting program) at Beal College in Bangor, Maine. Barbara's professional affiliations include membership in the American Association of Medical Assistants (AAMA) and American Association of Professional Coders. She is also a surveyor for the Medical Assistant Education Review Board.

Expert Reviewer

Cheryl Goretti, M.A. Biological Sciences; B.S. Medical Technology. Cheryl is Professor/Coordinator of Medical Assisting and other Allied Health Programs at Quinebaug Valley Community College in Danielson, Connecticut. Cheryl's professional affiliations include membership in a variety of organizations including American Society of Clinical Pathologists, Northeast Association of Clinical Microbiology and Infectious Disease, and American Association of Medical Assistants.

MEDICAL
ASSISTANT EXAM

Other Titles of Interest from LearningExpress

Becoming a Healthcare Professional
Health Occupations Entrance Exams

Manuscript developed by MTM Publishing, Inc.
www.mtmpublishing.com

President: Valerie Tomaselli
Project Editor: Cynthia Yazbek
Project Coordinator: Zach Gajewski

MEDICAL ASSISTANT EXAM ▶

Preparation for the CMA and RMA Exams

Second Edition

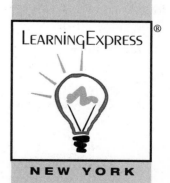

LEARNINGEXPRESS®

NEW YORK

Library of Congress Cataloging-in-Publication Data

Medical assistant exam : preparation for the CMA and RMA exams.—2nd ed.
     p. ; cm.
  ISBN 978-1-57685-924-7
  I. LearningExpress (Organization)
  [DNLM: 1. Medical Assistance—Examination Questions.   W 18.2]
  610.76—dc23

                                                          2013001028

Printed in the United States of America

9 8 7 6 5 4 3 2 1

ISBN-13: 978-1-57685-924-7

For more information or to place an order, contact LearningExpress at:
        80 Broad Street
        Suite 400
        New York, NY 10004

Or visit us at:
        www.learningexpressllc.com

CONTENTS

MEDICAL
ASSISTANT EXAM

CHAPTER 1

THE MEDICAL ASSISTANT PROFESSION

CHAPTER SUMMARY

A medical assistant is a trained, multi-skilled medical professional who performs administrative and clinical tasks in a wide variety of settings, such as medical offices, clinics, and hospitals. Medical assistants can work under the direct supervision of a physician, an office manager, or another healthcare practitioner. One of the fastest growing healthcare careers, the medical assisting profession is expected to continue growing because of the expansion of the healthcare industry and the increasing health needs of the aging U.S. population. These factors make medical assisting a stable career option in the healthcare field.

Medical assisting offers a challenging career to individuals who enjoy working with people and want to be involved in helping people lead healthier lives. A medical assistant has the opportunity to be actively involved in patient care not only by performing many administrative and clinical procedures, but also by providing moral support and comfort to patients of all ages. Working as a medical assistant is a rewarding profession that can provide personal satisfaction by fulfilling a vital role in the medical office.

Background and History of the Profession

A profession is a calling or a vocation founded on specialized educational training. Historically, medical assistants were trained on the job, because no structured educational facilities were available to teach students the administrative and clinical skills needed in the physician's office. Over the years, because of advancements in technology, an increased need for qualified medical assistants, an increase in malpractice lawsuits, and a lack of consistency with on-the-job training, various types of medical assisting educational programs emerged. In 1956, medical assisting was designated a profession and a national organization, the American Association of Medical Assistants (AAMA), was formed. Another medical agency, the American Medical Technologists, a national certifying agency for laboratory professionals since 1939, began offering a certification examination for medical assistants in the early 1970s. These professional organizations were instrumental in shaping the educational requirements needed for medical assisting programs and listing the skills for the administrative and clinical areas of medical assisting.

The duties of a medical assistant may vary depending on the place of employment, the size of the medical practice, and the specialty of the practitioner. Although a medical assistant may work in a variety of medical facilities, the majority work in physicians' offices and other outpatient facilities. The medical assistant is an important team member in such offices and facilities and is responsible for their smooth and proper operation.

The Working Environment

Many medical assistants work a 40-hour workweek, Monday through Friday, although the type of facility where the medical assistant is employed may require medical assistants to work some evenings, weekends, and even holidays. For example, walk-in centers and hospitals are open seven days a week and 24 hours a day, and need medical assistants to work various shifts to cover these hours.

The environments in which medical assistants work are usually busy and involve constant interactions with many people, as medical assistants often serve as a liaison between the patient and the physician. Administrative medical assistants typically work in the front office and perform a number of administrative duties. These tasks include:

- greeting patients
- answering the phone and triaging (screening) incoming calls
- taking phone messages
- collecting patient data during registration
- setting up and maintaining patient records
- scheduling patient appointments
- billing and payment collection
- posting patient charges and payments
- handling correspondence
- processing outgoing mail
- scheduling inpatient and outpatient diagnostic procedures and laboratory tests

WHAT'S IN A NAME?

A patient calls to you, a medical assistant, as you walk down the hall of the medical office, "Nurse, Nurse." What should the medical assistant do? He or she should respond to the patient, but also should inform the patient that the medical assistant is not a nurse. If the patient is not corrected—and is left to believe that he or she is speaking with a nurse and not a medical assistant—a charge of the illegal use of the title *nurse* may be brought against the medical assistant. This is a felony punishable by law.

SPECIALIZED MEDICAL ASSISTANTS

Although medical assistants are trained in both administrative and clinical skills, some medical assistants prefer to specialize in areas such as podiatry, a field of medicine relating to the care of the foot, or ophthalmology, a field of medicine relating to the care of the eye. A podiatric medical assistant earns a certifying credential from the American Society of Podiatric Medical Assistants and may be trained to make castings of the feet, assist in surgery, and take and process X-rays. An ophthalmic medical assistant earns a certifying credential from the Joint Commission on Allied Health Personnel in Ophthalmology and may be trained to perform vision tests using an eye chart, assist in surgery, and educate patients on inserting, removing, and caring for contact lenses. There are three levels of certification for ophthalmic medical assistants. An entry-level ophthalmic medical assistant has a salary range of $23,000 to $32,000, according to "Your Career as an Ophthalmic Medical Assistant" (http://www.cccti.edu/healthsci/oma_main.htm).

A medical administrative specialist is a multi-skilled practitioner in front office management including records management, insurance processing, and basic office management tasks, and is responsible for coordinating administrative functions in the healthcare setting. A medical administrative specialist may be a graduate of a medical assisting program, may have earned an RMA credential, and must have worked as an administrative specialist for at least five years in the field before applying for the Certified Medical Administrative Specialist (CMAS) credential awarded by the certification agency and professional organization American Medical Technologists (AMT).

- maintaining inventory
- ordering supplies
- handling correspondence
- processing insurance claims

The administrative medical assistant sets the tone of the medical office. He or she should provide a warm, friendly environment for all patients. The medical assistant is usually the first person to make contact with a patient, either by phone or when the patient arrives for his or her appointment. First impressions are important, and a skilled medical assistant is trained to project a warm personality, making patients feel welcome and confident in the medical care they are to receive.

Clinical medical assisting skills include:

- taking medical histories
- measuring vital signs
- performing diagnostic procedures such as electrocardiograms
- preparing patients for examinations

- assisting physicians in medical and surgical procedures
- changing dressings
- removing sutures
- preparing and administering medications (depending on state laws and regulations)
- drawing blood (phlebotomy)
- collecting and processing laboratory specimens
- providing patient education

The working environment in a medical facility demands much interaction and communication with patients and their families and with other members of the healthcare team. A medical assistant needs critical thinking skills, a wide range of administrative and clinical skills, and good communication skills. The skills performed will vary depending on the type of facility.

Salary and Benefits

The salary for a medical assistant depends on several factors: the medical assistant's skill level, his or her years of experience in the field, the existence of a certifying credential (CMA or RMA), the location of the facility, and the type of facility at which the medical assistant is employed. Facilities employing a large number of employees tend to offer a higher salary range than smaller facilities.

According to the Bureau of Labor Statistics, as reported at the website CollegeGrad.com (http://www.collegegrad.com/careers/servi07.shtml), state government facilities constituted the highest paying sector, with a mean (average) annual wage of $36,430. According to Salary.com (as reported by Allied Health Schools at http://www.alliedhealthschools.com/faqs/medical-assistant-salary.php), data showed that, in 2011, 50 percent of medical assistants in the middle of the salary range earned between $27,350 and $32,833, and those in the top 10 percent earned $35,389 or more. Some sources quote the salary range of an experienced medical assistant as more than $40,000 per year.

Medical assistants often receive higher salaries for work in medical practices that have higher earning power. For instance, specialty physicians in areas such as gynecology, cardiology, and hematology are paid more than primary care physicians for their services, and all physicians performing some type of surgery also earn more than primary care physicians.

Fringe benefits, also known as employee benefits, are the various types of non-wage compensation offered to employees of a facility in addition to their normal wages or salaries. Fringe benefits—often a key ingredient in attracting and retaining medical assisting employees—are generally not taxable to the employee. These benefits may add significantly to a medical assistant's total compensation, depending on the type of benefits offered. The medical assistant should be aware of benefit packages offered by perspective employers and, when evaluating potential job offers, should consider not only benefits that could be used immediately, such as a health insurance plan, but also long-term benefits, such as a retirement plan. Fringe benefits will vary from office to office and may include:

- health insurance, including medical, vision, and dental plans
- tuition reimbursement or free continuing education
- retirement benefits, including 401(k) plans, simple IRA plans, and other plans
- lunch vouchers
- uniform expense allowance
- paid parking
- paid vacation
- paid sick days
- paid holidays

Medical Assisting Education and Training

Medical assistant programs are typically taught at junior and community colleges, privately owned colleges, or secondary education vocational schools. A graduate from one of these programs can earn a diploma, a certificate, or an associate degree in applied science, depending on the length of the program and the content of the program. Diplomas are given to students after completion of specified educational requirements. Certificates are different from diplomas because they are usually given when a student completes a specific course of study and has mastered particular skills usually required for a specific job. Often the terms *diploma* and *certificate* are used interchangeably by colleges although the knowledge acquired is the same.

Types of Programs

A certificate program and an associate degree may open up many opportunities for the graduate and help in the advancement of a career. Because each program is different, the student must understand the difference between the programs offered and make a decision based on which program will meet his or her needs and goals.

- A **certificate program** usually takes one year or less to complete. Some certificate programs require that an applicant have some type of experience in the field of the certificate since the program often enhances the skills already acquired by the applicant. Many times a student will complete a certificate program and work in the field as he or she works toward an associate degree.
- It usually takes two years to complete the required credits for an **associate degree**. Students entering the degree program do not need to have experience in the chosen field. Earning an associate degree may be a stepping stone to earning higher academic degrees, such as a bachelor's degree or a master's degree.

A prospective medical assistant should give some thought to the course of his or her education and individual career goals before selecting the type of program in which to enroll. If a prospective student enjoys studying and decides to pursue a higher degree, the certificate program may not be the best choice; enrolling in a two-year associate program may be the better option. If the student's goal is to complete a program as quickly as possible and get out into the workforce, the certificate program may be a better choice.

Medical Assisting Courses

Courses offered in a medical assisting program may vary slightly depending on whether the program is a certificate or degree program. Degree programs require general education courses during the first year, with the medical assisting courses offered in the second year. Courses cover a wide range of material, including:

- anatomy and physiology: normal structures and workings of the human body
- pathophysiology: diseases and conditions affecting the human body
- medical terminology: jargon used in the medical field
- psychology: psychological growth and development, methods of communication, and so on
- keyboarding and knowledge of computer programs such as PowerPoint, Excel, and Word
- pharmacology: classification of drugs, calculation of dosages, preparation of medications, and administration of oral and parenteral medications (depending on state laws)
- clinical laboratory theory: learning and performing various lab tests used in medical offices, phlebotomy techniques, and so on
- CPR and first aid, such as the use of an automated external defibrillator (AED) for infants, children, and adults
- topics in health care law: various laws pertaining to the medical field, employment laws, and state and federal regulations
- ethics, including the "Patients' Bill of Rights"; the importance of honesty, integrity, caring, and freedom of choice for patients; informed consent; and patients' right to privacy and confidentiality in the use of their personal information
- administrative office procedures: medical records management, billing and collection, insurance claim processing, diagnostic and procedural coding, electronic submission of insurance claims, banking procedures, payroll procedures, and inventory and supply orders
- clinical skills and an internship experience

Two-year degree programs also require courses in English composition, advanced mathematics, and communication; elective courses in psychology, sociology, languages, history, art, music, and advanced computer skills are also available for the degree student.

Medical Assisting Credentials and Accreditation Agencies

Gaining medical assisting credentials is usually based on attending an educational program with proper accreditation. Medical assisting education programs are accredited by one of the two national accrediting agencies for medical assisting: the Commission on Accreditation of Allied Health Education Programs (CAAHEP) and the Accrediting Bureau of Health Education Schools (ABHES).

Certified Medical Assistant (CMA) Credentials

One route by which a medical assistant can gain credentials is through the Certified Medical Assistant exam. Only graduates from a CAAHEP- or ABHES-accredited medical assistant program are eligible to sit for the national CMA certification examinations offered by the American Association of Medical Assistants. Upon successfully passing the exam, the graduate medical assistant earns the CMA credential, which is recognized in every state and is valid for five years.

The accrediting agencies require that a CMA apply for recertification in two ways, either by retaking the national exam or by earning continuing education units (CEUs) in order to keep current with advances in the medical assisting profession and to retain the privilege of using the CMA credential. The AAMA requires 60 CEUs every five years divided between the administrative, clinical, and general areas of medical assisting. The 60 CEUs must include ten administrative, ten clinical, and ten general. The remaining 30 CEUs may include some combination of these three categories.

A CMA must also maintain a current CPR certificate and provide a photocopy of the card plus a written description of the type and length of the course to the AAMA. The CPR course taken must meet or exceed the requirements of the American Red Cross or the American Heart Association in order to be accepted by the AAMA.

The national organization of the AAMA comprises local chapters in more than 40 states. Membership is encouraged to keep current on changes in the healthcare field, to earn CEUs, and to network with other medical assistants. Local chapters offer continuing education, state chapters offer yearly conventions, and the national organization has a nationwide convention offering numerous opportunities for earning CEUs.

Registered Medical Assistant (RMA) Credentials

The medical assistant can also gain credentials by taking the Registered Medical Assistant (RMA) exam, offered by the American Medical Technologists. To be eligible for the RMA exam, an applicant must have successfully completed a medical assisting program accredited by CAAHEP or ABHES; must have graduated from a medical assisting program in an institution (postsecondary school or college) that has been accredited by a regional accrediting commission or national accrediting agency approved by the U.S. Department of Education; or must have worked in the medical assisting profession for at least five years. Upon passing the national RMA exam, the medical assistant automatically becomes a member of AMT and receives the quarterly magazine of the organization, among other benefits. AMT requires that an RMA earn 30 points within a three-year period in order to retain the RMA credential. The points may be earned through continuing education, employer evaluations, and professional and formal education.

The Value of Credentials and Accreditation

The purpose of accrediting medical assisting programs is to ensure that a program offers an education that will provide a graduate with the skills needed for an entry-level position in the medical assisting profession. Medical assisting programs choose to be accredited because many physicians prefer to hire a

CMA OR RMA?

Which credential should the medical assisting student seek: a CMA or an RMA? The accreditation of programs is more closely regulated than the accreditation of institutions, so it could be argued that the CMA is part of a more rigorous regulatory environment. Also, the CAAHEP and ABHES are the only two nationally programmatic accrediting agencies for medical assisting. However, once the graduate earns a credential—be it the CMA or RMA—it is accepted nationally. Personal preference and availability of medical assisting programs to meet a range of personal needs—such as location, size of institution, and the like—may influence the type of program and the type of credential sought upon graduation. Both the RMA and the CMA perform the same skills in the medical office, and both enjoy the rewarding experience of being a professional medical assistant.

graduate from an accredited program. Accreditation of a program by a national accrediting agency ensures that the medical assisting program has met the educational requirements set forth by the accrediting agency, as well as the requirements for entry-level skill competencies and responsibilities needed by the graduate to be a success in the working environment.

Medical assisting programs offer classroom instruction as well as a laboratory experience to practice both administrative and clinical skills, along with an unpaid internship experience in a medical facility. The internship experience, also referred to as an externship or a practicum, offers the student a time to practice and gain experience and confidence in the workplace before graduation, while still under the guidance and supervision of the educational facility and the medical facility.

There are many benefits to graduating from an accredited medical assisting program and earning the

CMA or RMA credential. An accredited program not only ensures the graduate a quality education, but also provides physicians and other recruiters with the confidence that they will be hiring a prepared, knowledgeable medical assistant.

About the National Exams

Two exams are offered through which the medical assistant can obtain certification: the Certified Medical Assistant exam and the Registered Medical Assistant exam.

Certified Medical Assistant Exam

The Certified Medical Assistant exam offers three eligibility categories.

1. Graduates from a CAAHEP or ABHES medical assisting program: Students in this category may take the exam up to 30 days prior to graduation after completing all requirements for graduation including the internship experience. No documentation is needed for graduating students, but the program director must verify that the applicant is a recent graduate who has met all the requirements of the program.
2. Non-recent graduates of a CAAHEP or ABHES medical assisting program: This category covers graduates applying for the exam later than 12 months after graduation. An official transcript from the medical assisting program of the applicant must be sent in with the application for the exam.
3. CMAs who need to be recertified: This category consists of medical assistants who already have a CMA and need only to be recertified. A photocopy of the CMA credential must be sent in with the application as well as a copy of the CPR and first aid certificate. If the applicant is unable to perform CPR because of physical disabilities, a note signed by a physician on official

letterhead must be sent in with the application for documentation.

Fees for the exam are nonrefundable and are nontransferable, meaning the scheduled date cannot be changed. Personal checks are not accepted, although the applicant may pay by credit card, debit card, or cashier's or certified check. Once the payment has cleared, the applicant will be notified within 45 days of mailing the payment that he or she is now eligible to take the exam. Information will be sent on the policies and procedures in effect at the test center.

Certain candidate information may not be divulged without written permission of the candidate, such as the exam score, the number of times the candidate has taken the exam, or any personal information about the candidate.

The CMA exam consists of 200 multiple-choice questions covering general knowledge, administrative knowledge and skills, and clinical knowledge and skills, with 180 questions being scored and the remaining 20 questions used as sample questions for future exams. The score is based on the number of correct answers to scored questions, not to the sample questions. The time allotment for the test is three hours. A nonofficial pass/fail grade will be given immediately after the exam, and the official score will be sent in approximately ten weeks.

Registered Medical Assistant Exam

The Registered Medical Assistant exam eligibility standards require that the applicant fit one of the following categories:

1. A recent graduate of a CAAHEP or ABHES medical assisting program
2. A graduate from a postsecondary institution or college that has institutional accreditation from a regional accrediting commission approved by the U.S. Department of Education
3. A current medical assistant with a minimum of five years' experience working in the profession

The RMA exam consists of 200 to 210 multiple-choice questions covering the same subject areas as the CMA exam. The questions are presented in no particular order and are allotted among the subject areas according to the following breakdown: general medical assisting knowledge, 41 percent; administrative medical assisting, 24 percent; and clinical medical assisting, 35 percent. The exam is offered at more than 200 Pearson VUE locations in the United States almost every day of the year, except on weekends and holidays.

After an application is completed and sent to the AMT registrar, the applicant will receive notification of acceptance and given information about the date, time, and place of the exam. Photo ID is needed for verification of identity before taking the exam. The medical assistant has two hours to take the exam. Results from the computer-based RMA exam are immediate.

Job Readiness and Seeking Employment

Graduating from an accredited medical assisting program provides graduates with the knowledge and training needed to enter the professional workplace with confidence. Gaining credentials by passing either national certification examination—the Certified Medical Assistant exam or the Registered Medical Assistant exam—will indicate to potential employers that the graduate has met a set of high professional standards. This credential, and the ongoing education required by the agencies to keep credentials current, may help with career advancement and financial compensation throughout a medical assistant's professional life.

Resume and Cover Letters

The most important tools of a medical assistant's job search are the resume and cover letter. A resume is a written description of work experience, skills, and

EXAMPLE OF A COVER LETTER

January 26, 2011

Mary Jane Smith
166 Elm Street
Goshen, CT 06145

Dale Evans, Office Manager
Mid-State Urgent Care
465 Terryville Avenue
Bristol, CT 06010

Dear Ms. Evans,

I am interested in a position as a medical assistant in your urgent care center. I have worked as a medical assistant for the past seven years and enjoy working with patients and helping them with their medical care.

I believe that my varied experience and skills would make me a valuable member of your healthcare team. I have worked in both the clinical and administrative medical assisting areas. My most recent position allowed me to gain extensive experience in helping patients of all ages and to manage triage in a busy walk-in facility.

Please call me at (860) 583-1465 to schedule an interview and further discuss my qualifications for the position available. I may also be reached at mjsmith@polcast.net. I look forward to hearing from you.

Sincerely,

Mary Jane Smith

Mary Jane Smith, CMA
Enclosure: resume

---

educational background that qualifies one for a particular job. It is a marketing tool used to inform a prospective employer about the applicant's good qualities, previous job experiences, and volunteer activities, and to help the employer decide whether or not to offer an interview. A cover letter is usually sent with a resume and should summarize information—either noted in the resume or not—that relates specifically to the position being offered.

Resumes should be accurate, concise, grammatically correct, and, if possible, limited to one page. There are different styles used to prepare a resume, and the medical assistant should use the style that best describes his or her qualifications for a specific job.

- A **chronological resume** summarizes an applicant's background in reverse chronological order, meaning that the most recent information is listed first. This type of resume may be used when emphasizing education and work experiences related to the offered position.
- A **targeted resume** is written specifically for an advertised job. It emphasizes the education and experiences that are directly related to fulfilling the expectations listed for the offered position.
- A **functional resume** emphasizes the most valuable experiences and skills that the applicant can bring to the job. In a functional resume, information is not necessarily arranged in chronological order, but rather focuses on learned skills that

would make the applicant the right person for the job.

References should not be listed on a resume, although a statement saying "References available on request" may be added to the resume, usually at the end. The medical assistant should ask permission before listing someone as a reference. Coworkers, former teachers, former employers, or anyone who knows the applicant's strengths and abilities would make a good reference. Applicants should avoid using family members as references.

Methods of Job Searching

A job search is the process of locating potential employers, understanding what the employers need, and providing information that shows each employer how his or her facility will benefit from hiring the applicant. There are many methods that may be used to help in the job search:

- **Networking.** Networking is the cultivation of relationships for business purposes or for job searching. Job seekers should "advertise" their skills, telling everyone in their networks—including teachers, relatives, neighbors, friends, and previous coworkers—that they are looking for a position as a medical assistant. Often, jobs are advertised by word-of-mouth and networking can help the job seeker find out about such opportunities.
- **Research on the Internet.** There are many job-hunting websites that list local and national job opportunities. Government agencies and private employers often list position openings on job boards. General job-hunting websites such as http://www.monster.com or http://www.career builder.com may be useful in locating available positions.
- **Professional organizations.** Many professional organizations offer employment information, list jobs, and may even offer job placement services.

The medical assistant should consider becoming a member of the AAMA or the AMT, as well as the local chapters of these organizations, which offer networking and professional development to medical assistants.

- **Placement offices at college or school.** Many colleges and schools offer continuing job placement services to students and alumni. Placement offices may produce job fairs to which recruiters are invited to conduct interviews with students on site. The medical assistant seeking a position should have his or her information listed with the college or school placement office.
- **Employers.** Contacting individual employers— either in person or by sending a resume and cover letter—is another method for finding a job.
- **Classified ads.** Checking the "Help Wanted" ads in the local newspaper can alert the medical assistant to a job opening.
- **Internship experience.** Many medical assistants find employment at the site of their internship experiences. This is a ideal way to gain a position because both the facility and the medical student have already gotten a chance to try each other out. Having been trained in the specific procedures and policies of an office, the medical assistant intern can more easily fit into a new position should one become available.

Interviewing

Getting ready for a job interview takes much preparation. The medical assistant should learn as much about the medical facility to which he or she is applying as possible before the job interview. In addition, the applicant should prepare for the interview by reviewing his or her qualifications and by practicing answering sample questions on general topics that may be asked.

Other pointers for job interviews include:

- Dress conservatively, use good hygiene, and have a positive attitude.

- Arrive early for the interview; being late will give the prospective employer the impression that you will likely not be able to be on time for work.
- Always be polite and courteous to everyone you encounter at the facility on the day of the interview, even those employees you think have no input on hiring decisions.
- Make eye contact, appear enthusiastic, and show a genuine interest in the position.
- Avoid questions about salary and benefits during a first interview.
- At the completion of the interview, thank the interviewer and shake hands.
- Send thank-you notes to everyone involved in the interview process.

Reaching your goal of becoming a professional medical assistant will lead you to a rewarding and satisfying career. Use the guidance and information in this book to prepare you to earn your credentials in this productive and challenging profession!

ANTICIPATING POSSIBLE INTERVIEW QUESTIONS

Try to anticipate the kind of questions that you will be asked in a job interview and to prepare for them. Possible interview questions might include:

- "Why should I hire you?"
- "Why do you want this position?"
- "What makes you the best person for this position?"
- "List some of your strengths and weaknesses."

Anticipating possible questions and being prepared with answers will instill confidence and help you to make a good impression on the employer.

2 ▶ THE LEARNINGEXPRESS TEST PREPARATION SYSTEM

CHAPTER OVERVIEW

Taking any written exam can be tough, and a top score demands a lot of preparation. The LearningExpress Test Preparation System, developed exclusively for LearningExpress by leading test experts, gives you the discipline and attitude you need to be a winner.

Taking this written exam is no picnic, and neither is getting ready for it. Your future career in medical assisting depends on whether you pass the test, and there are all sorts of pitfalls that can keep you from doing your best on this all-important exam. Here are some of the obstacles that can stand in the way of your success:

- Being unfamiliar with the format of the exam
- Being paralyzed by test anxiety
- Leaving your preparation to the last minute or not preparing at all
- Not knowing vital test-taking skills: how to pace yourself through the exam, how to use the process of elimination, and when to guess
- Not being in tip-top mental and physical shape
- Messing up on exam day by having to work on an empty stomach or shivering through the exam because the room is cold

What's the common denominator in all these test-taking pitfalls? One word: *control*. Who's in control, you or the exam?

The LearningExpress Test Preparation System puts you in control. In just nine easy-to-follow steps, you will learn everything you need to know to make sure that you are in charge of your preparation and your performance on the exam. Other test takers may let the exam get the better of them; other test takers may be unprepared or out of shape, but not you. After completing this chapter, you will have taken all the steps you need to get a high score on the medical assistant exam.

Here's how the LearningExpress Test Preparation System works: Nine easy steps lead you through everything you need to know and do to get ready for this exam. Each of the following steps includes both reading about the step and one or more activities. It's important that you do the activities along with the reading, or you won't be getting the full benefit of the system. Each step tells you approximately how much time that step will take you to complete.

Step 1: Get Information (30 minutes)

Step 2: Conquer Test Anxiety (20 minutes)

Step 3: Make a Plan (50 minutes)

Step 4: Learn to Manage Your Time (10 minutes)

Step 5: Learn to Use the Process of Elimination (20 minutes)

Step 6: Know When to Guess (20 minutes)

Step 7: Reach Your Peak Performance Zone (10 minutes)

Step 8: Get Your Act Together (10 minutes)

Step 9: Do It! (10 minutes)

Total time for complete system: 180 minutes— 3 hours

We estimate that working through the entire system will take you approximately three hours. It's perfectly okay if you work at a faster or slower pace. If you can spend a whole afternoon or evening working, you can work through the whole LearningExpress Test Preparation System in one sitting. Otherwise, you can break it up, and do just one or two steps a day for the next several days. It's up to you—remember, you are in control.

Step 1: Get Information

Time to complete: 30 minutes

Activities: Read Chapter 1, "The Medical Assistant Profession"

Knowledge is power. The first step in the Learning-Express Test Preparation System is finding out everything you can about the two types of medical assisting exams offered: the Certified Medical Assistant exam and the Registered Medical Assistant exam. Both exams test the same body of knowledge, with minor variations in how they approach certain topics. Take some time to familiarize yourself with the preparation material made available by the organizations that sponsor and administer both tests (see Resources, page 367). The more information you have, the more in control you will feel.

This book includes practice exams for both the CMA and RMA credentials. Even after you decide on which exam you'll take, you can use both sample tests to practice, since they cover virtually the same material.

What You Should Find Out

The more details you can discover about the exam, the more efficiently you will be able to study. Here's a list of some things you might want to find out about your exam:

- Will your test be computer-based, or use a paper booklet and answer sheet?
- What skills are tested?
- How many sections are on the exam?
- How many questions are in each section?
- Are the questions ordered from easy to hard, or is the sequence random?

- How much time is allotted for each section?
- Are there breaks between sections?
- What is the passing score, and how many questions do you have to answer correctly in order to get that score?
- Does a higher score give you any advantages?
- How is the exam scored, and is there a penalty for incorrect answers?
- Are you permitted to go back to a prior section or move on to the next section if you finish early?
- Can you write in the exam booklet for a paper test? Will you be given scratch paper?
- What should you bring with you on exam day?

Step 2: Conquer Test Anxiety

Time to complete: 20 minutes
Activity: Take the Test Anxiety Quiz (page 17)

Having complete information about the exam is the first step in getting control of it. Next, you have to overcome one of the biggest obstacles to test success: test anxiety. Test anxiety can not only impair your performance on the exam itself, but can even keep you from preparing properly. In Step 2, you will learn stress management techniques that will help you succeed on your exam. Learn these strategies now, and practice them as you work through the questions in this book, so they'll be second nature to you by exam day.

Combating Test Anxiety

The first thing you need to know is that a little test anxiety is a good thing. Everyone gets nervous before a big exam—and if that nervousness motivates you to prepare thoroughly, so much the better. It's said that Sir Laurence Olivier, one of the foremost British actors of the twentieth century, was ill before every performance. And younger actors—including Zac Efron and Claire Danes—also get the jitters. Their stage fright doesn't impair their performances, though; in fact, it probably gives them a little extra edge—just the kind of edge you need to do well, whether on a stage, in a film, or in an examination room.

On page 17 is the Test Anxiety Quiz. Stop now and answer the questions on that page to find out whether your level of test anxiety is something you should worry about.

Stress Management before the Exam

If you feel your level of anxiety is getting the best of you in the weeks before the exam, here is what you need to do to bring the level down again:

- **Get prepared.** There's nothing like knowing what to expect and being prepared for it to put you in control of test anxiety. That's why you're reading this book. Use it faithfully, and remind yourself that you're better prepared than most of the people taking the exam.
- **Practice self-confidence.** A positive attitude is a great way to combat test anxiety. This is no time to be humble or shy. Stand in front of the mirror and say to your reflection, "I'm prepared. I'm full of self-confidence. I'm going to ace this exam. I know I can do it." Say it into a recorder, and play it back once a day. Or type it into a text message and send it to yourself. It may feel a little weird, but if you hear it or see it often enough, you will believe it.
- **Fight negative messages.** Every time someone starts telling you how hard the exam is or how it's almost impossible to pass the test, start telling them the self-confidence messages you've been practicing. If the person delivering the negative messages is you—telling yourself that you don't do well on exams, that you just can't do it—don't listen. Turn on your recorder, or reread your text messages, and listen to yourself expressing confidence in your own abilities.

- **Visualize.** Imagine yourself reporting for duty on your first day of medical assisting. Think of yourself wearing your uniform with pride and learning skills you will use for the rest of your life. Visualizing success can help make it happen—and remind you of why you're doing all this work preparing for the exam.
- **Exercise.** Physical activity helps calm down your body and focus your mind. Besides, being in good physical shape can actually help you do well on the exam. Go for a run, lift weights, go swimming—and do it regularly.

Stress Management on Exam Day

There are several ways you can bring down your level of test stress and anxiety on exam day. They'll work best if you practice them in the weeks before the exam, so you know which ones work best for you.

- **Deep breathing.** Take a deep breath while you count to five. Hold it for a count of one, and then let it out on a count of five. Repeat several times.
- **Move your body.** Try rolling your head in a circle. Rotate your shoulders. Shake your hands from the wrist. Many people find these movements very relaxing.
- **Visualize again.** Think of the place where you are most relaxed: lying on the beach in the sun, walking through the park, or whatever relaxes you. Now, close your eyes and imagine you're there. If you practice in advance, you will find that you need only a few seconds of this exercise to experience a significant increase in your sense of well-being.

When anxiety threatens to overwhelm you during the exam, there are still things you can do to manage your stress level:

- **Repeat your self-confidence messages.** You should have them memorized by now. Say them quietly to yourself, and believe them!

- **Visualize one more time.** This time, visualize yourself moving smoothly and quickly through the exam, answering every question correctly and finishing just before time is up. Like most visualization techniques, this one works best if you've practiced it ahead of time.
- **Find an easy question.** If the test format allows, skim over the test until you find an easy question, and answer it. Completing even one question gets you into the test-taking groove.
- **Take a mental break.** Everyone loses concentration once in a while during a long exam. It's normal, so you shouldn't worry about it. Instead, accept what has happened. Say to yourself, "Hey, I lost it there for a minute. My brain is taking a break." Put down your pencil, close your eyes, and do some deep breathing for a few seconds. Then, you're ready to go back to work.

Try these techniques ahead of time, and see if they work for you!

Step 3: Make a Plan

Time to complete: 50 minutes
Activity: Construct a study plan, using Schedules A–D (pages 18–20)

Many people do poorly on exams because they forget to make a study schedule. The most important thing you can do to better prepare yourself for your exam is to create a study plan or schedule. Spending hours the day before the exam poring over sample test questions not only raises your level of anxiety, but also is not a substitute for careful preparation and practice over time.

Don't cram. Take control of your time by mapping out a study schedule. There are four examples of study schedules on pages 18–20, based on the amount of time you have before the exam. If you're the kind of person who needs deadlines and assignments to motivate you for a project, here they are. If you're the kind

TEST ANXIETY QUIZ

You need to worry about test anxiety only if it is extreme enough to impair your performance. The following questionnaire will provide a diagnosis of your level of test anxiety. In the blank before each statement, write the number that most accurately describes your experience.

0 = Never   1 = Once or twice   2 = Sometimes   3 = Often

_____ I have gotten so nervous before an exam that I simply put down the books and didn't study for it.

_____ I have experienced disabling physical symptoms such as vomiting and severe headaches because I was nervous about an exam.

_____ I have simply not showed up for an exam because I was scared to take it.

_____ I have experienced dizziness and disorientation while taking an exam.

_____ I have had trouble filling in the little circles because my hands were shaking too hard.

_____ I have failed an exam because I was too nervous to complete it.

_____ **Total: Add up the numbers in the blanks above.**

Your Test Anxiety Score

Here are the steps you should take, depending on your score. If you scored:

- **Below 3,** your level of test anxiety is nothing to worry about; it's probably just enough to give you that little extra edge.

- **Between 3 and 6,** your test anxiety may be enough to impair your performance, and you should practice the stress management techniques listed in this chapter to try to bring your test anxiety down to manageable levels.

- **Above 6,** your level of test anxiety is a serious concern. In addition to practicing the stress management techniques listed in this chapter, you may want to seek additional, personal help. Call your local high school or community college and ask for the academic counselor. Tell the counselor that you have a level of test anxiety that sometimes keeps you from being able to take the exam. The counselor may be willing to help you or may suggest someone else you should talk to.

SCHEDULE A: THE LEISURE PLAN

This schedule gives you at least five months to sharpen your skills and prepare for your exam. The more prep time you give yourself, the more relaxed you'll feel.

Time	Preparation
5 months before the test	Read the Introduction and Chapters 1 and 2. Start going to the library once every two weeks to read books or magazines about medical assisting. Start gathering information about working as a medical assistant. Find other people who are preparing for the exam, and form a study group with them.
4 months before the test	Read Chapter 3 and work through the practice questions. Use at least one of the additional resources for each chapter.
3 months before the test	Read Chapter 4 and work through the practice questions. You're still continuing with your reading, aren't you?
2 months before the test	Read Chapter 5 and work through the practice questions.
1 month before the test	Use your scores from the practice questions in Chapters 3, 4, and 5 to help you decide where to concentrate your efforts this month. Go back to the relevant chapters and review challenging topics. Continue working with your study group.
1 week before the test	Take and review the sample exams in Chapters 6 and 7. See how much you've learned in the past months. Concentrate on what you've done well, and decide not to let any areas where you still feel uncertain bother you.
1 day before the test	Relax. Do something unrelated to the medical assistant exam. Eat a good meal and go to bed at your usual time.

SCHEDULE B: THE JUST-ENOUGH-TIME PLAN

If you have three to four months before your exam, that should be enough time to prepare. This schedule assumes four months; stretch it out or compress it if you have more or less time.

Time	Preparation
3 months before the test	Read the Introduction and Chapters 1 and 2. Start going to the library once every two weeks to read books or magazines about medical assisting. Start gathering information about working as a medical assistant. Find other people who are preparing for the exam, and form a study group with them.
2 months before the test	Read Chapters 3, 4, and 5, and work through the exercises.
1 month before the test	Take one of the sample exams in Chapters 6 and 7. Use your score to help you decide where to concentrate your efforts this month. Go back to the relevant chapters and review challenging topics, or get the help of a friend or teacher.
1 week before the test	Review the sample exams in Chapters 6 and 7. See how much you have learned in the past months. Celebrate what you've done well, and decide not to let any areas where you still feel uncertain bother you.
1 day before the test	Relax. Do something unrelated to the medical assistant exam. Eat a good meal and go to bed at your usual time.

SCHEDULE C: MORE STUDY IN LESS TIME

If you have three weeks to one month before the exam, you still have enough time for some concentrated study that will help you improve your score.

Time	Preparation
3 weeks before the test	Read the Introduction and Chapters 1 through 5. Work through the practice questions in Chapters 3, 4, and 5. Review the areas in which you're weakest.
2 weeks before the test	Take one of the sample exams in Chapter 6 and 7. Then, score your exam and read the answer explanations until you're sure you understand them. Review the areas where you score the lowest.
1 week before the test	Review the sample exams, concentrating on the areas where a little work can help the most.
1 day before the test	Relax. Do something unrelated to the medical assistant exam. Eat a good meal and go to bed at your usual time.

SCHEDULE D: THE CRAM PLAN

If you have two weeks or less before the exam, you really have your work cut out for you. Carve half an hour out of your day, *every day*, for study. This schedule assumes you have the whole two weeks to prepare; if you have less time, you'll have to compress the schedule accordingly.

Time	Preparation
2 weeks before the test	Read the Introduction and Chapters 1 through 5. Work through the review questions in Chapters 4 and 5. Review areas where you show weakness.
1 week before the test	Evaluate your performance on the review questions. Review the parts of Chapters 3–5 where you had the most trouble. Get a friend or teacher to help you with the section you found to be the most difficult.
2 days before the test	Take the sample exams in Chapters 6 and 7. Review your results. Make sure you understand the answer explanations.
1 day before the test	Relax. Do something unrelated to the medical assistant exam. Eat a good meal and go to bed at your usual time.

of person who doesn't like to follow other people's plans, you can use the suggested schedules to construct your own.

Even more important than making a plan is making a commitment. You can't review everything you learned in your medical assisting program in one night. You have to set aside some time every day for studying and practice. Aim for at least 20 minutes a day. Twenty minutes daily will do you more good than two hours crammed into a Saturday.

If you have months before the exam, you're lucky. Don't put off your study until the week before the exam. Start now. Even ten minutes a day, with half an hour or more on weekends, can make a big difference in your score—and in your chances of becoming a medical assistant.

Step 4: Learn to Manage Your Time

Time to complete: 10 minutes to read, many hours of practice
Activities: Practice these strategies as you take the sample exams

Steps 4, 5, and 6 of the LearningExpress Test Preparation System put you in charge of your exam by showing you test-taking strategies that work. Practice these strategies as you take the sample exams in Chapters 6 and 7. Then, you will be ready to use them on exam day.

First, you will take control of your time on the exam. The first step in achieving this control is to find out the format of the exam you're going to take. The CMA exam has different sections that are each timed separately. You will want to practice using your time wisely on the practice exams and trying to avoid mistakes while working quickly. The RMA exam doesn't have separately timed sections. So, just practice pacing yourself on the practice exams so you don't spend too much time on difficult questions.

- **Listen carefully to directions.** By the time you get to the exam, you should know how the test works, but listen just in case something has changed.
- **Pace yourself.** Glance at your watch every few minutes, and compare the time to how far you've gotten in the section. Leave some extra time for review, so that when one quarter of the time has elapsed, you should be more than one quarter of the way through the section, and so on. If you're falling behind, pick up the pace.
- **Keep moving.** Don't spend too much time on one question. If you don't know the answer, skip the question and move on. Circle the number of the question in your test booklet in case you have time to come back to it later.
- **Keep track of your place on the answer sheet.** If you skip a question, make sure you skip it on the answer sheet, too. Check yourself every five to ten questions to make sure the question number and the answer sheet number match.
- **Don't rush.** You should keep moving, rushing won't help. Try to keep calm and work methodically and quickly.

Step 5: Learn to Use the Process of Elimination

Time to complete: 20 minutes
Activity: Complete the worksheet on Using the Process of Elimination (page 23)

After time management, the next most important tool for taking control of your exam is using the process of elimination wisely. It's standard test-taking wisdom that you should always read all the answer choices before choosing your answer. This helps you find the correct answer by eliminating incorrect answer choices. And, sure enough, that standard wisdom applies to this exam, too.

Let's say you are facing a medical assisting knowledge question that goes like this:

"Biology uses a binomial system of classification." In this sentence, the word *binomial* most nearly means
a. understanding the law.
b. having two names.
c. scientifically sound.
d. having a double meaning.

If you happen to know what *binomial* means, of course you don't need to use the process of elimination, but let's assume you don't. So, you look at the answer choices. "Understanding the law" sure doesn't sound very likely for something having to do with biology. So you eliminate choice **a**—and now you have only three answer choices to deal with. Mark an X next to choice **a**, so you never have to read it again.

Now, move on to the other answer choices. If you know that the prefix *bi-* means *two,* as in *bicycle,* you will flag choice **b** as a possible answer. Mark a check mark beside it, meaning "good answer, I might use this one."

Choice **c**, "scientifically sound," is a possibility. At least it's about science, not law. It could work here, though, when you think about it, having a "scientifically sound" classification system in a scientific field is kind of redundant. You remember the *bi-* in *binomial,* and probably continue to like choice **b** better. But you're not sure, so you put a question mark next to **c**, meaning "well, maybe."

Now, choice **d**, "having a double meaning." You're still keeping in mind that *bi-* means *two,* so this one looks possible at first. But then you look again at the sentence the word belongs in, and you think, "Why would biology want a system of classification that has two meanings? That wouldn't work very well!" If you're really taken with the idea that *bi-* means *two,* you might put a question mark here. But if you're feeling a little more confident, you'll put an X. You already have a better answer picked out.

Now your question looks like this:

"Biology uses a binomial system of classification." In this sentence, the word *binomial* most nearly means
X a. understanding the law.
✓ b. having two names.
? c. scientifically sound.
? d. having a double meaning.

You've got just one check mark for a good answer. If you're pressed for time, you should simply mark choice **b** on your answer sheet. If you have the time to be extra careful, you could compare your check-mark answer to your question-mark answers to make sure that it's better. (It is: The *binomial* system in biology is the one that gives a two-part genus and species name, like *Homo sapiens.*)

It is good to have a system for marking good, bad, and maybe answers. We recommend this one:

X = bad
✓ = good
? = maybe

If you don't like these marks, devise your own system. Just make sure you do it long before test day—while you are working through the practice exams in this book—so you won't have to worry about it during the test.

Even when you think you are absolutely clueless about a question, you can often use the process of elimination to get rid of at least one answer choice. If so, you are better prepared to make an educated guess, as you will see in Step 6. More often, you can eliminate answers until you have only two possible answers. Then you are in a strong position to guess.

Try using your powers of elimination on the questions in the worksheet on page 23, Using the Process of Elimination. The questions are not about medical assisting; they are just designed to show you how the process of elimination works. The answer

Use the process of elimination to answer the following questions.

1. Ilsa is as old as Meghan will be in five years. The difference between Ed's age and Meghan's age is twice the difference between Ilsa's age and Meghan's age. Ed is 29. How old is Ilsa?
   a. 4
   b. 10
   c. 19
   d. 24

2. "All drivers of commercial vehicles must carry a valid commercial driver's license whenever operating a commercial vehicle."
   According to this sentence, which of the following people need NOT carry a commercial driver's license?
   a. a truck driver idling his engine while waiting to be directed to a loading dock
   b. a bus operator backing her bus out of the way of another bus in the bus lot
   c. a taxi driver driving his personal car to the grocery store
   d. a limousine driver taking the limousine to her home after dropping off her last passenger of the evening

3. Smoking tobacco has been linked to
   a. increased risk of stroke and heart attack.
   b. all forms of respiratory disease.
   c. increasing mortality rates over the past ten years.
   d. juvenile delinquency.

4. Which of the following words is spelled correctly?
   a. incorrigible
   b. outragous
   c. domestickated
   d. understandible

Answers

Here are the answers, as well as some suggestions as to how you might have used the process of elimination to find them.

1. d. You should have eliminated choice **a** off the bat. Ilsa can't be four years old if Meghan is going to be Ilsa's age in five years. The best way to eliminate other answer choices is to try plugging them in to the information given in the problem. For instance, for choice **b**, if Ilsa is 10, then Meghan must be 5. The difference in their ages is 5. The difference between Ed's age, 29, and Meghan's age, 5, is 24. Is 24 two times 5? No. Then choice **b** is wrong. You could eliminate choice **c** in the same way and be left with choice **d**.

2. c. Note the word *not* in the question, and go through the answers one by one. Is the truck driver in choice **a** "operating a commercial vehicle"? Yes, idling counts as "operating," so he needs to have a commercial driver's license. Likewise, the bus operator in choice **b** is operating a commercial vehicle; the question doesn't say the operator has to be on the street. The limo driver in choice **d** is operating a commercial vehicle, even if it doesn't have a passenger in it. However, the cabbie in choice **c** is not operating a commercial vehicle, but his own private car.

3. a. You could eliminate choice **b** simply because of the presence of the word *all*. Such absolutes hardly ever appear in correct answer choices. Choice **c** looks attractive until you think a little about what you know—aren't fewer people smoking these days, rather than more? So how could smoking be responsible for a higher mortality rate? (If you didn't know that *mortality rate* means the rate at which people die, you might keep this choice as a possibility, but you would still be able to eliminate two answers and have only two to choose from.) And choice **d** is unlikely, so you could eliminate that one, too. You are left with the correct choice, **a**.

4. a. How you used the process of elimination here depends on which words you recognized as being spelled incorrectly. If you knew that the correct spellings were outrageous, domesticated, and understandable, then you were home free.

explanations for this worksheet show one possible way you might use the process to arrive at the right answer.

The process of elimination is your tool for the next step, which is knowing when to guess.

Step 6: Know When to Guess

Time to complete: 20 minutes
Activity: Complete Worksheet on Your Guessing Ability (pages 26–27)

Armed with the process of elimination, you're ready to take control of one of the big questions in test taking: Should I guess?

The main answer is yes. The medical assistant exams don't use a so-called guessing penalty. Basically, the number of questions you answer correctly yields your score, and there's no penalty for wrong answers. So, you don't have to worry—simply go ahead and guess.

The more complicated answer depends on you, your personality, and your "guessing intuition."

When There Is No Guessing Penalty

As previously noted, the medical assistant exams don't have a guessing penalty. That means that, all other things being equal, you should always go ahead and guess, even if you have no idea what the question means. Nothing can happen to you if you're wrong. But all other things aren't necessarily equal. The other factor in deciding whether or not to guess, besides the guessing penalty, is you. There are two things you need to know about yourself before you go into the exam:

- Are you a risk taker?
- Are you a good guesser?

Your risk-taking temperament matters most on exams with a guessing penalty. Without a guessing penalty, even if you're a play-it-safe person, guessing is

perfectly safe. Overcome your anxieties, and go ahead and mark an answer.

But what if you're not much of a risk taker, and you think of yourself as the world's worst guesser? Complete the Your Guessing Ability worksheet on pages 26–27 to get an idea of how good your intuition is.

Step 7: Reach Your Peak Performance Zone

Time to complete: 10 minutes to read; weeks to complete!
Activity: Complete the Physical Preparation Checklist (page 28)

To get ready for a challenge like a big exam, you also have to take control of your physical, as well as your mental, state. Exercise, proper diet, and rest will ensure that your body works with, rather than against, your mind on test day, as well as during your preparation.

Exercise

If you don't already have a regular exercise program going, the time during which you're preparing for an exam is an excellent time to start one. And if you're already keeping fit—or trying to get that way—don't let the pressure of preparing for an exam fool you into quitting now. Exercise helps reduce stress by pumping wonderful good-feeling hormones called endorphins into your system. It also increases the oxygen supply throughout your body, including your brain, so you will be at peak performance on exam day.

A half hour of vigorous activity—enough to break a sweat—every day should be your aim. If you're really pressed for time, every other day is okay. Choose an activity you like and get out there and do it. Jogging with a friend always makes the time go faster, as does running with a radio or MP3 player.

But don't overdo it. You don't want to exhaust yourself. Moderation is the key.

Diet

First, cut out the junk. Go easy on caffeine, and try to eliminate alcohol and nicotine from your system at least two weeks before the exam.

What your body needs for peak performance is simply a balanced diet. Eat plenty of fruits and vegetables, along with protein and complex carbohydrates. Foods that are high in lecithin (an amino acid), such as fish and beans, are especially good "brain foods."

The night before the exam, you might "carbo-load" the way athletes do before a contest. Eat a big plate of spaghetti, rice and beans, or whatever your favorite carbohydrate is.

Rest

You probably know how much sleep you need every night to be at your best, even if you don't always get it. Make sure you do get that much sleep, though, for at least a week before the exam. Moderation is important here, too. Too much sleep will just make you groggy.

If you're not a morning person and your exam will be given in the morning, you should reset your internal clock so that your body doesn't think you're taking an exam at three a.m. You have to start this process well before the exam. The way it works is to get up half an hour earlier each morning, and then go to bed half an hour earlier that night. Don't try it the other way around; you will just toss and turn if you go to bed early without having gotten up early. The next morning, get up another half an hour earlier, and so on. How long you will have to do this depends on how late you're used to getting up. Use the Physical Preparation Checklist on page 28 to make sure you're in tip-top form.

Step 8: Get Your Act Together

Time to complete: 10 minutes to read; time to complete will vary

Activity: Complete Final Preparations worksheet (page 30)

You're in control of your mind and body; you're in charge of your test anxiety, your preparation, and your test-taking strategies. Now, it's time to take charge of external factors, like the exam site and the materials you need to take the exam.

Find Out Where the Exam Is and Make a Trial Run

The testing agency or your medical assistant exam instructor will notify you when and where your exam is being held. Do you know how to get to the exam site? Do you know how long it will take to get there? If not, make a trial run, preferably on the same day of the week at the same time of day. Make note, on the Final Preparations worksheet on page 30, of the amount of time it will take you to get to the exam site. Plan on arriving 10 to 15 minutes early so you can get the lay of the land, use the bathroom, and calm down. Then, figure out how early you will have to get up that morning, and make sure you get up that early every day for a week before the exam.

Gather Your Materials

The night before the exam, lay out the clothes you will wear and the materials you have to bring with you to the exam. Plan on dressing in layers; you won't have any control over the temperature of the examination room. Have a sweater or jacket you can take off if it's warm. Use the checklist on the Final Preparations worksheet on page 30 to help you pull together what you will need.

YOUR GUESSING ABILITY

The following are ten really hard questions. You are not supposed to know the answers. Rather, this is an assessment of your ability to guess when you don't have a clue. Read each question carefully, just as if you did expect to answer it. If you have any knowledge of the subject, use that knowledge to help you eliminate wrong answer choices.

1. September 7 is Independence Day in
   a. India.
   b. Costa Rica.
   c. Brazil.
   d. Australia.

2. Which of the following is the formula for determining the momentum of an object?
   a. $p = MV$
   b. $F = ma$
   c. $P = IV$
   d. $E = mc^2$

3. Because of the expansion of the universe, the stars and other celestial bodies are all moving away from each other. This phenomenon is known as
   a. Newton's first law.
   b. the big bang.
   c. gravitational collapse.
   d. Hubble flow.

4. American author Gertrude Stein was born in
   a. 1713.
   b. 1830.
   c. 1874.
   d. 1901.

5. Which of the following is NOT one of the Five Classics attributed to Confucius?
   a. *I Ching*
   b. *Book of Holiness*
   c. *Spring and Autumn Annals*
   d. *Book of History*

6. The religious and philosophical doctrine that holds that the universe is constantly in a struggle between good and evil is known as
   a. Pelagianism.
   b. Manichaeanism.
   c. neo-Hegelianism.
   d. Epicureanism.

7. The third chief justice of the U.S. Supreme Court was
   a. John Blair.
   b. William Cushing.
   c. James Wilson.
   d. John Jay.

8. Which of the following is the poisonous portion of a daffodil?
   a. the bulb
   b. the leaves
   c. the stem
   d. the flowers

9. The winner of the Masters golf tournament in 1953 was
   a. Sam Snead.
   b. Cary Middlecoff.
   c. Arnold Palmer.
   d. Ben Hogan.

10. The state with the highest per capita personal income in 1980 was
   a. Alaska.
   b. Connecticut.
   c. New York.
   d. Texas.

Answers

Check your answers against the following correct answers.

1. c.
2. a.
3. d.
4. c.
5. b.
6. b.
7. b.
8. a.
9. d.
10. a.

How Did You Do?

You may have simply gotten lucky and actually known the answers to one or two questions. In addition, your guessing was probably more successful if you were able to use the process of elimination on any of the questions. Maybe you didn't know who the third chief justice was (question 7), but you knew that John Jay was the first. In that case, you would have eliminated choice **d** and therefore improved your odds of guessing right from one in four to one in three.

According to probability, you should get two and a half answers correct, so getting either two or three right would be average. If you got four or more right, you may be a really terrific guesser. If you got one or none right, you may be a poor guesser.

Keep in mind, though, that this is only a small sample. You should continue to keep track of your guessing ability as you work through the sample questions in this book. Circle the numbers of questions you guess on as you make your guess; or, if you don't have time while you take the practice tests, go back afterward and try to remember which questions you guessed at. Remember, on a test with four answer choices, your chance of guessing correctly is one in four. So keep a separate "guessing" score for each exam. How many questions did you guess on? How many did you get right? If the number you got right is at least one-fourth of the number of questions you guessed on, you are at least an average guesser—maybe better—and you should always go ahead and guess on the real exam. If the number you got right is significantly lower than one-fourth of the number you guessed on, you would be safe in guessing anyway, but maybe you would feel more comfortable if you guessed only selectively, when you can eliminate a wrong answer or at least have a good feeling about one of the answer choices.

Because the medical assistant exams have no guessing penalty, even if you are a play-it-safe person with lousy intuition, you are still safe guessing every time.

PHYSICAL PREPARATION CHECKLIST

For the week before the test, write down what physical exercise you engaged in and for how long, and what you ate for each meal. Remember, you're trying for at least half an hour of exercise every other day (preferably every day) and a balanced diet that's light on junk food.

Exam minus 7 days

Exercise: _____ for _____ minutes
Breakfast: _____
Lunch: _____
Dinner: _____
Snacks: _____

Exam minus 6 days

Exercise: _____ for _____ minutes
Breakfast: _____
Lunch: _____
Dinner: _____
Snacks: _____

Exam minus 5 days

Exercise: _____ for _____ minutes
Breakfast: _____
Lunch: _____
Dinner: _____
Snacks: _____

Exam minus 4 days

Exercise: _____ for _____ minutes
Breakfast: _____
Lunch: _____
Dinner: _____
Snacks: _____

Exam minus 3 days

Exercise: _____ for _____ minutes
Breakfast: _____
Lunch: _____
Dinner: _____
Snacks: _____

Exam minus 2 days

Exercise: _____ for _____ minutes
Breakfast: _____
Lunch: _____
Dinner: _____
Snacks: _____

Exam minus 1 day

Exercise: _____ for _____ minutes
Breakfast: _____
Lunch: _____
Dinner: _____
Snacks: _____

Don't Skip Breakfast

Even if you don't usually eat breakfast, do so on exam morning. A cup of coffee doesn't count. Don't choose doughnuts or other sweet foods, either. A sugar high will leave you with a sugar low in the middle of the exam. A mix of protein and carbohydrates is best. Cereal with milk or eggs with toast will do your body a world of good.

Step 9: Do It!

Time to complete: 10 minutes, plus test-taking time
Activity: Ace the medical assisting exam!

Fast forward to exam day. You're ready. You made a study plan and followed through. You practiced your test-taking strategies while working through this book. You're in control of your physical, mental, and emotional state. You know when and where to show up and what to bring with you. In other words, you're better prepared than most of the other people taking the medical assistant exam with you. You're psyched.

Just one more thing. When you're done with the exam, you will have earned a reward. Plan a celebration. Call up your friends and plan a party, or have a nice dinner for two, or pick out a movie to see—whatever your heart desires. Give yourself something to look forward to.

And then do it. Go into the exam, full of confidence, armed with test-taking strategies you've practiced until they're second nature. You're in control of yourself, your environment, and your performance on the exam. You're ready to succeed. So do it. Go in there and ace the exam. And look forward to your future career as a medical assistant.

FINAL PREPARATIONS

Getting to the Exam Site

Location of exam site: _____

Date: _____

Departure time: _____

Do I know how to get to the exam site?   Yes ___   No ___   (If no, make a trial run.)

Time it will take to get to exam site: _____

Things to Lay Out the Night Before

Clothes I will wear   ___

Sweater/jacket   ___

Watch   ___

Photo ID (*one form for CMA; two forms for RMA*)   ___

Four #2 pencils (*if taking paper-based exam*)   ___

Scheduling permit (*for CMA exam only*)   ___

Other Things to Bring/Remember

_____   _____

_____   _____

_____   _____

_____   _____

3 ▶ GENERAL MEDICAL ASSISTING KNOWLEDGE

Medical Terminology

Terminology used in the medical field is a specialized language; in fact, much of it is based on words that originated in Greek and Latin. Learning a few key aspects of those languages—prefixes, suffixes, and roots, for example—is a critical part in the training of any medical assistant and a key area to review for your RMA or CMA exam.

Word Parts

The three key parts, or components, of most medical terms are the root, the prefix, and the suffix.

- **root:** the main stem, or fundamental part, of the word; the part of the word that conveys the most meaning; often describes the body part or system
  Example: *Cutane* is a root word meaning skin. By adding the prefix *sub* before the root and the suffix *ous* after the root, the word subcutaneous is formed. This new word means situated or applied under the skin.

- **prefix:** the part added to the front of the root word, often indicating location, time, number, or status

  Example: When the prefix *dys*, which means bad, painful, or difficult, is placed before the root word *uria*, which means urine, the term *dysuria* is formed. This new word means painful, difficult urination.

- **suffix:** the part added to the end of the root word; often indicates a procedure, condition, disorder, or disease

  Example: When the suffix *dynia*, which means pain or swelling, is added to the end of the root word *pharyngo*, which means throat, the term *pharyngodynia* is created. This new word means pain in the throat.

Common Roots

Here are some of the most common roots for medical terms. The letter following the slash indicates a letter added when the root is combined with a suffix beginning with a consonant.

Example: *hist* (meaning *tissue*) + *o* (the combining vowel) + *logy* (meaning *the study of*) = *histology*, which means *the study of tissues.*

ROOT	MEANING	ROOT	MEANING
adren	gland	fibr/o	connective tissue
angi/o	blood vessel	gastr/o	stomach
arteri/o	artery	gingiv/o	gum
arthr/o	joint	glyc/o	sugar
articul/o	joint	gon/o	genitals
audi/o	hearing	gyn(ec)/o	woman
blephar/o	eyelid	hepat/o	liver
bronch/i	bronchus (air passage)	hist/o	tissue
bucc/o	cheek	hyster/o	womb, uterus
burs/o	bursa	ir/o	iris
calc/i	stone	kal/i	potassium
carcini/o	cancer	kary/o	nucleus
cardi/o	heart	labi/o	lip
cervi/o	neck	lacrim/o	tear
chem/o	drug, or chemistry	laper/o	abdomen
cholechyst/o	gallbladder	laryng/o	larynx
colon/o	colon	leuk/o	white
cost/o	rib	lip/o	fat
crani/o	skull	litho	stone
cutane/o	skin	lymph/o	lymph
cyst/o	bladder	mamm/o	breast
cyt/o	cell	mast/o	breast
dactyl/o	finger, toe	mening/o	membrane
derm/o	skin	men/o	menstruation
dors/o	back	my/o	muscle
encephal/o	brain	nephr/o	kidney
enter/o	intestine	neur/o	nerve
fasci/o	fibrous tissue	ocul/o	eye

ROOT	MEANING	ROOT	MEANING
onc/o	tumor	rect/o	rectum
opt/o	vision	retin/o	retina
ot/o	ear	rhin/o	nose
orchi/o	testes	spleno	spleen
oste/o	bone	synovi/o	lining the joint
path/o	disease	tend/o	tendon
pector/o	chest	thorac/i or /o	rib cage
pharyng/o	pharynx	thromb/o	blood clot
phleb/o	blood	urethr/a	urethra
pleur/o	rib	uter/o	uterus, womb
pneumon/o	air	ven/o	vein
psych/o	mind	vesic/o	bladder
pulmon/o	lung		

Common Prefixes

Here are some of the most common prefixes used in medical terms.

PREFIX	MEANING	PREFIX	MEANING
a, an	absence of	inter	between
ab	away from	intra	within
ad	toward	iso	equal
aniso	unequal	mal	bad
ante	before	mega	large
anti	against	meso	middle
auto	self	meta	beyond
bi	both, two	micro	tiny
bio	life	mono	one
circum	around	multi	many
con	with	myel/o	relating to bone marrow
contra	against, opposite	neo	new
cryo	cold	pachy	thick
dis	apart	para	alongside, abnormal
dys	painful, bad	per	through
ec	out	peri	surrounding
ecto	outside of	poly	many
en	in	post	after
endo	inside of	pre	before
epi	on, before	primi	first
eu	good	retro	behind
ex	out	semi	half
hemi	half	sub	beneath
hemo	pertaining to blood	super	in excess
homeo	similar	supra	above
hyper	high	syn	with
hypo	low, below	tachy	fast
idio	one's own	uni	one

Common Suffixes

Here are some of the most common suffixes used in medical terms. Note that some suffixes have the same meaning.

SUFFIX	MEANING	SUFFIX	MEANING
ad	toward	oid	resembling, like
al	pertaining to	oma	tumor
algia	pain	osis	condition of
ary	pertaining to	ous	pertaining to
cele	hernia, swelling	pathy	disease
centesis	puncture in order to aspirate	penia	deficiency
cidal	destroying of	pexy	fixation or suspension
desis	binding	phagia	eating, swallowing
dynia	pain	phil or philia	abnormal attraction
ectomy	removal of	phobia	abnormal fear
ectasis	expansion of	plasia	development
emesis	vomiting	plasty	surgical repair
genic, genesis	producing	plegia	paralysis
graph	recording device	poiesis	production
graphy	recording process	ptosis	drooping, falling
iasis	abnormal condition	osis	abnormal condition
iatric	treatment of	rrhage	bursting forth, excessive flowing
iatry	field of medicine	rrhaphy	surgical suturing
ic	relating to	rrhexis	rupture
ism	condition of	rrhea	discharge, flowing
ite	resembling, like	rrhoea	discharge, flowing
itis	inflammation	sis	condition of
lepsis	seizure, attack	stasis	stop
logist	specialist in the study of	stenosis	narrowing
logy	study of	scope	viewing device
lysis	destruction of	scopy	process using a scope
malacia	softening	stomy	making a surgical incision
megaly	enlargement	tic	pertaining to
meter	measurement tool	tomy	incision, or cutting, into

Common Abbreviations

Here are some of the most common abbreviations used in medical terminology.

ABBREVIATION	MEANING	ABBREVIATION	MEANING
A	anterior	AIDS	acquired immunodeficiency syndrome
Abd, Abdo	abdomen	AML	acute myeloblastic leukemia
Ac	acute	Anat	anatomy
AF, A fib, Afib	atrial fibrillation	AP	appendectomy or appendicitis

ABBREVIATION	MEANING	ABBREVIATION	MEANING
ASCVD	arteriosclerotic cardiovascular disease	LH	luteinizing hormone
BM	bone marrow, bowel movement	LMP	last menstrual period
BMI	body mass index	LUQ	left upper quadrant
BOM	bilaterial otitis media	MET, met	metastasis
BSE	breast self examination	MG	myasthenia gravis
CA, Ca	cancer, cardiac arrest, carcinoma, chronological age	Na	sodium
CFS	chronic fatigue syndrome	N/G	nasogastric (tube)
CD	communicable disease	NIDDM	non-insulin-dependent diabetes mellitus
CH, chr	chromosomes	Noc, noct	night
COPD	chronic obstructive pulmonary disease	NPO	nothing by mouth
Cyt	cytology	NSAID	nonsteroidal anti-inflammatory drug
DG, Dg, Diag, DX, Dx	diagnosis	Oa	osteoarthritis
D	dorsal	OB, Obs	obstetrics
DNR	do not resuscitate	OM	otitis media
DOB	date of birth	PA, Pa, path	pathology
DPT	diphtheria, pertussis, and tetanus vaccine	PERRLA	pupils equal, round, reactive to light and accommodation
DVT	deep vein thrombosis	PFT	pulmonary function test
EBV	Epstein-Barr virus	Prog, progn, Prx, Px	prognosis
ECG, EKG	electrocardiogram	PSA	prostate specific antigen
ENT	ear, nose, and throat	SIDS	sudden infant death syndrome
FBS	fasting blood sugar	SOB	shortness of breath
FOBT	fecal occult blood test	SQ, SC	subcutaneous
FX, Fx	fracture	Sx	symptom
GTT	glucose tolerance test	TB	tuberculosis
H&H	hemoglobin and hematocrit	TIA	transient ischemic attack
HBV	hepatitis B virus	TPR	temperature, pulse, and respiration
He	hemorrhage	Umb	umbilical
HIS, Histo, histol	histology	URI	upper respiratory infection
IDDM	insulin-dependent diabetes mellitus	UTI	urinary tract infection
IM	intramuscular	V, vent, ventr	ventral
K	potassium	V fib, VF	ventricular fibrillation
KOH	potassium hydrocholoride	WBC	white blood count

Names for Common Medical Specialties and Specialists

The following list includes terms associated with the most common medical specialties. Note the root words used in these terms—some of which are not included in the previous root word list—to reinforce your knowledge of medical terminology.

Skeletal System

- **chiropractor:** a medical professional with an advanced degree who specializes in the manipulative treatment of disorders originating from the misalignment of the spine
- **orthopedic surgeon:** a physician who specializes in diagnosing and treating diseases and disorders involving the bones, joints, and muscles
- **osteopath:** a physician who holds a Doctor of Osteopathy (DO) degree and uses traditional forms of medical treatment in addition to specializing in treating health problems by spinal manipulation
- **podiatrist:** a physician who specializes in diagnosing and treating disorders of the foot

Muscular System

- **neurologist:** a physician who specializes in physical medicine and rehabilitation with the focus on restoring function
- **rheumatologist:** a physician who specializes in the diagnosis and treatment of arthritis and disorders such as osteoporosis, fibromyalgia, and tendonitis

Cardiovascular System

- **cardiologist:** a physician who specializes in diagnosing and treating abnormalities, diseases, and disorders of the heart
- **hematologist:** a physician who specializes in diagnosing and treating abnormalities, diseases, and disorders of the blood and blood-forming tissues

Lymphatic and Immune System

- **allergist:** a physician who specializes in diagnosing and treating conditions of altered immunologic reactivity such as allergic reactions
- **immunologist:** a physician who specializes in diagnosing and treating disorders of the immune system
- **oncologist:** a physician who specializes in diagnosing and treating malignant disorders such as tumors and cancer

Respiratory System

- **otolaryngologist:** a physician who specializes in the diagnosing and treatment of diseases and disorders of the ears, nose, and throat and related structures of the head and neck; also known as an ENT
- **pulmonologist:** a physician who specializes in diagnosing and treating diseases and disorders of the lungs and associated tissues

Digestive System

- **bariatrics:** the branch of medicine concerned with the prevention and control of obesity and associated diseases
- **dentist:** a physician who holds a Doctor of Dental Surgery (DDS) or Doctor of Medical Denistry (DMD) degree and specializes in diagnosing and treating diseases and disorders of the teeth and tissues of the oral cavity
- **gastroenterologist:** a physician who specializes in diagnosing and treating diseases and disorders of the stomach and intestines
- **orthodontist:** a dental specialist who prevents or corrects malocclusion of the teeth and related facial structures
- **peridontist:** a dental specialist who prevents or treats disorders of the tissues surrounding the teeth
- **proctologist:** a physician who specializes in disorders of the colon, rectum, and anus

Urinary System

- **nephrologist:** a physician who specializes in diagnosing and treating diseases and disorders of the kidneys
- **urologist:** a physician who specializes in diagnosing and treating diseases and disorders of the urinary system of females and the genitourinary system of males

Nervous System

- **anesthesiologist:** a physician who specializes in administering anesthetic agents before and during surgery
- **anesthetist:** a medical professional who specializes in administering anesthesia, but is not a physician
- **neurologist:** a physician who specializes in diagnosing and treating diseases and disorders of the nervous system
- **neurosurgeon:** a physician who specializes in surgery of the nervous system
- **psychiatrist:** a physician who specializes in diagnosing and treating chemical dependencies, emotional problems, and mental illness
- **psychologist:** a medical professional who holds an advanced degree, but is not a medical doctor; this specialist evaluates and treats emotional problems and mental illness

Eyes and Ears

- **ophthalmologist:** a physician who specializes in diagnosing and treating diseases and disorders of the eyes and vision
- **optometrist:** a physician who holds a Doctor of Optometry degree and specializes in measuring the accuracy of vision to determine whether corrective lenses are needed
- **audiologist:** a technologist with an advanced degree who specializes in the measurement of hearing function and in the rehabilitation of people with hearing impairments

Integumentary System

- **dermatologist:** a physician who specializes in diagnosing and treating diseases and disorders of the skin
- **cosmetic surgeon:** a physician who specializes in the surgical restoration and reconstruction of body structures

Endocrine System

- **endocrinologist:** a physician who specializes in diagnosing and treating diseases and malfunctions of the endocrine glands

Reproductive System

- **urologist:** a physician who specializes in diagnosing and treating disease and disorders of the urinary system
- **gynecologist:** a physician who specializes in diagnosing and treating disease and disorders of the female reproductive system
- **obstetrician:** a physician who specializes in providing medical care to women during pregnancy, childbirth, and the postpartum period
- **neonatologist:** a physician who treats and diagnoses disorders of newborns
- **pediatrician:** a physician who specializes in diagnosing, treating, and preventing disorders and diseases of children

Names for Common Surgical Procedures

The following list includes terms associated with the most common medical surgical procedures. The term is taken apart, showing the components, to help you see the meaning of the term. You will find some word components that are not on the previous lists of roots, prefixes, and suffixes, so you can add them to the growing list of word parts with which you are familiar.

Skeletal System

- **arthrodesis:** *arthr/o* means "joint" and *desis* means "surgical fixation"
- **arthrolysis:** *arthr/o* means "joint" and *lysis* means "loosening or setting free"
- **bursectomy:** *burs* means "bursa" and *ectomy* means "surgical removal"
- **chondroplasty:** *chondr/o* means "cartilage" and *plasty* means "surgical repair"
- **synovectomy:** *synov* means "synovial membrane" and *ectomy* means "surgical removal"
- **laminectomy:** *lamin* means "lamina" and *ectomy* means "surgical removal"
- **craniectomy:** *crani* means "skull" and *ectomy* means "surgical incision"
- **osteorrhaphy:** *oste/o* means "bone" and *rrhaphy* means "surgical suturing"

Muscular System

- **myectomy:** *my* means "muscle" and *ectomy* means "surgical removal"
- **myoplasty:** *my* means "muscle" and *plasty* means "surgical repair"
- **myorraphy:** *my* means "muscle" and *rraphy* means "surgical suturing"
- **myotomy:** *my* means "muscle" and *otomy* means "surgical incision"

Cardiovascular System

- **atherectomy:** *ather* means "plaque" and *ectomy* means "surgical removal"
- **carotid endarterectomy:** the surgical removal of the lining of a portion of a clogged carotid artery, which leads to the brain
- **coronary artery bypass graft:** also known as bypass surgery, in which a vein from the leg or chest is implanted in the heart to replace a blocked coronary artery to improve the flow of blood to the heart
- **aneurysmorrhaphy:** *aneurysm* stands for itself and *rrhaphy* means "surgical suturing"

- **valvoplasty:** *valv/o* means "valve" and *plasty* means "surgical repair"

Lymphatic and Immune System

- **lumpectomy:** the surgical removal of only the cancerous tissue, assuming the surrounding tissue is normal
- **mastectomy:** *mast* means "breast" and *ectomy* means "surgical removal"

Respiratory System

- **lobectomy:** *lob* means "lobe" and *ectomy* means "surgical removal" (can relate to other body systems)
- **pleurectomy:** *pleur* means "pleura," a membrane in the lungs, and *ectomy* means "surgical removal"
- **pneumonectomy:** *pneumon* means "lung" and *ectomy* means "surgical removal"
- **thoracentesis:** *thor/a* means "chest" and *centesis* means "surgical puncture to remove fluid"

Digestive System

- **colectomy:** *col* means "colon" and *ectomy* means "surgical removal"
- **diverticulectomy:** *diverticul* means "diverticulum," an abnormal pouch, usually in the intestines, and *ectomy* means "surgical removal"
- **gastroduodenostomy:** *gastr/o* means "stomach," *duoden* means "first part of the small intestine," and *ostomy* means "surgically creating an opening"
- **proctopexy:** *proct/o* means "rectum" and *pexy* means "surgical fixation"

Urinary System

- **nephrolithotomy:** *nephr/o* means "kidney," *lith* means "stone," and *otomy* means "surgical incision"
- **nephropexy:** *nephr/o* means "kidney" and *pexy* means "surgical fixation"
- **pyeloplasty:** *pyel/o* means renal "pelvis" and *plasty* means "surgical repair"

- **cystorrhaphy:** *cyst/o* means "bladder" and *rrhaphy* means "surgical suturing"
- **urethrostomy:** *urethra/o* means "ureter" and *ostomy* means "creating an opening"
- **transurethral prostatectomy:** the removal of an overgrowth of tissue from the prostate gland through a resectoscope; referred to as TURP

Nervous System

- **lobectomy:** the surgical removal of a portion of the brain to treat brain cancer or seizure disorders
- **thalamotomy:** *thalam* means "thalamus," part of the brain, and *otomy* means "surgical incision"
- **neuroplasty:** *neur/o* means "nerve" and *plasty* means "surgical repair"
- **neurorrhaphy:** *neur/o* means "nerve" and *rrhaphy* means "surgical suturing"
- **neurotomy:** *neur/o* means "nerve" and *otomy* means "surgical incision"

Integumentary System

- **lipectomy:** *lip* means "fat" and *ectomy* means "surgical removal"
- **liposuction:** *lip* means "fat," so a liposuction is the process of removing fat by a suctioning method
- **rhytidectomy:** *rhytid* means "wrinkle" and *ectomy* means "surgical removal"

Eyes

- **laser iridotomy:** *irid* means "iris" and *otomy* means "surgical incision"
- **orbitotomy:** *orbit* means "bony socket" (which houses the eye), and *otomy* means "surgical incision"
- **tarsorrhaphy:** *tars/o* means "eyelid" and *rrhaphy* means "surgical suturing"
- **conjunctivoplasty:** *conjunctiv* means "conjunctiva," the mucous membrane lining the eyelid, and *plasty* means "surgical repair"
- **iridectomy:** *irid* means "iris" and *ectomy* means "surgical removal"

- **vitrectomy:** *vitr* means "vitreous fluid" and *ectomy* means "removal"
- **lensectomy:** *lens* means "lens" and *ectomy* means "surgical removal"
- **blepharoplasty:** *blephar/o* means "eyelid" and *plasty* means "surgical repair"
- **retinopexy:** *retin/o* means "retina" and *pexy* means "surgical fixation"
- **LASIK:** an abbreviation for laser-assisted in situ keratomileusis: *kerat/o* means "cornea" and *mileuis* means "carving"

Ears

- **otoplasty:** *ot/o* means ear, and *plasty* means surgical repair
- **mastoidectomy:** *mastoid* means mastoid process and *ectomy* means surgical removal
- **myringotomy:** *myring/o* means eardrum and *otomy* means surgical incision
- **tympanostomy:** *tympan/o* means eardrum, and *ostomy* means creating an opening
- **tympanoplasty:** *tympan/o* means eardrum, and *plasty* means surgical repair

Endocrine System

- **laparoscopic adrenalectomy:** *adrenal* means "adrenal gland," and *ectomy* means "surgical removal;" *laparoscopic* indicates a type of minimally invasive surgical procedure
- **pancreatectomy:** *pancreat* means "pancreas," and *ectomy* means "surgical removal"
- **thymectomy:** *thym* means "thymus" and *ectomy* means "surgical removal"
- **pinealectomy:** *pineal* means "pineal gland" and *ectomy* means "surgical removal"

Reproductive System

- **ovariectomy:** *ovari* means "ovary" and *ectomy* means "surgical removal"
- **salpingectomy:** *salping* means "fallopian tube" and *ectomy* means "surgical removal"

- **salpingoophorectomy:** *salping* means "one or both fallopian tubes," *oophor* means "ovary," and *ectomy* means "surgical removal"
- **orchiectomy:** *orchi/o* means "testicle" and *ectomy* means "surgical removal"
- **orchiopexy:** *orchid/o* means "testicle" and *pexy* means "surgical fixation"
- **colpopexy:** *colp/o* means "vagina" and *pexy* means "surgical fixation in place"
- **colporrhaphy:** *colp/o* means "vagina" and *rrhaphy* means "surgical suturing"
- **myomectomy:** *myom* means "muscle tumor" and *ectomy* means "surgical removal"
- **hysterectomy:** *hyster* means "uterus" and *ectomy* means "surgical removal"
- **mastopexy:** *mast/o* means "breast" and *pexy* means "surgical fixation"
- **vasectomy:** *vas* means "vas deferens," part of the male reproductive system, and *ectomy* means "surgical removal"

Names for Common Diagnostic Procedures and Treatments

The following list includes terms associated with the most common diagnostic procedures and treatments. This list includes only a few notations and reminders about the meaning of word parts, as many of the terms discussed in this section are not based on the Latin and Greek word parts. They are nevertheless important terms for the medical assistant to recognize and understand.

Skeletal System

- **radiograph:** also known as an X-ray; is used to visualize bone fractures and other abnormalities
- **arthroscopy:** *arthro* means "joint"; the visual examination of the internal structure of a joint
- **magnetic resonance imaging (MRI):** used to take pictures of soft tissue structures, such as the interior of complex joints
- **bone density test:** used to determine losses or changes in bone density

Muscular System

- **electromyography:** *myo* means "muscle"; a diagnostic test that measures the electrical activity within a muscle fibers in response to nerve stimulation
- **electroneuromyography:** *neuro* means "nerve" and *myo* means "muscle"; a diagnostic procedure for testing and recording neuromuscular activity by the electric stimulation for the nerve trunk that carries fibers to and from the muscle
- **range of motion:** a diagnostic procedure to evaluate joint mobility and muscle strength

Cardiovascular System

- **angiography:** *angio* means "blood vessel"; a radiographic study of the blood vessels after the injection of a contrast medium
- **cardiac cauterization:** *cardio* means "heart"; a diagnostic procedure in which a catheter is passed into a vein or artery and then guided into the heart
- **digital subtraction angiography:** *angio* means "blood"; the combination of an angiography with computerized components to clarify the view of the area of interest by removing the soft tissue and bones from the images
- **duplex ultrasound:** a diagnostic procedure to image the structures of the blood vessels and the flow of blood through the vessels
- **electrocardiogram:** *cardio* means "heart"; a record of the electrical activity of the myocardium, the muscle layer lining the wall of the heart
- **stress test:** a test that assesses cardiovascular health and function during and after stress (exercise)
- **thalium stress test:** a test that evaluates how well blood flows through the coronary arteries of the heart muscle during exercise

Lymphatic and Immune System

- **mammography:** *mammo* means "breast"; a radiographic examination of the breasts to detect the presence of tumors or precancerous cells
- **scratch test:** a diagnostic test to identify commonly troublesome allergens, such as tree pollen and ragweed
- **chemotherapy:** *chemo* means "drugs or chemicals"; the use of chemical agents and drugs in combinations selected to destroy malignant cells and tissues

Respiratory System

- **bronchoscopy:** the visual examination of the bronchi, or air passages, using a bronchoscope
- **laryngoscopy:** the visual examination of the larynx using a laryngoscope inserted through the mouth and placed into the pharynx to examine the larynx
- **polysomnography:** *somno* means "sleep"; a measurement of physiological activity during sleep, most often performed to detect nocturnal defects in breathing associated with sleep apnea
- **pulmonary function tests:** *pulmon* means "lung"; a group of tests that measure volume and flow of air by utilizing a spirometer
- **spirometer:** a recording device that measures the amount of air inhaled or exhaled and the length of time required for each breath
- **pulse oximeter:** an external monitor placed on the patient's finger or earlobe to measure oxygen saturation level in the blood
- **tuberculin skin test:** a screening test for tuberculosis (TB) during which the skin of the arm is injected with a harmless antigen extracted from TB bacteria

Digestive System

- **abdominal computed tomography (CT):** a radiographic procedure that produces a detailed cross-section of the tissue structure within the abdomen

- **cholangiography:** a radiographic examination of the bile ducts with the use of a contrast medium
- **esophagogastroduodenoscopy:** an endoscopic procedure that allows direct visualization of the upper GI (gastrointestinal) tract, which includes the esophagus, stomach, and upper duodenum
- **hemoccult:** *hemo* means "blood"; a laboratory test for hidden blood in the stool; also known as the fecal occult blood test

Urinary System

- **urinalysis:** the examination of urine to determine the presence of abnormal elements
- **bladder ultrasound:** the use of a handheld transducer to measure the amount of urine remaining in the bladder after urination
- **cystography:** *cysto* means "bladder"; a radiographic examination of the bladder after instillation of a contrast medium via a urethral catheter
- **cystoscopy:** *cysto* means "bladder"; the visual examination of the urinary bladder using a cystoscope
- **intravenous pyelogram:** a radiographic study of the kidneys and ureters
- **KUB:** stands for kidney, ureters, bladder; a radiographic study of these structures without the use of a contrast medium

Nervous System

- **carotid ultrasonography:** an ultrasound study of the carotid artery
- **echoencephalography:** the use of ultrasound imaging to diagnose a shift in the midline structures of the brain
- **myelography:** a radiographic study of the spinal cord after the injection of a contrast medium through a lumbar puncture
- **lumbar puncture:** the process of obtaining a sample of cerebrospinal fluid by inserting a needle into the subarachnoid space of the lumbar region to withdraw fluid

Eyes and Ears

- **tympanometry:** the use of air pressure in the ear canal to test for disorders of the middle ear
- **binaural testing:** testing that involves both ears
- **monoaural testing:** testing that involves one ear
- **audiometry:** the use of an audiometer to measure hearing acuity

Integumentary System

- **laser:** a means of light amplification by stimulated emission of radiation; used to treat skin conditions and other disorders of the body
- **biopsy:** the removal of a small piece of living tissue for examination to confirm or establish a diagnosis
- **exfoliative cystology:** a technique in which cells are scraped from the tissue and examined under a microscope

Endocrine System

- **thyroid-stimulating hormone (TSH) test:** a blood test to measure the circulating blood levels of thyroid-stimulating hormones
- **thyroid scan:** a test that measures thyroid function; a form of nuclear medicine
- **chemical thyroidectomy:** the administration of radioactive iodine to destroy thyroid cells
- **lobectomy:** the surgical removal of one lobe of the thyroid gland
- **synthetic thyroid hormone:** a therapy hormone used to replace lost thyroid function
- **fasting blood sugar:** a measurement of glucose levels after the patient has not eaten for eight to 12 hours
- **fructosamine test:** a blood test that measures average glucose levels over the past three weeks
- **hemoglobin A1c:** a blood test that measures the average blood glucose level over the previous three to four months
- **cortisone:** the synthetic equivalent of corticosteroids produced by the body; administered to suppress inflammation; an immunosuppressant

- **epinephrine:** a synthetic hormone used as a vasoconstrictor to treat conditions such as heart dysrhythmias and asthma attacks

Reproductive System

- **testicular exam:** a manual exam useful in early detection of testicular cancer
- **colposcopy:** a direct visual exam of the tissues of the cervix and vagina
- **endometrial biopsy:** the removal of a small amount of tissue from the lining of the uterus for the purpose of microscopic examination
- **hysterosalpingography:** a radiographic examination of the uterus and fallopian tubes
- **Papanicolaou test (Pap smear):** an exfoliative biopsy for the detection of conditions that may be early indicators of cervical cancer
- **chorionic villus sampling:** the examination of cells retrieved from the chorionic villi, which are minute, vascular projections on the chorion
- **amniocentesis:** a surgical puncture with a needle to obtain a specimen of amniotic fluid
- **episiotomy:** a surgical incision made through the perineum to enlarge the vaginal orifice to prevent tearing of the tissue as the infant moves out of the birth canal during delivery
- **episiorrhaphy:** the surgical suturing to repair an episiotomy

Anatomy and Physiology

Anatomy is the study of the structures of the body, while *physiology* is the study of the functions of the body and its structures.

Structural Units of the Human Body

The human body is a complex organism composed of various levels of structure. The levels of structure include cells, tissues, organs, system, and organism. Each structure has a specific function that aids in the overall function of the human body.

Cells

Cells are the structural and functional units of the human body. The study of cells is called **cytology**. **Homeostasis**, or the tendency of the body toward a state of equilibrium, depends on the interaction between the cell and its environment. During development, cells become specialized in size, shape, characteristics, and function, resulting in a large variety of types of cells in the body.

Every cell in the body is enclosed by a plasma **cell membrane**. The plasma membrane separates the material outside of the cell (extracellular) from the material inside the cell (intracellular). It maintains the integrity of the cell; if the plasma cell membrane ruptures or is broken, the cell dies. The plasma cell membrane determines what can go into or out of the cell. The main structural components of the plasma cell membrane are phospholipids and proteins.

The **cytoplasm** is the gel-like fluid inside the cell. The cytoplasm has numerous small structures, called **organelles**, suspended in it. These organelles are the functional machinery of the cell, and each organelle type has a specific role in the metabolic reactions that take place in the cytoplasm.

The cytoplasm consists primarily of liquid known as the intracellular fluid. Intracellular fluid is made up of a complex mix of substances dissolved in water. About two-thirds of the water in the body is in the cytoplasm of cells. The intracellular fluid contains dissolved electrolytes, metabolic waste products, and nutrients such as amino acids and simple sugars.

The **nucleus** is the control center that directs the activities of the cell. All cells have at least one nucleus at some time during their existence; some, however, such as red blood cells, lose their nucleus as they mature. Other cells, such as skeletal muscle cells, have multiple nuclei.

The nucleus is a relatively large, spherical body that is usually located near the center of the cell. It is enclosed by a double-layered nuclear membrane that separates the cytoplasm of the cell from the nucleoplasm, the fluid portion inside the nucleus.

The nucleus contains the genetic material of the cell. In the nondividing cell, the genetic material deoxyribonucleic acid (DNA), is present as long, slender, filamentous threads called chromatin. When the cell starts to divide or replicate, the chromatin condenses and becomes tightly coiled to form short, rod-like chromosomes.

Tissues

Tissues are groups of cells that are similar in structure and function. The study of tissues is called histology. The four major types of tissues of the body are epithelial, connective, muscle, and nervous.

Epithelial Tissue

Epithelial tissue covers organ surfaces; lines cavities, vessels, and canals; and provides the secreting portions of glands. Its function is to protect, absorb, secrete, and filtrate.

Connective Tissue

Connective tissue includes bones, cartilage, blood cells, and fat cells. Its function is to protect, support, and connect other tissues and organs.

Muscle Tissue

Muscle tissue contracts to produce movement. The three types of muscle tissue are skeletal, cardiac, and smooth. Skeletal muscle is attached to bones and causes voluntary movement of body parts. Cardiac muscle is located only in the heart and causes involuntary heart contractions. Smooth muscle also involves involuntary contractions, but within the walls of hollow organs and blood vessels.

Nervous Tissue

Nervous tissue consists of neurons that receive and conduct electrochemical impulses.

Organs

Organs are body structures that consist of several tissues and perform specialized functions. Organs include structures such as the brain, stomach, skin, nose, nasopharynx, bladder, heart, liver, lungs, spleen, thymus, thyroid, kidney, uterus, intestines, gall bladder, ovaries, prostate, and testes.

Systems

A system is an organized grouping of structure, including the integumentary system, musculoskeletal system, cardiovascular system, respiratory system, digestive system, urinary system, reproductive system, endocrine system, sensory system, and the nervous system.

- The **integumentary system** includes the skin and its appendages, hair, nails, and glands. This system protects the body from potentially harmful external elements and helps to regulate the body's temperature, among other functions.
- The **musculoskeletal system** is comprised of muscles, tendons, and associated structures. This system makes movement possible, moves body fluid, and generates body heat.
- The **cardiovascular system** consists of the heart, arteries, veins, capillaries, and blood. This system circulates blood throughout the body to transport oxygen and nutrients to cells and to carry waste products to the kidneys, where waste is removed by filtration.
- The **respiratory system** consists of the nose, pharynx, trachea, larynx, and lungs. This system brings oxygen into the body for transportation to the cells. It also removes carbon dioxide and some water waste from the body.
- The **urinary system** consists of the kidneys, ureters, urinary bladder, and urethra. This system filters blood to remove waste and maintains the electrolyte and fluid balance within the body.

- The **male reproductive system** consists of the penis and testicles. The **female reproductive system** consists of the ovaries, uterus, and vagina. The reproductive system produces new life.
- The **endocrine system** consists of the adrenal glands, gonads, pancreas, parathyroids, pineal, pituitary, thymus, and thyroid. This system is responsible for integrating all body functions.
- The **digestive system** consists of the mouth, esophagus, stomach, small intestine, large intestine, liver, and pancreas. This system is responsible for the digestion of food, so that nutrients from the food can be absorbed into the bloodstream and waste can be eliminated.
- The **sensory system** consists of the organs of sight, hearing, smell, taste, and touch. This system is responsible for sight, hearing, taste, and sensations.
- The **nervous system** consists of the nerves, brain, and spinal cord. This system is responsible for coordinating the reception of stimuli.

Anatomical Divisions

Observing the relative locations and organization of internal body parts requires sectioning the body along various regions.

- **hypochondriac region:** upper lateral regions beneath the ribs
- **epigastric region:** middle lateral regions
- **umbilical region:** region of the navel
- **inguinal regions:** lower lateral groin regions
- **hypogastric region:** region below the navel

Positions and Directions

Directional terms are used to describe the relative position of one part of the body to another.
- **Superior** means that one part is above another part or closer to the head. The nose is superior to the mouth.

- **Inferior** means that one part is below another part or closer to the feet. The heart is inferior to the neck.
- **Anterior** means toward the front surface. The heart is anterior to the vertebral column.
- **Posterior** means toward the back. The heart is posterior to the sternum.
- **Medial** means toward or nearer the midline of the body. The nose is medial to the ears.
- **Lateral** means toward or nearer the side, away from the midline. The ears are lateral to the eyes.
- **Proximal** means that one part is closer to a point of attachment, or closer to the trunk of the body, than another part. The elbow is proximal to the wrist.
- **Distal** means that one part is farther away from a point of attachment than another part is. The fingers are distal to the wrist.
- **Superficial** means located on or near the surface. The superficial layer of the skin is the epidermis.
- **Deep** means away from the surface. Muscles are deep to the skin surface.
- **Visceral** pertains to internal organs or the covering of the organs. The visceral pericardium covers the heart.
- **Parietal** refers to the wall of a body cavity. The parietal peritoneum lines the wall of the abdominal cavity.

Body Planes

To aid in visualizing the spatial relationships of internal body parts, anatomists use three imaginary planes, each of which cuts through the body in a different direction.

1. **Sagittal plane** refers to a lengthwise cut that divides the body into right and left portions; sometimes called a longitudinal section.

   Midsagittal, or **median, plane** refers to a cut that passes through the *midline* of the body that divides the body into *equal* right and left halves.

2. **Transverse plane**, or horizontal plane, is perpendicular to the sagittal plane and cuts across the body horizontally to divide it into superior and inferior portions. Sections cut this way are sometimes called cross sections.

3. **Frontal plane** divides the body into anterior and posterior portions. It is perpendicular to both the sagittal plane and the transverse plane; sometimes called a coronal plane.

Common Diseases and Pathology of Each Body System

Pathology is the study and diagnosis of disease through examination of organs, tissues, bodily fluids, and whole bodies (autopsies). Anything that upsets the normal structure or working of the body is considered a disease and is studied as the science of pathology.

Integumentary System

The integumentary system consists of the skin and its accessory organs. The skin, which is the largest organ in the body, is composed of three layers, the **epidermis**, **dermis**, and **subcutaneous**. The accessory organs include the **glands**, **hair**, and **nails**.

The functions of the skin and its accessory organs include:

- **Protection:** The skin protects the body from sunlight, microorganisms, and other harmful elements. In addition, hair in the nasal and ear cavities, as well as on the eyelids, helps protect against harmful microorganisms by trapping them and not allowing them to enter the body. Nails help protect the ends of the fingers and toes.
- **Secretion:** Sebaceous glands secrete sebum to help lubricate the skin, while sudoriferous glands secrete sweat to help cool the body when the environment is too hot.

- **Sensation:** The skin contains sensory touch receptors that allow the person to feel temperature, pain, and touch.
- **Temperature regulation:** The skin plays an important role in insulating the body and maintaining heat when the body is exposed to cold temperatures. The production of sweat by the sudoriferous glands aids in cooling off the body when the environment is too hot.

Related Conditions and Diseases

- **psoriasis:** a chronic inflammatory skin disease characterized by red or pink patches covered by thick, dry, silvery scales
- **urticaria:** an inflammatory skin eruption, usually caused by an allergic reaction, which is characterized by red patches called wheals; also known as hives
- **alopecia:** a partial or complete loss of hair, especially on the head
- **dermatitis:** an inflammation of the skin characterized by severe itching, redness, and the appearance of small skin vesicles
- **pediculosis:** an infestation of lice characterized by severe itching; commonly transmitted through the use of brushes, combs, or hats that have been used by an infected person
- **decubitis ulcers:** commonly known as bedsores or pressure sores; localized open sores, frequently seen over a bony prominence, due to persistent pressure and poor blood flow to the area
- **scabies:** a contagious infestation of the skin caused by the itch mite; characterized by severe itching and lesions
- **warts:** benign, circumscribed, raised lesions due to hypertrophy, or exaggerated growth, of the papillae and epidermis; commonly caused by the papilloma virus
- **shingles:** a painful, inflammatory skin condition characterized by the eruption of vesicles, or raised blisterlike protuberances; caused by the herpes zoster virus

- **skin cancer:** a cancer that is caused by overexposure to the ultraviolet rays of the sun as well as exposure to radiation. There are three forms: basal cell carcinoma, squamous cell carcinoma, and malignant melanoma.
- **hematoma:** the accumulation of blood under the skin due to a break in a blood vessel; also known as a bruise
- **impetigo:** an infectious skin infection caused by staphyloccocal and/or streptococal bacteria
- **schleroderma:** a chronic autoimmune disease characterized by hardening of the skin, which becomes taunt, firm, and edematous, or swollen

Musculoskeletal System

The musculoskeletal system consists of bones, cartilage, joints, muscles, ligaments, and tendons. Its function is to provide support and protection for the body's structures, as well as to allow for physical movement.

Related Conditions and Diseases

- **kyphosis:** abnormal outward curvature of the spine
- **scoliosis:** abnormal sideward curvature of the spine
- **lordosis:** abnormal inward curvature of the spine
- **osteoporosis:** metabolic bone disease characterized by decreased bone mass
- **osteomyelitis:** infection of the bone-forming tissue, characterized by inflammation and swelling over the affected bone
- **fracture:** a break in the bone characterized by swelling, pain, and tenderness at and around the site of the injury, possible deformity, and limited range of motion
- **rheumatoid arthritis:** a chronic connective tissue disease characterized by painful and swollen joints that may result in deformities and immobility

- **gout:** a form of arthritis characterized by the accumulation of uric acid crystals in various joints
- **bursitis:** inflammation of the bursa commonly affecting areas such as the shoulder, arm, and elbow
- **tendonitis:** inflammation of the tendon commonly affecting the shoulder rotator cuff, hip, or hamstring
- **sprain:** an injury to a ligament that causes pain and limited range of motion
- **myasthenia gravis:** a chronic autoimmune neuromuscular disease characterized by muscle weakness and abnormal fatigue
- **carpal tunnel syndrome:** compression of the median nerve in the hand and wrist that is characterized by pain, tingling, and numbness; usually seen in patients who perform repetitive motion tasks or jobs
- **muscular dystrophy:** a progressive congenital disorder characterized by the wasting of skeletal muscle tissue

The Nervous System

The nervous system controls the body's response to stimuli and helps maintain homeostasis. It helps control both voluntary and involuntary functions. The nervous system has two major parts:

- The **central nervous system**, which consists of the brain and spinal cord. The function of the central nervous system is to receive and process information and to regulate all bodily activity.
- The **peripheral nervous system**, which consists of 31 pairs of spinal nerves and 12 cranial nerves. The function of the peripheral nervous system is to transmit nerve signals to and from the central nervous system.

Related Conditions and Diseases

- **migraine headaches:** severe, pulsating headaches that are usually accompanied by vision and gastrointestinal disturbances
- **concussion:** a trauma or blow to the head causing the brain to strike the skull; may cause confusion and temporary unconsciousness
- **hemiplegia:** a spinal cord injury in which there is paralysis on one side of the body
- **paraplegia:** a spinal cord injury in which there is paralysis of the lower half of the body (trunk and legs)
- **quadriplegia:** a spinal cord injury in which there is paralysis of all four extremities and usually the trunk of the body
- **cerebrovascular accident:** a vascular injury to the brain characterized by a sudden loss of neurological function; also known as a stroke
- **transient ischemic attack:** a brief disruption of blood flow to the brain, causing temporary impairment of neurological function
- **epilepsy:** abnormal electrical discharges within the brain causing recurrent seizures, sensory disturbances, abnormal behavior, and/or loss of consciousness
- **meningitis:** inflammation of the meninges and cerebral spinal fluid commonly caused by an infectious agent such as bacteria or viruses
- **encephalitis:** inflammation of the brain commonly caused by an infectious agent such as bacteria or viruses
- **Bell's palsy:** a condition of temporary weakness or paralysis of one side of the face
- **Alzheimer's disease:** a form of pre-senile dementia, characterized by memory loss, deterioration of intellectual function, disorientation, and emotional instability
- **Parkinson's disease:** a chronic progressive disease of the central nervous system characterized by movement disorders and changes in mood and cognition

■ **multiple sclerosis:** a chronic disease of the central nervous system characterized by the degeneration of the myelin sheath that covers nerve fibers

The Cardiovascular, Hematopoietic, and Lymphatic Systems

The **cardiovascular system** consists of the heart and related blood vessels (arteries, veins, and capillaries), also known as the **circulatory system**. The function of the cardiovascular system is to pump and distribute blood throughout the body and deliver oxygen and other nutrients to every organ, tissue, and cell of the body.

The **hematopoietic system** consists of the blood cells produced by the bone marrow. These cells consist of the **erythrocytes, leukocytes,** and **thrombocytes.** In the hematopoietic system, each of the blood cells has its distinct function. The erythrocyte is responsible for transporting oxygen throughout the body and for transporting carbon dioxide to the lungs to be expelled by the body. Leukocytes are responsible for fighting off infection and for producing antibodies. Thrombocytes are responsible for blood clotting and play a role in the coagulation process.

The **lymphatic system** consists of the tissue fluid called lymph, lymph vessels, and lymph nodes. Organs related to the lymph system include the **thymus gland** and **spleen.** The lymphatic system has three primary functions:

■ to transport immune cells to and from the lymph nodes
■ to remove interstitial fluid from tissues
■ to filter harmful substances such as viruses and bacteria from the lymph nodes

Related Conditions and Diseases

■ **myocardial infarction:** occlusion of blood flow within a coronary artery, which in turn causes damage to the heart muscle; also known as a heart attack

■ **coronary artery disease:** a narrowing or blockage of any of the coronary arteries that supply blood to the heart
■ **congestive heart failure:** inability of the heart to pump efficiently, causing fluid to build up the lungs or peripheral body areas
■ **angina pectoris:** chest pain or pressure around the heart caused by a deficiency of oxygen supply to the heart muscle
■ **endocarditis:** inflammation of the endocardium, the membrane lining the heart cavities, and the heart valves
■ **hypertension:** high blood pressure
■ **aneurysm:** weakness in an artery wall that causes the artery to bulge and/or rupture
■ **arteriosclerosis:** thickening of an artery wall
■ **atherosclerosis:** the accumulation of cholesterol in the artery wall
■ **thrombophlebitis:** inflammation of a vein combined with clot formation
■ **iron deficiency anemia:** a decrease in the number of red blood cells resulting from a decrease in iron
■ **aplastic anemia:** decreased production of red blood cells by the bone marrow
■ **sickle cell anemia:** anemia due to an abnormal red blood cell morphology and function, in which the cells are shaped like a sickle
■ **lymphedema:** abnormal accumulation of fluid due to obstruction of lymph vessels
■ **Hodgkin's lymphoma:** a type of cancer affecting the lymph nodes and eventually spreading throughout the lymphatic system to affect the spleen and bone marrow
■ **leukemia:** malignancy of the blood and blood-forming tissues; characterized by the blood cell being affected and also classified as chronic or acute

The Respiratory System

The respiratory system consists of the upper respiratory tract and the lower respiratory tract. The function of the respiratory system is to facilitate breathing and to provide for gas exchange to all parts of the body.

- The **upper respiratory tract** includes the nose and nasal cavities, pharynx, larynx, and upper trachea.
- The **lower respiratory tract** includes the lower trachea, bronchi, and lungs.

Related Conditions and Diseases

- **epistaxis:** nosebleed
- **pneumonia:** an inflammatory condition of the lungs commonly caused by infectious microorganisms
- **bronchitis:** inflammation of the bronchi of the lungs
- **sinusitis:** inflammation of the sinuses
- **acute pharygitis:** inflammation of the throat characterized by pain and redness, and commonly caused by streptococcal bacteria
- **pneumothorax:** air in the chest cavity
- **hemothorax:** blood in the chest cavity
- **pleurisy:** an inflammation of the lining of the lungs that causes pain during breathing or coughing
- **emphysema:** a chronic progressive disease of the lungs characterized by shortness of breath
- **tuberculosis:** an infection of the lungs caused by mycobacterium; characterized by chronic cough, blood-tinged sputum, weight loss, and night sweats
- **croup:** inflammation of the upper airways; characterized by a barking cough
- **pulmonary embolism:** a sudden blockage in a lung artery, usually caused by a blood clot

The Digestive System

The digestive system consists of the digestive tract and the accessory organs of digestion. The digestive tract contains structures such as the mouth, tongue, teeth, gums, uvula, and esophagus. Organs associated with the digestive tract include the stomach, small intestine, large intestine, rectum, and anus. The accessory organs include the gall bladder, liver, and pancreas.

The functions of the digestive system include the breakdown of food, digestion of nutrients, and elimination of wastes.

Related Conditions and Diseases

- **gastritis:** inflammation of the stomach
- **gastroesophageal reflux disease (GERD):** a condition in which the liquid content of the stomach regurgitates (backs up or refluxes) into the esophagus; commonly referred to as acid reflux
- **gastroenteritis:** inflammation of the stomach and intestines
- **hiatal hernia:** a condition in which a portion of the stomach protrudes upward into the chest, through an opening in the diaphragm
- **peptic ulcer:** a hole in the lining of the stomach or duodenum characterized by abdominal pain and usually caused by the bacterium *Helicobacter pylori*
- **celiac disease:** an autoimmune disease in which the lining of the small intestine is damaged from eating gluten and other proteins found in wheat, barley, rye, and possibly oats
- **irritable bowel syndrome:** a disorder of the lower intestinal tract characterized by abdominal pain, cramping, bloating, constipation, and diarrhea
- **Crohn's disease:** a chronic inflammation of the digestive tract, characterized by abdominal cramping, fever, fatigue, and persistent watery diarrhea
- **ulcerative colitis:** inflammation and ulcers of the lining of the colon and rectum characterized by abdominal pain and bloody diarrhea
- **acute appendicitis:** inflammation of the appendix
- **cholelithiasis:** gallstones
- **hepatitis:** inflammation of the liver, usually caused by viruses
- **pancreatitis:** inflammation of the pancreas
- **jaundice:** yellowish coloring of the skin because of an increase of bilirubin in the bloodstream

- **hemorrhoids:** condition in which the veins around the anus or lower rectum are swollen and inflamed

The Urinary System

The urinary system consists of the **kidneys, ureters, urinary bladder**, and **urethra.** The functions of the urinary system are to filter the blood, regulate fluid and electrolytes, and excrete wastes.

Related Conditions and Diseases

- **glomerulonephritis:** inflammation of the glomeruli of the kidney
- **polycystic disease:** genetic disorder characterized by the growth of numerous cysts in the kidneys
- **uremia:** presence of urine in the bloodstream
- **nephrotic syndrome:** a syndrome caused by various disorders that damage the kidneys and characterized by protein in the urine
- **renal calculi:** painful condition of stones in the kidney, characterized by blood in the urine and severe pain radiating from the back, down the flank, and into the groin
- **cystitis:** inflammation of the bladder, usually caused by a bacterial infection
- **urethritis:** inflammation of the urethra
- **neurogenic bladder:** condition in which the bladder does not empty properly due to a neurological problem
- **end-stage renal disease:** irreversible kidney failure

The Reproductive System

The female reproductive system consists of the **breasts, ovaries, fallopian tubes, uterus, cervix**, and **vagina.** The function of the reproductive system is to bear offspring. The male reproductive system consists of the **penis, urethra, testes, scrotum**, and **prostate gland.** The function of the male reproductive system is the production and transportation of sperm for the purpose of reproduction.

Related Conditions and Diseases—Female Reproductive System

- **premenstrual syndrome (PMS):** a condition characterized by anxiety, mood swings, fatigue, depression, headaches, vertigo, bloating, acne, swollen breasts, and changes in appetite that typically occur seven to ten days prior to menstruation and end a few days after the onset of menstruation
- **amenorrhea:** absence of menstruation
- **dysmenorrhea:** pain during menstruation
- **ovarian cysts:** benign fluid-filled sacs that form on the ovary
- **endometriosis:** an abnormal condition of endometrial tissue occurring and growing outside the endometrium
- **pelvic inflammatory disease (PID):** a condition resulting from the extension of infections from the reproductive organs into the pelvic cavity; often involves the peritoneum
- **menopause:** the cessation of menstruation; usually occurs in women between the ages of 40–58
- **cervical cancer:** cancer of the cervix typically caused by the human papillomavirus (HPV)
- **sexually transmitted diseases (STDs):** diseases such as gonorrhea, chlamydia, herpes, syphilis, and AIDS that are caused by various infectious microorganisms and are contracted during sexual activity; affects both male and female reproductive systems

Related Conditions and Diseases—Male Reproductive System

- **prostatitis:** inflammation of the prostate
- **epididymitis:** inflammation of the epididymis
- **orchitis:** inflammation of the testes
- **cryptorchism:** condition of the testes in which the testes have not descended properly into the scrotum
- **benign prostatic hyperplasia:** a progressive condition characterized by enlargement of the prostate and obstruction of the urethra

- **prostatic cancer:** malignant tumor of the prostate gland
- **testicular cancer:** malignant tumor of a testis
- **hydrocele:** swelling of the testes
- **impotence:** inability to sustain an erection

The Endocrine System

The endocrine system is responsible for regulating the body's metabolic activities through the secretion of hormones by various glands within the system. The endocrine glands include the **hypothalamus, pineal gland, thryroid gland, parathyroid glands, thymus glands, pancreas, adrenal glands, ovaries,** and **testes.**

Related Conditions and Diseases

- **thyroiditis:** inflammation of the thyroid gland
- **hyperthyroidism:** overactive thyroid gland characterized by the oversecretion of thyroid hormones; also known as Graves disease
- **hypothyroidism:** underactive thyroid gland characterized by the undersecretion of thyroid hormones; also known as myxedema
- **hyperparathyroidism:** excessive secretion of parathyroid hormone that affects phosphate and calcium metabolism
- **hypoparathyroidism:** undersecretion of parathyroid hormone resulting in hypocalcemia
- **diabetes mellitus:** a chronic disorder of carbohydrate metabolism resulting from inadequate amounts of insulin, characterized by increased glucose in the bloodstream and urine
- **hypoglycemia:** abnormal decrease in blood glucose levels characterized by acute fatigue, malaise, irritability, and weakness
- **Cushing's disease:** hormone disorder caused by high levels of glucocorticoids secreted by the adrenal cortex
- **Addison's disease:** decrease in production of steroid hormones by the adrenal glands
- **hyperpituitarism:** oversecretion of growth hormone by the pituitary gland

The Sensory System

The sensory system is responsible for vision, hearing, touch, taste, and smell. Organs within the system include the **eyes, ears, nose,** and **tongue.**

Related Conditions and Diseases

- **myopia:** nearsightedness
- **hyperopia:** farsightedness
- **presbyopia:** a form of farsightedness that occurs with age
- **astigmatism:** a defect in sight caused by changes in the curvature over certain portions of the cornea and lens of the eye
- **conjunctivitis:** inflammation of the conjunctiva, the membrane lining the inside of the eyelid; typically caused by a microorganism
- **blepharitis:** inflammation of the eyelids
- **glaucoma:** damage to the retina and optic nerve because of an increase in fluid pressure within the eye
- **macular degenerative disease:** a degenerative disease of the retina (a thin layer of nerve cells that lines the back of the eyeball) that causes progressive loss of central vision
- **cataract:** clouding of the eye lens, causing a decrease in visual acuity
- **otitis media:** inflammation of the inner ear
- **otitis externa:** inflammation of the external ear
- **otosclerosis:** abnormal condition causing the formation of spongy bone in the ear resulting in a progressive loss of hearing
- **Meniere's disease:** progressive condition characterized by ringing in the ears, dizziness, and a sensation of pressure in the ears
- **presbycusis:** impairment of hearing that occurs with age
- **deafness:** complete or partial loss of hearing
- **tinnitus:** ringing in the ear
- **vertigo:** a disturbance in equilibrium characterized by the feeling of moving around in space

Psychology

Medical assistants routinely deal with patients in a variety of encounters, and patients respond to medical care differently, depending on their developmental stage, their psychological well-being, and the nature of their health status. This section discusses the principles of psychology and human behavior that are most pertinent to medical assistants in their dealings with patients.

Psychological Theories

Psychiatrists, psychologists, and other researchers have developed a range of theories to explain human thought, emotion, and behavior. While the medical assistant is not required to know the details of these theories, a broad understanding of the approaches taken by researchers will allow them to be more informed about the entire medical field and human behavior in general.

Psychoanalytical Theory

Developed by Austrian physician Sigmund Freud in the early 1900s, this theory was founded largely upon Freud's research into and thinking about the unconscious mind and the structure and development of "personality."

According to Freud, an individual's personality is composed of the id, the ego, and the superego, which are explained here.

- **id:** the collection of basic drives and impulses that arises from our preoccupation with and concerns about survival, preservation, and the procreation of life; this component is largely buried in an individual's subconscious.
- **ego:** the aspect of an individual's personality that, in a way, sits above the id, in the realm of awareness, and is comprised of perception, cognition, and action. Through the ego, an individual most directly interacts with other individuals and his or her environment.

- **superego:** the part of "personality" that functions, again as in the relationship between the id and the ego, above the ego. It arises from elements outside the individual, in the realm of family relationships, societal values, social mores, and the like. It is in the realm of the superego that a person's moral standards and conscience reside.

Psychotherapy, based on Freud's ideas about personality, involves what is sometimes called "talk therapy," in which a psychoanalyst guides a patient in probing conversation and free association aimed at uncovering aspects of the patient's personality buried in the subconscious.

Behaviorism

Behaviorism largely arose out of criticism of Freud's approach in analyzing personality. Theorists John B. Watson in the 1920s and later B. F. Skinner in the 1950s, among others, developed the idea that observable behavior, rather the subconscious, was the more important aspect of personality to explore. A person's response to external conditions was the core to understanding what underlay his or her behavior.

From these theories came behavior therapy, or behavior modification, which was popularized in the 1950s and 1960s. Rather than uncovering unconscious motivations, thoughts, and feelings, this approach concerned itself with modifying behavior that could be observed and then changing that behavior.

Humanistic Psychology

Humanistic psychology developed as a means to understand and analyze the whole person, not just the components of personality that psychoanalytical theory employed and not just the more scientifically observable aspects of behavior that behavioral theory employed. It focused less on pathology and more on efforts toward growth.

One of the main theorists—Abraham Maslow—established what he described as a hierarchy of human needs. This "pyramid" approach explained how the most basic physiological human needs, such as the need for food and shelter, must be met before more advanced requirements— security, social interaction, self-esteem, and self-actualization—could be achieved.

Cognitivism

Developed by a range of researchers, including those from the information sciences field, in the latter part of the twentieth century, cognitive psychology focuses on how an individual learns and processes information. It is particularly concerned with these questions as they help to shape a person's behavioral patterns.

Cognitive therapy, with its focus on cognition, is a popular style of treatment style for certain disorders, such as depression and anxiety. The patient is encouraged to explore and uncover errors in their thinking that arise from "irrational beliefs." Such irrationality can exist in thinking that is outside the realm of possibility. For instance, a student may feel that the only way to achieve self-worth is through attaining the highest grades in his or her class in every subject studied; while this goal may be attainable in some cases and at some times, it is not truly sustainable. Uncovering such cognitive errors helps an individual adapt to more realistic expectations and adjust their behavior and emotional responses to events accordingly.

Terminally Ill Patients and the Process of Grieving

Severely and terminally ill patients—and their loved ones—face a set of emotions and psychological challenges not typical of other patients. Specialized research and treatment have been developed to assist those individuals.

Elizabeth Kübler-Ross's Five Stages of Grief

Elizabeth Kübler-Ross, a Swiss-born psychiatrist who lived and worked for much of her life in the United States, developed a model that described the pattern that dying patients go through in dealing with their impending death. Known as the five stages of grief, they are:

- **Denial:** Behavior in this stage is characterized by a refusal to accept the severity of illness and the fact that death is inescapable. Denial at this stage is a natural defense mechanism, as the patient is not emotionally equipped or ready to face the idea of their own death.
- **Anger:** This stage is characterized by feelings of anger and outrage, often directed outwardly at loved ones, caregivers, and medical professionals encountered during treatment.
- **Bargaining:** In this stage, individuals are often given to expressions of desperate hope that the grave situation they face will reverse itself. Behaviors can include seeking drastic alternative treatments, for instance, or promising to change behavior patterns that are thought to have brought on the condition.
- **Depression:** At this stage, individuals begin to face the reality of their own death. In doing so, typical signs of depression, such as withdrawal and crying, are normal.
- **Acceptance:** This final stage completes the emotional journey of the previous stage: As the individual faces reality, he or she comes to accept his or her situation and start to "let go." Patients become less emotionally wrought and more accepting of their situation.

Terminally ill patients do not always undergo these stages in the same order or, of course, in exactly the same way. Also, the stages have come to be applied not just to terminally ill patients, but to individuals who have suffered the loss of a loved one or who have undergone any type of serious trauma and loss, such as a grave illness that results in incapacitation or a massive change in lifestyle.

The medical assistant may be required to deal with terminally ill patients and their loved ones. It is useful, therefore, that they understand these patterns of behavior associated with grief and respond appropriately. For instance, understanding that a patient's anger about his or her illness may be directed outwardly at healthcare professionals should help the medical assistant react calmly, without becoming defensive or angry.

Hospice Care

Largely because of Kübler-Ross's work, as well as the English physician Cecily Saunders, the hospice care movement developed. Hospice is a method of attending to the needs of terminally ill patients that treats the whole patient, not just the physical illness. Treatment and care administered under hospice programs are based on the acceptance of the terminal nature of a patient's illness and therefore are focused on easing the effects of the illness, including not just physical symptoms such as pain, but the emotional and psychological aspects as well.

This method of care, frequently delivered by trained volunteers in community-based organizations and agencies, applies not just to patient but to loved ones and caregivers, to help reduce the emotional and practical stress involved in taking care of a dying patient. The medical assistant will often be asked to give terminally patients and their loved ones information about hospice care and to help contacting the community organizations that offer such services.

Defense Mechanisms

Defense mechanisms are strategies individuals use to avoid difficult or painful feelings. They are means to submerge upsetting emotions into an individual's subconscious. There are a range of defense mechanisms patients use to deal with their illnesses and health conditions. Here are some of the most common.

- **denial:** A complete rejection of a difficult fact or feeling, this strategy was previously discussed as one of the five stages of grief. This refusal to accept one's circumstances can indeed apply to patients who are less than terminally ill.
- **suppression:** While not completely in denial, a patient may push a fact or feeling to back of their conscious thought, thereby allowing them to escape uncomfortable feelings.

- **projection:** In this strategy, a person experiencing difficult or negative feelings or thoughts may accuse others of thinking or feeling the way they do, protecting or insulating an individual from his or her own negative thoughts and feelings.
- **rationalization:** A person uses this strategy when he or she makes excuses to justify inappropriate behavior. For example, when an employee takes a 45-minute lunch break, but puts only 30 minutes for lunch on his or her time card, he or she might rationalize this indiscretion by saying, "They don't pay me enough anyway."
- **intellectualization:** This strategy is a more intellectual form of rationalization. For instance, a patient, angry at insurance company's refusal to cover a specific treatment because he or she forgot to get a referral or put a claim in on time, may try to blame the entire health insurance industry or the heathcare policy of the country.

Medical assistants will be able to improve their interactions with patients if they are aware of these types of defense mechanisms. However, their primary role is to engage with patients in a calm and compassionate way, not try to diagnose psychological or emotional problems.

Professional Standards

Professionalism is a code of behavior and a set of qualities expected of the members of a profession. Medical assistants, like other professionals, are expected to live up to professional standards and a code of ethics emphasizing honesty, integrity, and service to society.

Displaying a Professional Attitude

A medical assistant is a multi-skilled professional capable of competently performing administrative and clinical tasks in a variety of outpatient or ambulatory care facilities. Characteristics of a professional medical assistant may include:

- **Genuinely liking people.** Ideally, the medical assistant should be a friendly, caring individual who enjoys being around people and shows a willingness to help others.
- **Dependability.** It is important for the medical assistant to be on time for work, to show up for work every day, and to shoulder his or her share of the work in an office.
- **Flexibility.** The daily schedule in a medical office often changes due to emergencies and extended appointment times. The medical assistant should be able to adjust to abrupt changes in the office environment.
- **Accuracy and attention to details.** The medical assistant must be able to manage details accurately in order to provide quality care to patients and to help maintain the efficient functioning of the medical practice.
- **Good manners.** The medical assistant should be courteous, tactful, and respectful, and should be able to represent the medical office favorably to patients and the public.
- **Personal accountability for his or her actions.** It is essential that the medical assistant admit to errors made or omissions that may have occurred in patient treatment.
- **Membership in a professional organization.** Medical assistants are encouraged to join and participate in the professional organizations that grant credentials to medical assistants—the American Association of Medical Assistants or American Medical Technologists.
- **Commitment to lifelong learning.** The national medical assisting organizations that grant credentials to medical assistants require continuing education to help medical assistants to keep their knowledge current.
- **Professional appearance.** The medical assistant should have impeccable hygiene and wear a limited amount of makeup, perfume, and jewelry. The medical assistant should dress conservatively, wearing clean, pressed clothing and comfortable, well-fitting, clean shoes.

FIRST IMPRESSIONS

As the saying goes, first impressions are made only once, and this is certainly true for the medical assistant. As the first representative of the medical facility with whom patients come into contact, the medical assistant should make a patient feel that he or she will get the best care possible. Often, a patient will judge an office by the manner in which the medical assistant answers the phone or responds to a question. All medical care—starting with the first time a patient calls the medical office—should be patient oriented, or an unsatisfied patient may seek medical treatment elsewhere.

- **Positive attitude.** The medical assistant should be a good team member by having a positive attitude, offering to help other team members of the team, and speaking only well about others.

Working as a Team to Achieve Goals

Each member of a healthcare team brings his or her individual experiences, knowledge, and expectations to the group. Group dynamics—the interacting forces among individuals in a group—are important to consider in order to become a responsible team player. These forces can include the personality of the members, the roles of team members, issues of power and control, and even friendships among the various team members.

A new medical assistant may feel intimidated by certain aspects of the group dynamics in his or her office. For instance, more experienced medical assistants or other healthcare personnel on the team may cause a new medical assistant to feel less important, and extroverts may be more vocal and overshadow the opinions of more introverted team members. All group issues must be recognized and individually dealt with in order for the healthcare team to fully understand the dynamics of the group and to come together when caring for patients. The team leader should focus the efforts of the team toward a common goal and should encourage communication between team members.

Communication

Communication is the exchange of information, both verbally and nonverbally. Oral communication relies on the spoken word and the tone and inflections of the voice. Communicating effectively with patients and their families is an essential skill needed by the medical assistant.

Four key attributes define professional communication and behavior.

- **Tact** is having a good sense of how to avoid offending or insulting an individual or being sensitive and considerate when choosing to discuss issues with patients or coworkers. The tone in which something is spoken is as important as the words used.
- **Diplomacy** allows the medical assistant to handle delicate situations between groups or individuals without arousing hostilities.
- **Courtesy** refers to treating individuals in a thoughtful and respectful manner, and is critical for all people the medical assistant comes into contact with (patients, physicians, and coworkers).
- **Responsibility** and **integrity** are also important traits for medical assistants. These traits increase patients' trust and create camaraderie among all the individuals in a healthcare team.

Verbal (spoken words) and nonverbal (gestures and facial expressions) communication are closely linked. The medical assistant is trained to be a good communicator, actively listening to the patient and asking various types of questions to elicit information or clarify the message from the patient, and providing feedback to the patient (that is, a response to his or her question, comment, or concern).

How skilled a medical assistant is at interviewing patients also plays a role in the information received verbally from a patient. A skilled medical assistant may realize that the nonverbal message the patient is communicating is not the same as the words being spoken.

Nonverbal Communication

Nonverbal communication is the exchange of information without exchanging words. Nonverbal communication is made up of body gestures and poses and is often referred to as *body language.*

The study of body language is called **kinesics**. According to Alton Barbour, author of *Louder Than Words: Nonverbal Communication*, the total impact of a message breaks down as follows: 7% verbal (words), 38% vocal (volume, pitch, rhythm), and 55% body movements (mostly facial expressions). Clearly, nonverbal communication plays an important role in a patient-healthcare team relationship. Observing a patient's nonverbal messages is just as important as hearing the words he or she is saying. The medical assistant should also be aware of his or her own body gestures, as well as the messages those gestures may be sending to patients or coworkers.

Listening Skills

Listening skills should be used by the medical assistant in all area of conversations with patients and coworkers. Nonverbal messages are sent even when someone is just listening to a conversation. Glancing away from the speaker, looking at the clock on the wall, or placing one's hand on the doorknob of the examining room's exit may indicate impatience or lack of interest in what is being discussed.

Eye Contact

Eye contact is a means of nonverbal communication that can strongly reinforce the spoken word. Eye contact can send a message of honesty and confidence. Some people may feel a person is not telling the truth if he or she is having trouble keeping eye contact. Others may believe that avoiding eye contact shows that a person is shy or nervous. However, most people agree that it is rude to stare at someone.

Adapting Communication to an Individual's Needs

Speech, hand signals, writing, behaviors, body gestures, and tone of speech are a few examples of the many ways humans communicate. The medical assistant must have a basic understanding of these various communication tools and be aware of the need for adapting communication according to an individual's needs.

Roadblocks to communication may include a variety of physiological, emotional, or psychological impairments; cultural differences; age-related difficulties; or language barriers. The medical team should be prepared to adapt communication to meet address these roadblocks. Individuals who may need some type of adjustment in communication include:

- **The visually impaired.** The medical assistant should ask before assuming that a visually impaired person needs help. Also, the patient should be informed when the medical assistant is leaving the room. Braille signs should be available on doorways and on elevator control panels.

- **The hearing impaired.** When communicating with a patient with a hearing impairment, the medical assistant should face the person directly because some hearing impaired people read lips, and facing the patient directly helps his or her comprehension. Writing down instructions is another way to communicate effectively with a hearing-impaired patient.

- **The elderly.** An elderly patient's ability to see, hear, and respond coherently should be assessed by the medical assistant before automatically assuming the patient has a physical or psychological impairment. However, some elderly patients may be a little slower to comprehend or to remember details of instructions, so the medical assistant should state instructions in a clear, concise manner, eliminating extra steps and unnecessary details. Elderly patients should be addressed in a respectful manner, not with terms such as "Gramps" or "honey."

HANDLING EMOTIONAL BARRIERS IN PRE-OP PATIENTS

Emotional barriers might arise when the medical assistant is trying to discuss pre-op instructions with a patient. The patient may not be able to absorb what is being said because he or she is so worried about the danger of the surgery or about how to find the money to pay out-of-pocket expenses.

The medical assistant should ask the patient about his or her major concerns about the surgery prior to discussing the pre-op directions. The medical assistant should also offer to discuss a payment plan with the accounting office or to set up a time for the patient to discuss his or her concerns about the dangers of the surgery with the physician. These actions may help remove the emotional barrier and allow the patient to concentrate on the important information relayed by the medical assistant.

- **Children.** Children should be treated with the same respect as adults. Children experience the same fears and apprehension that adults feel when going to a medical facility. The medical assistant must gain the confidence of the child in order to establish a positive relationship. Also, it is important to be honest with the child. For example, a child should not be told that an injection won't hurt. The medical assistant should reassure the child that it will hurt for only a moment and provide comfort immediately after the injection.

- **Seriously ill patients.** Seriously ill patients and their family members are suffering and may need someone to listen to their concerns. The medical assistant should allow these patients to express their feelings, and provide comfort and solutions to their problems when possible. The medical assistant should also encourage a patient to speak with a psychologist or mental health professional who has been trained to deal with problems beyond the expertise of the medical assistant and the rest of the staff in the medical office.

- **The mentally impaired.** Respect and patience are needed for communicating with mentally challenged individuals. The medical assistant should speak directly to the individual, observing facial expressions that would indicate the level of comprehension. Using simple terms and repeating explanations can help mentally impaired patients feel involved in their own care.

- **Illiterate patients.** If a patient is illiterate, verbal explanations and directions may be used. An illiterate patient may have difficulty taking prescription medication properly or remembering detailed instructions. If it is agreeable to the patient, a family member may be asked to read any written instructions given to the patient.

- **Non-English-speaking patients.** The medical assistant may have to communicate with patients who do not speak English or who speak very limited English. The medical assistant should try to communicate with these patients as effectively as is possible. For instance, it is often possible to communicate greetings, directions, or simple instructions through nonverbal communication.

- **Anxious patients.** An anxious patient may have difficulty understanding or remembering verbal instructions or information because his or her thoughts are focused on other issues. The medical assistant can help relieve a patient's anxiety by being friendly and calm and by encouraging the patient to discuss the issues or concerns that are causing the anxiety.

- **Angry or distraught patients.** When an angry or distraught patient calls the office, the first thing the medical assistant should do is listen. Listening closely to what the patient is saying can help identify the problem and help the medical assistant to work with the patient toward a solution.

TECHNIQUES FOR ACTIVE LISTENING

When actively listening, the medical assistant should spend more time listening than talking, giving the patient 100 percent of his or her attention. The medical assistant should show that he or she is listening by looking directly at the patient and acknowledging that he or she understands what the patient is saying. The medical assistant should allow the patient to finish speaking before interjecting any opinions, and provide feedback by asking questions to clarify the patient's message. The medical assistant should also be aware of his or her body language.

- **Culturally diverse patients.** A medical practice may have many culturally diverse patients, people from various ethnic, racial, and socioeconomic groups. The personnel of a medical facility may also be culturally diverse. Individuals from different cultures may have established value systems that do not match the value systems of the medical assistant. The medical assistant who has some knowledge of cultural customs may be able to prevent misunderstandings with patients or coworkers that are a result of cultural differences.

Barriers to Communication

Barriers to communication can be physical, emotional, or psychological.

- **Physical barriers** to communication may include visual, auditory, or speech impairment. Physical barriers to communication may also apply to the workplace itself. Closed office doors, barrier screens within the office, environmental noise, and even a glass partition between the reception area and the front office where the medical assistant sits can all create obstacles to communication.

- **Emotional barriers** that hinder open and free communication often stem from fear, mistrust, and suspicion. As children, we are often taught to keep our feelings to ourselves. Emotional barriers may also consist of fear, mistrust, or suspicions. The medical assistant should be able to identify the emotional needs of others and be aware of emotional barriers that may interfere with patients' listening and understanding.
- **Psychological barriers** are closely related to emotional barriers and may include fear of losing independence, fear of the stigma attached to certain conditions or diseases, or fear of not wanting be dependent on others. Psychological and emotional barriers may prevent a patient from seeking medical attention. Patients under stress may see situations differently than they would if they were not under stress. When a patient is under stress, he or she may blow a small issue out of proportion. For example, the patient may have less patience about waiting for an appointment or for a lab result than he or she normally would.

Cultural Factors in Communications

A person's cultural background may influence how he or she interprets a situation. **Perception**, or how another individual sees a situation or an individual, is often based on past experiences, biases, and stereotyping.

- A **bias** is a predetermined slant or attitude about a person or situation that may interfere with one's impartial judgment—for example, the belief that male patients should be treated only by male physicians or that female patients should be treated only by female physicians.
- **Prejudice** also involves making predetermined conclusions or judgments without knowledge, thought, or reason. A prejudice may be expressed as a negative comment against a group of individuals based on their culture, religion, or nationality.

- A **stereotype** is a generalized assumption about a group of individuals that can be either positive or negative. For example, it would be a stereotype to say that all elderly patients are hearing impaired or to say that all teenagers take illegal drugs. It would also be a stereotype to say that girls are smarter than boys. Medical assistants must be able to identify their own personal biases and prejudices so that they can avoid stereotyping patients and coworkers.

Maintaining a Therapeutic Relationship

The term *therapeutic relationship* refers to the relationship that the medical assistant and other members of the healthcare staff have with a patient. In a positive therapeutic relationship, the patient is made to feel accepted and respected. Some factors in developing positive therapeutic relationships with patients are:

- treating all patients impartially by avoiding prejudice, bias, and stereotypes
- having an understanding of emotional behavior—such as stress, anger, and fear—during times of stress and illness
- having and expressing **empathy** for the patient and his or her circumstances. Empathy is putting yourself into someone else's shoes, understanding how an individual feels while keeping the focus on that person. **Sympathy** involves a more emotional response and may result in a lack of objectivity on the part of the medical assistant.

Patient Interviewing Techniques

Different questioning techniques can be used to gather information needed from a patient. Questions should be exploratory in nature, geared toward eliciting information about the patient's understanding his or her condition, of the treatment, and of the patient's feelings about them. Exploratory questions, or open-ended questions, require the patient to answer in more than one word, encouraging the patient to provide information. Asking a patient a closed question will often result in a yes-or-no answer, limiting the response and information received. For example, if the medical assistant asks the patient, "Are you following your low-sodium diet, Mr. Smith?" he could simply answer, "Yes" or "No." If the medical assistant asks the question in an open-ended way, such as, "Mr. Smith, what foods you are eating on your low-sodium diet?" the patient will likely respond with more detail.

Evaluating the Effectiveness of Communication

Evaluating the effectiveness of their communication with patients, and adjusting their techniques accordingly during conversations, are important to medical assistants' communication with patients. The communication process involves a **sender**, the person sending the message; a **receiver**, the person receiving the message; and a **message**, the content or information being transferred.

Channels are part of the communication process and include various types of verbal and nonverbal methods, such as speaking, writing, and body language, to convey messages. More than one channel may be used to send information and to help clarify the message being sent.

Feedback, the final part of the communication process, is the response given to the sender of the message. Feedback allows the sender to evaluate whether the receiver correctly understood the message sent. Feedback also gives the sender an opportunity to correct any misunderstandings in the message. For example, the medical assistant may respond to a worried-looking patient's statement "I can't wait to get this operation over with" by rephrasing the statement as "You seem to be nervous about the surgery. Is that right?" Being aware of the patient's concern, the medical assistant may ask more questions to find out the patient's exact fears, answer any questions the patient may have, or refer the patient to the correct person.

Active Listening

Active listening is more than just hearing another person talk. When a medical assistant actively listens

CEUs

The medical assistant has the responsibility to keep his or her credentials current. Continuing education units, or CEUs, may be obtained by taking continuing education courses, attending approved lectures and conferences, and reading approved articles in magazines such as *CMA Today*. Often, reimbursement for continuing education courses and conferences may be available from the employer. The medical assistant must accurately keep track of earned CEUs in order to be sure that the appropriate number and types of credits earned will be applied to the recertification of the credential.

to a patient, he or she is interpreting the message being sent and paying close attention to the words used in the conversation as well as the tone of the words spoken.

Legal Restrictions

When interviewing patients, the medical assistant must remember that the patient's medical record is confidential. Before the patient interview begins, the medical assistant should inquire if the patient has any questions. Balancing the need-to-know details of a patient's condition and history with respect for the patient's privacy is one of the challenges of the patient interview.

Medical history is the basis for all patient care; therefore, it needs to be detailed and complete. The medical assistant must be sensitive to the feelings of the patient when he or she is asking the patient personal questions. Often, if a patient is initially reluctant to answer a question, the medical assistant may readdress the topic later in the interview, when the patient is more relaxed.

Accurate documentation during a patient interview is also important because the medical record is a legal document. There are no legal restrictions on questions asked during a patient interview, as long as the questions relate to or are necessary for the patient's medical problem or care.

Care must be taken to ask questions about sensitive topics such as sexual activity or drug or alcohol use in a matter-of-fact tone and to accept answers in a nonjudgmental manner. The patient should be reassured that all conversations will remain confidential.

Medicolegal Guidelines and Requirements

In a medical office, established guidelines govern the physician-patient relationship. The patient has the right to expect quality care, confidentiality of personal information, respectful treatment, and the right to make his or her own healthcare decisions. The physician and medical staff members have the right to protect themselves against lawsuits.

Medical assistants must be aware of current federal and state laws regulating many issues in a medical facility. Failure to be compliant with federal regulations and standards may lead to legal actions against the medical facility and against the medical assistant.

Medical Practice Acts

The Medical Practice Acts are **statutes**, or laws designed to protect patients from harm. Each state has its own set of regulations that oversee the licensing of physicians, the physician-patient relationship, standards of care, professional liability (malpractice), rules of confidentiality, and professional behavior and record management.

The medical assistant in a medical facility is under the direct supervision of the physician and acts on the physician's behalf when performing many procedures and clerical tasks and, therefore, may be held responsible for failure to comply with state and federal regulations or failure to act within the scope of medical assisting education and training.

Tort Law

Failure to comply with the provisions of the Medical Practice Acts may result in committing a **tort**. A tort is a wrongful act, other than a breach of contract, which results in the injury of another person, who may seek compensation for damages that may have occurred as a result of the act. A tort falls under **civil law,** and the penalties for committing a tort can range from monetary fines to imprisonment, depending on the violation.

A common tort at issue in medical practice is negligence, which implies low standards or poor conduct. Negligence indicates a failure to exercise care and treatment that correspond to reasonable professional standards.

A medical assistant may be charged with breach of duty if he or she performed with low standards or poor conduct and if the patient or his or her family feel that the medical assistant provided a poor standard of care that resulted in physical or emotional harm to the patient. Even though the medical assistant is under the supervision of a physician, the medical assistant is responsible for adhering to a standard of conduct established by medical assistant professional organizations.

Licenses and Certifications

Most professions have some type of regulation to ensure the competency of their members. Professionals may be licensed, certified, or registered.

The Licensing of Physicians

Physicians must be licensed in the state in which they are practicing. Qualifications to take the licensing exam for physicians include graduating from an approved medical school, completing an approved residency program, and reaching the age of majority (the legal age of adulthood).

Once licensed, a physician may choose to work in another state and obtain a license for that state through the process of reciprocity rather than taking the licensing exam for the second state. **Reciprocity** is the mutual exchange of privileges between states, meaning that if a physician holds a license in one state and has equal or higher qualifications than those required by the state in which they are applying, that state will grant a license without requiring the physician to take that state's licensing exam.

Revocation and Suspension of a Physician's License

A physician's license must be renewed every two years. In every state, physicians must also complete an annual five-hour training session for **risk management** and show proof that continuing education has been done. It is illegal to practice medicine without a valid license. The law does not differentiate between a person who practices with a lapsed license and a person who never qualified for a license.

The physician who does not comply with federal and state regulations may be fined or charged with a **felony**, which is a serious crime usually punishable by prison time. A physician may also have his or her medical license revoked if convicted of a crime.

Fraud is an intentional deception usually made for personal gain, such as billing for procedures and services never performed or falsifying medical records. Fraud is considered less serious than a felony and may be considered a **misdemeanor**, depending on the crime committed.

A physician may have his or her medical license revoked because of unprofessional conduct such as:

- substance abuse—addiction to legal or illegal drugs or alcohol
- impersonating another physician or falsifying credentials
- providing substandard care—practicing medicine in a manner that harms or may harm a patient
- prescribing controlled substances for reasons other than the accepted therapeutic purposes
- inappropriate billing practices

Certification and Registration for the Medical Assistant

Certification and registration are voluntary for the medical assistant. The medical assistant may earn either a CMA or an RMA certification after completing the national exam offered by one of the two national accrediting agencies for medical assisting. Credentialing is important for the graduate of a medical assistant program; many medical facility employers prefer to hire certified or registered medical assistants because certification demonstrates competency in the medical assisting areas. To remain certified or registered, the medical assistant must complete continuing education units (CEUs) as required by the national organizations. (See Chapter 1, "The Medical Assistant Profession," for more information on certification and registration.)

Legislation

Various legislation has been passed to cover medical-legal issues that have arisen over the years as a result of breakthroughs in technology, advancements in patient care, and the desire to make the patient an active decision-maker in his or her medical care. The information that comes to a medical office from many different sources provides data regarding tax regulations, updates to controlled substances, or even changes in employment laws. The medical assistant has the responsibility to be aware of these federal and state regulations.

Advance Directives

Advance directives are legal directions that provide an individual with a way to communicate his or her decisions about end-of-life care to family, physicians, and healthcare professionals. Specifically, an advance directive is a document signed by the patient that outlines what types of treatments that patient authorizes in the event that he or she becomes incapacitated or unable to make decisions. When the patient spells out and legally documents his or her decisions, there is no confusion as to what the patient wants.

- A **living will** is a limited type of advance directive: It covers only the decisions an individual has made about life-sustaining procedures in the event that death is imminent or that the individual is in a permanent vegetative state with no hope of recovery. An advance directive is more encompassing than a living will. For instance, it allows an individual to select a healthcare agent to make healthcare decisions if and when the individual cannot make the necessary decisions.

- A **durable power of attorney for healthcare** is a document that names the person a patient has chosen to represent him- or herself. This selected person, called a healthcare agent, will be responsible to make the final decisions about the individual's end-of-life healthcare. The chosen person should be a trusted family member, friend, or attorney.

An advance directive does not have to be prepared by a lawyer, but the individual should get some information about the types of life-sustaining treatments that are available and may be used in his or her care. For example, the patient must decide if he or she is willing to be put on a dialysis machine or a respirator, if CPR should be administered if the heart or breathing stops, or if a feeding tube may be inserted. Decisions about organ donation should also be considered.

The medical assistant should place a copy of any advance directives in the individual's medical file for safekeeping, making sure that it exists in a prominent place in the patient's records. A copy of the advance directives should be given to the healthcare agent of the individual.

Each state has its own guidelines for advance directives. Once the advance directive is prepared its signing must be witnessed by two adults. Although state laws vary, it is recommended that at least one witness be someone who is not affiliated with the individual's healthcare facility and the other witness be a physician.

Anatomical Gifts

The Uniform Anatomical Gift Act governs the making of anatomical gifts after death (and sometimes before death) for either organ donation for transplants or cadaver donation to medical schools to be used for educational purposes. An individual must be at least 18 years of age to complete an organ donation form, although the law allows a surviving spouse or relative to make an organ donation decision upon the death of an individual. Tissue, cells, and body fluids may be used for donation and may include some of the following: kidney, lung, pancreas, liver, skin, intestines, stomach, testis, hand, cornea, blood vessels, bone, blood transfusions, islets of Langerhans, or heart.

Some organs may not be suitable for donation if the patient had certain infectious diseases or some types of cancer. The medical team in charge of the transplant will make the final decision of whether an organ is acceptable for transplant. There is no specific age limit for organ donation. Many sources state that donations may be accepted from newborns to about age 70 for cadaver organ donations. Tissue and cornea donations may come from older individuals (up to 80 years old), and there is no cutoff age for skin donation. When an individual decides to become an organ donor, he or she can donate as many organs or as few organs as desired. There is no charge to an organ donor or his or her family.

Reportable Incidences

Reportable incidences may include communicable diseases, substance abuse, chemical dependencies, wounds resulting from violence, and certain statistical information such as births and deaths. Reporting allows for the gathering of important statistics regarding how often specific diseases or conditions occur. These statistics give researchers the ability to identify trends, including any increase or decrease in disease outbreaks, with the hope of controlling future outbreaks. Statistics gathered about chemical dependencies and substance abuse can also be used to research treatment and prevention areas.

Birth and Death Data

Reporting of births and deaths to the State Center for Health Statistics is important in compiling **infant mortality rates** based on the infant's birth weight, mother's age, prenatal care, smoking and alcohol use during pregnancy, mother's education, and any other area deemed important to measure. In many states, details about stillbirths are reportable. Information gained from analyzing these statistics may be helpful in identifying risk areas for fetuses and newborns, which may then be prevented through education.

Statistics gathered from adult mortality rates provide insight into the types of diseases and conditions causing deaths in the United States. This statistical information may be used to report on the progress of curing or managing diseases (thus prolonging life), such as early cancer detection and the identification or treatment of diseases and conditions that are increasing (e.g., diabetes and obesity).

Communicable Diseases

Communicable diseases are classified as infectious diseases that may be transmitted from one individual to another. It is the responsibility of the healthcare provider to report the diseases to the state or local health agencies.

Acts of violence such as stabbings, gunshot wounds, and poisoning—whether accidental, suspicious, or unexplained—need to be reported to the local police department. Statistics from violence reporting can provide information used for prevention and education, in the hopes of decreasing violent activity or injury.

Occupational Safety and Health Act

The Occupational Safety and Health Act (OSHA) was legislation passed in 1971 to ensure employee safety and health in the working environment. The goal of OSHA was to make working environments safer and healthier by employing fair and effective enforcement of its regulations, setting safety and health standards, establishing training and education for employers and employees, and providing compliance assistance to worksites.

OSHA safety regulations include standards to regulate noise and exposure to hazardous substances such as lead, toxic chemicals, asbestos, and pesticides.

Workplace safety issues addressed by OSHA of specific concern to medical facilities are discussed in Chapter 5, in the "Infection Control" section.

Food and Drug Administration

The Food and Drug Administration (FDA) is an agency within the U.S. Public Health Service, which is a part of the Department of Health and Human Services. The Food and Drug Administration was created when Congress passed the Pure Food and Drug Act of 1906, the first in a series of acts designed to regulate foods and patent medicines. The Pure Food and Drug Act requires that all drugs marketed in the United States meet minimal standards for purity, strength, and quality. The act requires that any drug containing morphine be labeled appropriately and identify the ingredients. The Pure Food and Drug act also established two references that listed officially approved drugs—the United States Pharmacopeia (USP) and the National Formulary (NF), which are now combined into one reference book.

Enacted over time, federal legislation established stricter and more specific guidelines that prevented tampering with drugs, required accurate labels and warning labels for side effects such as drowsiness on certain products, and designated which drugs need a prescription and which can be sold over the counter without a physician's prescription.

Controlled Substances Act of 1970

The Controlled Substances Act of 1970 put a tighter control on the substances being abused by the public, such as narcotics, depressants, stimulants, anabolic steroids, and psychedelic drugs. This act isolates abused and addicting drugs into five schedules, or categories, indicating the potential for abuse and addiction. The higher the schedule number, the lower the potential for addiction and abuse. For example, Schedule I includes drugs that have the potential to be highly addictive and abused and that have no medicinal use, such as heroin; the drugs on Schedule V have the least or lowest potential for addiction and abuse, such as cough suppressants containing codeine.

The legislation sets strict security rules for anyone who dispenses, receives, sells, or destroys any of the controlled substances (drugs) listed in the five schedules. Physicians, pharmacists, hospitals, and drug companies fall into that category. The controlled substances are to be kept under double lock and key, and an exact inventory of each substance is to be kept with documentation of every dose dispensed. Inventory lists must be on file for two years. Any outdated or contaminated drug (those dropped on the floor, for example) must be returned to the pharmacy rather than discarded.

Limits are set on the number of prescription refills that are allowed in a six-month period, and dictate whether a specific controlled substance can be prescribed by phone to a pharmacy or whether the drug requires a written prescription. Some states may have stricter schedules than those set by the federal government. The act requires that each prescriber be registered with the Drug Enforcement Administration (DEA), a bureau of the Justice Department that was set up to enforce the provisions of the Controlled Substances Act. Each prescriber applies for and receives a registration number that has to be written on all prescriptions for controlled substances. The registration needs to be renewed every three years. The medical assistant may be responsible for the renewal of the physician's DEA registration number.

Keeping prescription pads out of sight and unavailable to patients and keeping all drugs safely locked away during and after office hours help to prevent unauthorized access to controlled substances. The drugs are kept under double lock and key; the medical assistant should be aware of the location of the key at all times.

Clinical Laboratory Improvement Act of 1988

The Clinical Laboratory Improvement Act (CLIA) of 1988 was passed by Congress to develop quality, comprehensive standards that would ensure the accuracy of laboratory testing in facilities that process human specimens for the purpose of diagnosis, prevention, and treatment of diseases. The goal of the standards is also to improve reliability and to decrease waiting times for test results, regardless of where the test is performed. In 1992, CLIA regulations were recategorized based on the complexity of the test method, with more stringent regulations being required for more complex tests. Laboratory tests are now divided into three categories: waived complexity, moderate complexity, and high complexity. Specific standards have been set for each level of testing category.

CLIA regulates laboratories in order to be sure that the standards are being met. A comprehensive quality assurance program for a laboratory is designed to analyze every aspect of the testing—from collection of the specimen to the final determination of the test results. The overall quality of the total testing process is evaluated. If an error is discovered in any part of the testing, then sequence corrective measures are instituted so that the goal of quality is achieved.

Americans with Disabilities Act

The Americans with Disabilities Act (ADA), established in 1991, protects the rights of people with physical and mental disabilities. This law applies to business that have 15 or more employees. Medical offices must comply with specific guidelines for easy accessibility to the medical facility for those with disabilities. (See Chapter 4, "Administrative Procedures: Maintaining the Office Environment: Americans with Disabilities Act," for more details about the specific guidelines of the ADA.)

Health Insurance Portability and Accountability Act

Enacted by Congress in 1996, HIPAA aims to improve the efficiency of the healthcare system. The main areas addressed by HIPAA regulations include:

- providing protection of healthcare coverage for workers and their families when they change or lose their jobs

- improving access to long-term care services and coverage
- simplifying the administration of health insurance
- promoting the use of medical savings accounts
- prohibiting discrimination against employees and their dependents based on health status
- guaranteeing renewal of health coverage
- providing security and privacy of health data

Regulations limit access to the medical records of patients. Insurance companies that pay for patient services through health plans; physicians, hospitals, nursing homes, pharmacists, and chiropractors who treat patients; and healthcare clearing houses that process insurance claims are among the healthcare entities allowed access to private patient information.

Not all organizations or agencies are required to follow the rules set by HIPAA. Carriers for life insurance and workers' compensation, state agencies such as child protective services, many law enforcement agencies, school districts, and employers are not governed by the HIPAA regulations. An employee personnel record, for instance, is not considered confidential even if it contains health-related issues. Because an employer is not regulated under the privacy rule, the employer has the right to ask an employee for a doctor's note to determine whether an employee may return to work or to determine an employee's status under a worker's compensation claim. The employer does not have the right to ask the physician for the note, and the physician has the right to deny the employer access to any of the patient's medical information without the patient's written permission, unless required to do so by law.

Drug Enforcement Administration

The Drug Enforcement Administration (DEA) is a bureau of the Justice Department that was set up to enforce the provisions of the Controlled Substances Act. The DEA is the lead agency for domestic enforcement of drug policy in the United States (sharing concurrent jurisdiction with the FBI) and is the sole agency responsible for pursuing U.S. drug

investigations abroad. Prescribers of drugs are required to be registered with the DEA. Information on the registration process is included in this chapter in the "Controlled Substances Act of 1970" section (page 64).

Internal Revenue Service

The W-2 and the W-4 are two forms issued and reviewed by the Internal Revenue Service (IRS) to determine the taxes due from individual workers. Both forms deal with employee wages but are used for different purposes.

The W-4 form contains identifying information about the employee such as his or her name, address, and social security number. The W-4 form allows the employee to report to the employer the number of allowances to be used in calculating payroll deductions for the employee. More information is available in Chapter 4, in the "Financial Practices" section.

The W-2 form is the document used by the employer to report the wages for a specific employee for the year and is filed once a year, usually by the end of January. The W-2 form contains identifying information about the employee and the employer. It also breaks down the wages and payroll deductions applied to the employee's past year of wages and withholdings. The employer is responsible for filing the W-2 to the IRS and the state taxing authority and for providing the employee with multiple copies to include with his or her income tax returns.

Equal Employment Opportunity Laws

The Federal Equal Employment Opportunity (EEO) laws prohibit discrimination against individuals seeking employment. Discrimination in the workplace means treating individuals differently based on factors other than individual merit and may include areas such as hiring and firing, compensation for work, promotions, recruiting, fringe benefits, and retirement plans. Discriminatory practices may include harassment, retaliation if complaints are made about discrimination, and denying employment opportunities based on age and gender. The federal Equal Employment Opportunity laws include the following acts:

- Title VII of the Civil Rights Act of 1964 prohibits discrimination for employment based on race, religion, gender, or national origin.
- The Equal Pay Act (EPA) of 1963 prohibits gender-based discrimination within a specific place of employment by requiring equal pay for equal work regardless of whether the employee is male or female.
- The Age Discrimination in Employment Act of 1967 (ADEA) prohibits discrimination against individuals age 40 and over. It is illegal to refuse to hire an individual based solely on his or her age. This discrimination law applies to all employers with 20 or more employees and includes both state and federal agencies.
- The Rehabilitation Act of 1973 prohibits discrimination against qualified employees with disabilities who are employed in the federal government.
- The Americans with Disabilities Act of 1990 prohibits employment discrimination against qualified applicants because of disabilities.
- The Civil Rights Act of 1991 provides compensation (which may be monetary) to individual victims of intentional employment discrimination.
- The Genetic Information Nondiscrimination Act of 2008 (GINA) prohibits discrimination against applicants or employees based on genetic information. (Genetic information may consist of an individual's genetic test results and information about any genetic diseases or conditions that may predispose this individual to a higher risk for getting a disease or condition in the future, such as an individual's risk for certain types of cancer.)

Workers' Compensation

Workers' compensation laws protect employees who are injured or disabled on the job or due to work performed. An individual may be entitled to recover medical fees, lost wages, and future wages depending on the severity of the injury. Workers' compensation laws include both state and federal laws (although federal compensation laws deal mainly with federal employees). In most states, employers are responsible for purchasing a workers' compensation insurance plan to cover injuries that occur on the job. Covered injuries do not necessarily have to be caused by a one-time accident (such as a burn or a laceration from a broken bottle). The injuries may occur gradually over time from repetitive behaviors—for example, a lung condition caused by exposure to toxic chemicals over time.

Certain conditions may prevent workers' compensation from covering an injury received at work. If the injury occurred from a violation of posted and known rules, workers' compensation would not cover the incident. For instance, if an individual did not wear the required personal protective equipment for a particular procedure, or if the injury occurred because the individual was intoxicated or using drugs that impaired his or her judgment, then coverage would not be available. Preexisting conditions may also be excluded from coverage, unless it can be proved that the current working environment exacerbated the symptoms.

Medical Records

Documentation of procedures, treatments, and care provided to patients is an essential function of the medical assistant. HIPAA regulations of patient privacy govern who has access to the documentation concerning patients.

Documentation in the medical record needs to be accurate, legible, and correct because the medical record is considered a legal document and may need to be used in a court of law. Proper procedure must be used when making a correction to a medical record. (For information about the proper procedure for correcting the medical record, see Chapter 4, "Administrative Procedures: Medical Records Management: Making Corrections to Medical Records.") Written patient consent is needed when information is to be reported, transferred, or released.

Personnel Records

Personnel records are usually kept so that the medical office has organized information about each employee available, if needed. Much of the information in the personnel record is required by federal and state government agencies for tax information.

Many states regulate who may have access to an employee's personnel record. All states seem to agree that an employee has the right to examine the contents of his or her own personnel record and may request copies of the information in the record; however, in some states the employer does not necessarily have to comply with the employee's request. Most states agree that the employer owns the personnel record and the contents within the record. Personnel records should be correct, and if an employee has the option to review his or her personnel record and finds an error or disagrees with its content, a written response by the employee may be included in the record stating the employee's version of the recorded situation.

Access to the personnel record should be limited to only those in the company who may need the information. Personnel records should be kept in a locked cabinet; employee authorization is needed before information can be sent or released to others inquiring about the employee.

The Personnel Record Review Act of 1990, used by some states to oversee the proper use of personnel records, dictates that employers cannot keep a record of an employee's activities, such as political activities or organizational membership, occurring off the premises of the place of employment. Although the law states that keeping personnel records is not mandatory, keeping information regarding job performance and work-related issues in the personnel record may be beneficial to the employer if, for instance, a disgruntled employee decides to sue for wrongful termination. The personnel record will help in the employer's defense.

TICKLER FILES

Tickler files are useful for keeping track of patient information such as lab test results or reminders to notify patients about appointments or other scheduled activities. An efficient tickler system may also be used to keep track of renewing important information. For example, the physician's licenses for practicing medicine, his or her license to prescribe controlled substances, and his or her malpractice insurance should not be allowed to lapse. A tickler system may help the busy medical assistant remember these important dates.

Performance Evaluations

Performance evaluations are regularly scheduled reviews of how well an employee is performing at his or her job. Performance evaluations provide the employee with a chance to learn what the employer feels his or her strengths are and what areas need improvement. Traits evaluated may include flexibility, dependability, and ability to work well with coworkers on the team.

The employee's performance evaluation is also a time when the employee can discuss issues of concern about the job. Many performance evaluations now include questions about the employees' goals for the future and accomplishments made during the year.

Although not all medical offices use a rigorous written evaluation policy, it is the best way to keep a record of employee evaluations. The written evaluation is presented to the employee, who has the right to make comments (whether oral or written) about the evaluation. The evaluation is then signed by both the employee and the employer and kept in the personnel record of the employee.

Consent

Three kinds of consent are possible in the course of a patient's medical care.

- **Implied consent** is an indirect acceptance, for example, when a patient may extend his or her arm for the medical assistant to measure the patient's blood pressure.
- **Expressed consent** is a spoken or written agreement that provides consent. Many times a non-verbal gesture such as a handshake is considered expressed consent.

SCOPE OF PRACTICE

Medical assistants are bound by law and ethics to perform only procedures and skills within their scope of practice. Scope of practice is the general term used to describe the procedures and tasks that a professional medical assistant can and cannot do. Scope of practice is limited by state laws, education and training, and level of experience. Because state laws vary, the medical assistant is responsible for knowing which skills may be performed in the state in which he or she practices.

Medical assistants should never diagnose a patient's condition or make independent medical assessments. Medical assistants should give medication only under the direct supervision of a physician (and only in states in which administration of medications by a medical assistant is allowed). Also, some state laws require special training and licensing to perform phlebotomy, take X-rays, or do an ultrasound.

The medical facility should clearly list its policies regarding which procedures are acceptable for a medical assistant to perform. Acting beyond the scope of practice can expose the medical assistant and the medical assistant's supervisor to a lawsuit.

- **Informed consent** is a written statement signed by the patient, agreeing to the procedure or treatment recommended by the physician only after receiving a detailed explanation of the procedure to be done, the reasons for the procedure, the risks involved, complications that may occur, and any alternate methods of treatment that may be used instead of the procedure being discussed. Many times a patient may be asked to write a description of what the procedure entails in his or her own words to be sure that there is a clear understanding of what will be done. A physician who fails to obtain informed consent from a patient may be charged with the crime of **battery**. Patients may also be asked to sign a written consent or a written authorization in order to release information to a third-party payer, such as an insurance carrier, for reimbursement procedures.

Releasing Medical Information

Rules and laws (such as HIPAA) have been established to protect patients' privacy and limit access to medical records of patients. The only individuals or entities allowed access to patients' information are:

- insurance companies that pay for patient services through health plans
- healthcare providers such as physicians, hospitals, nursing homes, pharmacists, and chiropractors who treat patients
- healthcare clearinghouses that process insurance claims

Even for these individuals or entities, certain conditions must be met in order to gain access to patient information. In some instances, written consent is required. Other parties, such as patients' friends and families or patients' attorneys, nearly always need patients' written consent before they may have access to patient information.

THE MEDICAL ASSISTANT AND CONFIDENTIALITY

The medical assistant must be careful not to repeat any information about a patient that may be overheard by others. Test results should not be left in a voicemail on a home phone, should never be given to a member of the patient's family (unless the patient has provided written consent allowing a member of the family to have access to the patient's medical records), and should never be faxed to a patient's place of employment or anywhere else unless the patient has requested it. Test results may end up in the hands of unauthorized individuals, revealing private information that the patient did not wish shared. Any specific instructions from the patient regarding test results should be documented in the patient's medical record, stating that the test results were faxed or left on the answering machine at the patient's request.

HIPAA requires medical facilities to identify in writing the policies regarding patient confidentiality and the release of patient information. The medical assistant has the responsibility to maintain the patient's confidentiality in all areas of patient care. Care must be taken so that private patient information is released only with the written permission of the patient, or as otherwise required by law.

Special Situations Concerning Release of Patient Information

Drug and Alcohol Treatment

Drug and alcohol rehabilitation records are protected by federal law and cannot be disclosed without the written authorization of the patient, except for a court order or to medical personnel in case of an emergency. The rehabilitation facility may not even acknowledge that an individual attended, is currently undergoing, or has completed a drug and alcohol rehabilitation program.

Public Health and Welfare Needs

Protected health information may be made available, even without the individual's authorization, to public officials in charge of dealing with serious public health issues, including, for instance, bioterrorism or disaster-relief efforts.

HIV-Related Issues

Human immunodeficiency virus (HIV)-related issues for medical assistants and healthcare practitioners in general may involve the authorization for release of information, patient confidentiality, and penalties if HIV information is released without proper authorization. Ethics and law agree that information disclosed to a physician providing care to a patient is confidential and should never be revealed or released without the express consent of the patient unless required to do so by law. The only exception to this rule is if the patient is threatening bodily harm to other people or to him- or herself.

There are two types of HIV testing: anonymous and confidential. Anonymous testing uses a number code and does not identify the patient by name. Anonymous testing is often done at a clinic for testing. Confidential testing includes a patient's name, address, date of birth, ethnic origin, and gender. Confidential testing is usually ordered by the patient's physician.

HIV is a reportable condition; therefore, positive test results, including the patient's personal data, are reportable to the state department of health. A breach of confidentiality occurs, however, when the physician releases confidential information to a third party, such as an insurance carrier, an employer, or the patient's family members without the patient's consent or without a court order. The release form used to obtain the written permission of the patient must clearly state that the release is for HIV-related information, and the form must identify specifically to whom the information is being sent.

The utmost care should be taken by the medical assistant before releasing HIV-related information to a third party. The medical assistant should be sure that written authorization to release HIV-related information is documented in the patient's medical record. HIV-related information may be recorded in electronic medical records because this information is an important part of the patient's medical history and medical care. Reported information includes the patient name (if given), date of birth, and ethnicity or race.

If a patient does not have the capability to make decisions for his or her own healthcare, the patient's healthcare agent may be given this information if he or she requests it and if it may affect decisions made on the patient's behalf. Penalties for releasing HIV-related information without proper authorization may be severe.

Subpoena Duces Tecum

A **subpoena duces tecum** is an order to appear in court and bring any papers, books, or information necessary to explain in detail the issue in question. The subpoena may indicate that the person testifying—the physician, office manager, or medical assistant—may be asked to discuss the material needed for court. Appearing before a court of law may be intimidating for any individual, but the individual is simply required to tell the facts.

Original records should never be handed over to the court, so the medical assistant may be asked to make photocopies of the material requested. The material copied should cover only the area requested by the subpoena. Physician approval must be obtained for copying material from the medical record, and the medical office may ask for a fee to compensate the time involved in preparing and copying the requested material.

Rescinding Authorization for Release

Rescinding authorization for release of information may be accomplished by putting the request in writing, dating the form, and submitting the signed form to the appropriate person or medical office. Unfortunately, material already disclosed cannot be rescinded.

Physician-Patient Relationship

The physician-patient relationship is based on mutual respect and trust, governed by contract law, and subject to certain rights and responsibilities.

THE MEDICAL ASSISTANT AS AN AGENT OF THE PHYSICIAN

The medical assistant is an agent of the physician and must follow the federal and state guidelines required for healthcare professionals because the behavior and actions of the medical assistant may have legal consequences for the physician. The physician may be found guilty of negligence based on the actions of the medical assistant because of a law stating that physicians are liable for the negligent actions of any employee working under their supervision.

Contract Law

Contract law governs agreements, either oral or written, between individuals. The contract establishing the physician-patient relationship is based on an agreement between two parties: The physician makes an offer to treat patients when he or she opens a medical office; the patient accepts the offer when an appointment is made and the patient arrives for the first visit, establishing an implied contract. Because the physician may select the patients he or she will treat, the physician is under no obligation to a person calling for information or care, unless that person is a patient of the physician or an appointment has been scheduled.

Once an individual has been accepted as a patient, the physician has a legal responsibility to provide care with the degree of competency similar to other physicians with comparable medical training. An individual should feel confident that a licensed physician has met the standards necessary to provide quality medical care.

Contracts—such as the one implied between patients and their physicians—are considered valid or legal only when they fulfill certain requirements. Valid contracts must be made by mutual consent between two mentally sound consenting adults or **emancipated minors**, used only for legal subject matter, and must be for a valid consideration, such as medical treatment. For example, individuals under the influence of drugs or alcohol and mentally impaired individuals are not considered mentally competent, and any contract made with one of these individuals would not be valid and binding. Contracts involving illegal activity, such as prescribing prescription drugs when not needed or selling signed prescription requisitions, are not considered legally binding or valid.

Responsibilities and Rights

Physicians and patients have rights regarding medical care. The physician has the right to select the patients he or she treats, the type of services provided, the office location, and the hours of operation. A physician also has the right to expect payment for the services provided.

The patient has the right to consent to or refuse treatments. If a patient consents to treatment, he or she expects that the treatment provided will be carried out by a competent, caring physician. Patients have the right to expect that all information disclosed in the physician-patient relationship will be kept confidential by the physician and members of the healthcare team. The patient has a financial obligation to the physician for the treatment received and is expected to pay the physician for the medical services rendered.

The medical assistant has a professional responsibility to perform tasks only within the realm of medical assisting knowledge and training. For example, the medical assistant should not offer medical advice to a patient, interpret EKGs, or prescribe medications, because these skills are not included in the standard of care for a medical assistant. The medical assistant is responsible for maintaining patient confidentiality, performing skills competently, keeping his or her skills current, and providing quality care to all individuals under the direct supervision of the physician.

Res ipsa loquitur, meaning "the thing speaks for itself," applies to the law of negligence. It means that the negligent action was so obvious, it needs no further examination or explanation.

Guidelines for Third-Party Agreements

A third party in the medical field is usually considered a party other than the patient that is responsible for payment of services rendered for medical care, such as an insurance carrier. The physician has the opportunity to join various third-party payers for patient reimbursement.

Before signing a payer agreement, the physician should carefully read the contract and understand its provisions. The medical assistant is often the individual in charge of requesting payments from such third parties, so he or she must be knowledgeable of third-party policies and procedures.

Professional Liability

Professional liability is a legal obligation that arises from errors, negligent acts, or omissions during the course of someone's professional practice. Negligence, or medical malpractice, is considered to be the improper treatment or the absence of needed treatment for a patient. Negligence implies that the physician did not act in a manner in which a prudent physician would act. For instance, if a physician performed a procedure in a manner not consistent with the way other competent physicians would have performed it, or failed to order an appropriate test or provide an appropriate treatment that other qualified physicians would have, the physician may be charged with negligence.

Negligence can be broken down into **malfeasance** (performing a wrong or unlawful act), **misfeasance** (improperly performing a legal act), and **nonfeasance** (omitting or failing to perform an act that should have been performed).

In order for the physician to be found guilty of malpractice, certain criteria—the "four Ds" of negligence—must be met:

1. **Duty**. The physician accepted the responsibility for the care of the patient when the initial physician-patient contract was established.
2. **Derelict**. The physician's failure to provide competent care is an example of dereliction of duty.
3. **Direct cause**. Proof must be established that the harm caused to the patient was a direct result of the physician's actions or lack of actions.
4. **Damages**. The court determines an amount of money that would be sufficient compensation for the patient's suffering, living expenses, and perhaps rehabilitation.

The **statutes of limitation** refer to the time period in which a legal malpractice claim may be filed in a court of law. Statutes of limitation laws vary from state to state. Statutes of limitation do not always start at the time of the negligent act; rather, they can start when the negligent act came to the attention of the patient. If the negligent damages involve a child patient, a representative of the court, or a **guardian *ad litem***, may assist in the lawsuit, or the lawsuit may be initiated when the child reaches maturity. The medical assistant should be aware of the specific number of years for the statutes of limitations in the state in which he or she is employed. Medical records should not be destroyed within that time frame because they may be needed for a court case.

Arbitration Agreements

Arbitration is a legal technique used to resolve disputes between parties (such as a physician and a patient) without going to court. A panel of neutral parties who are knowledgeable about the subject will listen to both sides of the dispute and will make an impartial judgment that both sides agree to obey.

Parties may choose arbitration over trying the case in court because the resolution to the dispute is more confidential, less expensive, more convenient and less time-consuming than a court case's, which could take years. Arbitration statutes apply the same measure of damages as a decision in a court case.

Affirmative Defense

An **affirmative defense** is one in which the **defendant** (the person being sued) is trying to win the lawsuit between the patient (the **plaintiff**) and the physician (the defendant) by acknowledging that he or she shares the blame for the injury received by the patient. **Contributory negligence** is one of the most common and effectives types of affirmative defense used in malpractice cases. The defense tries to show that the patient's behavior or negligence was partially responsible for the injury or complication that occurred, although the physician will admit to performing the procedure that led to the patient's injury. Consent forms could document that the patient was aware of the risks involved in the surgery that was performed and was willing to take those risks. Proving contributory negligence may lessen the damages collected by the plaintiff because he or she was found to be partially responsible for the injury incurred.

Termination of Medical Care

A physician may discontinue treatment of a patient for a variety of reasons. One may be that the patient is not following the physician's advice. Another may be that a personality conflict between the physician and the patient is interfering with the medical care provided. If, for any reason, the physician chooses to discontinue treating the patient, written notification must be sent to the patient, usually in the form of a certified letter with receipt requested. The certified letter should inform the patient that medical care is being terminated.

Although reasons or details for termination do not have to be listed, many physicians will explain the reason for terminating the physician-patient relationship in the letter. The patient should be given ample time—at least one month—to find another physician before medical care is terminated. The patient should be reassured that the physician will be available for emergency care until a new physician-patient relationship is established. The patient should be notified that his or her medical records will be transferred to the new physician upon written request.

A copy of the dismissal letter and the receipt from the certified letter sent to the patient should be kept in the patient's medical record as documentation of the patient's dismissal from the physician-patient contract. Without documentation, the patient may bring a lawsuit against the physician for abandonment.

The patient may terminate the physician-patient contract by requesting in writing that his or her medical records be transferred to another physician or simply by not making new appointments with the physician.

Performing within Ethical Boundaries

Professions have codes of behaviors that members of the profession should follow. Most professional codes include ethical and legal boundaries.

Ethical Standards

Ethics are a set of values—knowing what is right and wrong and acting appropriately. Many sources use the terms *ethics* and *morals* interchangeably. Ethics are not laws, although many laws are based on ethics (for example, the Equal Employment Opportunity laws, which make certain types of discrimination against individuals illegal). Principles of professional ethics may include:

- **objectivity and impartiality:** respecting all patients and providing equal treatment to all patients

- **openness and complete honesty:** providing all information necessary for treatment and the outcomes of treatment
- **confidentiality:** never repeating private personal information inappropriately
- **responsibility:** providing attention and quality care to every patient

The medical assistant's code of ethics is based on the code of ethics physicians are expected to follow. Being objective, treating patients with respect and confidentiality, and providing the best care possible are behaviors expected of a medical assistant.

Patient Rights

The Patient's Bill of Rights, developed by the American Hospital Association, is a list of rights that should be accorded to an individual seeking medical treatment.

Patient rights have been discussed in many areas of healthcare, such as patient confidentiality, right to informed consent, and HIPAA regulations for repeating and releasing private patient information. The Patient's Bill of Rights was adopted by the U.S. Commission on Consumer Protection and Quality in the Healthcare Industry in 1998, summarizing the rights and responsibilities of healthcare providers such as physicians and hospitals, as well as the rights and responsibilities of patients. The bill was designed to help patients feel more comfortable and confident in the healthcare they receive, to stress the importance of a good physician-patient relationship in promoting and maintaining good healthcare, and to emphasize the important role patients must play in the responsibility for their own healthcare.

Practice Questions

Medical Terminology

1. Which of the following terms means "surgical removal of the uterus"?
   a. appendectomy
   b. cholecystectomy
   c. hysterectomy
   d. nephrectomy
   e. splenectomy

2. Which of the following terms refers to an excessive amount of menstrual flow?
   a. amenorrhea
   b. dysmenorrhea
   c. menarche
   d. menorrhagia
   e. polymenorrhea

3. The prefix *myelo* means
   a. capillary.
   b. kidney.
   c. marrow.
   d. mucus.
   e. pancreas.

4. Which of the following suffixes means "softening"?
   a. *lithiasis*
   b. *malacia*
   c. *megaly*
   d. *ptosis*
   e. *sclerosis*

5. Which of the following terms means "abnormal enlargement of the liver"?
   a. hepatitis
   b. hepatomalacia
   c. hepatomegaly
   d. hepatorrhexis
   e. hemophilia

6. The prefix *pachy* means which of the following?
   a. dull
   b. fixed
   c. thick
   d. thin
   e. sharp

7. The instrument used to view the interior of the ear canal is known as
   a. an otoscope.
   b. an anoscope.
   c. an ophthalmoscope.
   d. a speculum.
   e. a laryngoscope.

8. The medical term that describes an inflammation of the brain is
   a. encephalitis.
   b. mastitis.
   c. meningitis.
   d. myelitis.
   e. nephritis.

9. Which suffix means "rupture"?
   a. *rrhage*
   b. *rrhapy*
   c. *rrhea*
   d. *rrhexis*
   e. *rrhestis*

10. Which word denotes the condition of total paralysis affecting only one side of the body?
 a. hemiparesis
 b. hemiplegia
 c. paraplegia
 d. quadriplegia
 e. otioplegia

11. The medical assistant instructed the patient to be NPO before the procedure. NPO means?
 a. no pizza or oils
 b. no solid food
 c. nothing to eat past one in the afternoon
 d. nothing by mouth
 e. nothing to eat past one in the morning

12. The physician orders a K level to be drawn. The K level is
 a. ketones.
 b. potassium.
 c. sodium.
 d. creatine.
 e. hematocrit.

13. The patient is diagnosed with COPD. What does COPD stand for?
 a. cardiac occlusive pulmonary disease
 b. cardiac occult phlebitis disease
 c. chronic obstructive pulmonary disease
 d. chronic occult physical disease
 e. crippling occurrence physical disease

14. The patient is being treated for an URI. What is a URI?
 a. urinary restrictive infection
 b. urinary reductive infection
 c. upper respiratory inclusion
 d. upper respiratory infection
 e. ureter restrictive infection

15. The patient's results were PERRLA. What does PERRLA stand for?
 a. physical examination, respiratory, reproductive, lungs and abdomen
 b. pupils equal, round, reactive to light and accommodation
 c. pupils even, round, reactive to light and accommodation
 d. physical examination, reproductive, respiratory and extremities
 e. patient examination results reactive to light and accommodation

Anatomy and Physiology

1. *Superior* means that a body part is
 a. toward the front.
 b. above another part, or closer to the head.
 c. toward the side.
 d. toward the back.
 e. toward the middle.

2. Which of the following is sometimes called the coronal plane?
 a. transverse plane
 b. midsagittal plane
 c. sagittal plane
 d. frontal plane
 e. visceral

3. Shingles is also known as
 a. alopecia.
 b. urticaria.
 c. psoriasis.
 d. herpes zoster.
 e. dermatitis.

4. Which of the following is a bruise?
   a. hematoma
   b. impetigo
   c. verruca
   d. furuncle
   e. schleroderma

5. Which of the following is a spinal cord injury in which paralysis is on one side of the body?
   a. multiple sclerosis
   b. encephalitis
   c. quadriplegia
   d. paraplegia
   e. hemiplegia

6. Which of the following is a myocardial infarction?
   a. weakness of an artery
   b. narrowing or blockage of arteries
   c. heart attack
   d. chest pain
   e. buildup of cholesterol in the artery wall

7. Which of the following is also known as myxedema?
   a. thyroiditis
   b. hyperthyroidism
   c. hypothyroidism
   d. hyperparathyroidism
   e. hypoparathyroidism

8. Which of the following is the gland that produces oily secretions that lubricate the skin?
   a. pineal
   b. sebaceous
   c. pituitary
   d. parathyroid
   e. adrenal

9. Which of the following describes a function of the respiratory system?
   a. hormone production
   b. movement
   c. transportation of elements
   d. waste removal
   e. air exchange

10. Which of the following terms means that the body is in a state of equilibrium or balance?
   a. anabolism
   b. homeostasis
   c. metabolism
   d. synergism
   e. catabolism

Psychology

1. Behavior modification is an application of which type of psychological theory?
   a. psychoanalytical theory
   b. cognitivism
   c. behaviorism
   d. humanistic psychology
   e. psychiatry

2. Uncovering irrational beliefs is an important part of what type of psychotherapy?
   a. cognitive therapy
   b. behavior therapy
   c. talk therapy
   d. psychoanalytical theory
   e. art therapy

3. Which of the following is not a defense mechanism?
   a. rationalization
   b. suppression
   c. projection
   d. anxiety
   e. intellectualization

4. Elizabeth Kübler-Ross's five stages of grief are:
  a. anxiety, anger, bargaining, depression, acceptance.
  b. denial, anger, bargaining, depression, acceptance.
  c. denial, anger, projection, depression, acceptance.
  d. denial, anger, outrage, bargaining, depression.
  e. denial, rationalization, anger, depression, acceptance.

Professional Standards

  1. Which term describes the set of values that dictates the behavior of professionals?
  a. civil law
  b. statutes of limitation
  c. criminal law
  d. ethics
  e. tort law

  2. The patient looks for all of the following attributes in a medical assistant EXCEPT
  a. dependability.
  b. clean appearance.
  c. courteousness.
  d. disinterest.
  e. flexibility.

  3. Which of the following describes the medical assistant's ability to adjust to abrupt changes in a medical office environment?
  a. dependability
  b. accountability
  c. flexibility
  d. respect
  e. positive attitude

4. All of the following statements are true about a credentialed medical assistant EXCEPT
  a. a credential builds self-esteem.
  b. a credential may help in career advancement and financial compensation.
  c. a credential indicates professional and technical competence.
  d. a credential guarantees a job.
  e. a credential gives the medical assistant confidence.

5. An example of providing privacy to a patient is
  a. knocking before entering the examination room.
  b. talking on the phone with a patient while the glass partition is open to the reception area.
  c. leaving the examination door slightly ajar so that the medical assistant will be able to hear if the physician needs him or her.
  d. discussing the registration form with a patient while he or she is sitting in the reception area.
  e. discussing financial issues with a patient at the reception desk.

6. All of the following are attributes of a professional EXCEPT
  a. having a professional code of ethics.
  b. being limited to jobs only in the medical field.
  c. requiring specialized training or knowledge.
  d. involving values and morals.
  e. having an organized group to regulate its members.

7. All of the following would be a breach of patient confidentiality by the medical assistant EXCEPT

   a. discussing a patient's condition in the elevator.

   b. telling the patient's physician about the abnormal test results just received from the lab.

   c. discussing the patient's illness with the patient's attorney.

   d. leaving the patient's medical record open on the front desk.

   e. calling the lab to request test results for a patient while another patient is standing at the desk waiting to speak with you.

8. Which of the following best describes active listening?

   a. helping the patient complete his or her thoughts

   b. interrupting the patient's conversation to add your comments

   c. recording all patient information on a voice recorder for later use

   d. restating what the patient has said to verify that you have understood him or her correctly

   e. writing information in the medical record as the patient is speaking

9. When communicating with a visually impaired patient, the medical assistant should

   a. speak louder.

   b. automatically take the patient's arm when directing him or her to the examining room.

   c. leave quietly when leaving a room so as not to distract the patient.

   d. introduce himself or herself to the patient when entering the room.

   e. tape every conversation for the patient to listen to at a later time.

10. Which of the following statements is true about all elderly patients?

   a. All elderly patients are hearing impaired.

   b. All elderly patients prefer to be treated with respect.

   c. All elderly patients like to be called by nicknames or endearments.

   d. All elderly patients have a loss of intelligence as they age.

   e. All elderly patients have physical impairments that make walking difficult for them.

11. All of the following statements about seriously ill patients are true EXCEPT

   a. seriously ill patients may respond differently to their illnesses.

   b. a seriously ill patient may be in denial about his or her condition.

   c. the family of a seriously ill patient may need comforting and referral to support groups.

   d. the medical assistant should encourage the patient to think about happier times and forget about his or her illness.

   e. a seriously ill patient should be encouraged to discuss his or her fears and concerns about the illness and the future.

12. All of the following statements about cultural diversity are true EXCEPT

   a. all cultures use the same nonverbal body gestures.

   b. some cultures find closeness and hugging impolite and overly familiar.

   c. some cultures find direct eye contact impolite.

   d. cultural diversity includes gender, race, ethnic, and socioeconomic backgrounds.

   e. knowledge of cultural diversity may decrease miscommunications between coworkers.

13. Mentally impaired patients
   a. are able to enter into contracts by themselves.
   b. should be spoken to directly in simple, easy-to-understand terms.
   c. should not be spoken to directly.
   d. should have directions explained only once to avoid confusion.
   e. are seen only by specialists who treat mentally impaired patients.

14. All of the following are barriers to communication EXCEPT
   a. closed doors.
   b. mistrust.
   c. fear.
   d. trust.
   e. stress.

15. When a child asks whether a procedure will hurt, the reply to the child should be
   a. referred to the parents to answer.
   b. answered by telling the child that the physician will explain everything later.
   c. answered in simple, honest terms.
   d. ignored by changing the subject.
   e. to tell the child not to worry about anything.

16. The various types of verbal and nonverbal methods that may be used to convey messages such as speaking, writing, and body language are referred to as
   a. receivers.
   b. feedback.
   c. channels.
   d. senders.
   e. messages.

17. Which of the following is the proper response a medical assistant should give to the statement "I can't wait until this operation is over"?
   a. "Don't worry about the operation. You'll be just fine."
   b. "You seem worried about the operation. Am I correct?"
   c. "Dr. Smith is the best. You'll be in great hands."
   d. "Don't think about tomorrow."
   e. "It doesn't do any good to worry about what will happen, so in my opinion, forget about it."

Answers and Explanations

Medical Terminology

1. c. Hysterectomy, because *hyster* means "uterus" and *ectomy* means "removal of."

2. d. Menorrhagia, because *meno* means "menstruation" and *rrhagia* means "excessive flow."

3. c. *Myelo* means "marrow."

4. b. *Melacia* means "softening."

5. c. Hepatomegaly, because *hepato* means "liver" and *megaly* means "enlargement."

6. c. *Pachy* means "thick."

7. a. An otoscope is used to look inside the ear canal.

8. a. Encephalitis, because *encephal* means "brain" and *itis* means "inflammation."

9. d. The suffix *rrhexis* means "rupture."

10. b. Hemiplegia, because *hemi* means "one-half" and *plegia* means "paralysis."

11. d. NPO means "nothing by mouth."

12. b. Potassium (sodium is Na)

13. c. COPD stands for "chronic obstructive pulmonary disease."

14. d. URI stands for upper respiratory infection.

15. b. PERRLA stands for "pupils equal, round, reactive to light and accommodation."

Anatomy and Physiology

1. b. *Superior* means that one body part is above another part, or closer to the head. *Anterior* means that one body part is closer to the front. *Lateral* means closer to the side. *Medial* means that one body part is closer to the middle. *Posterior* means that one body part is closer to the back.

2. d. The frontal plane is sometimes called the coronal plane. The transverse plane divides the body into upper and lower parts. The midsagittal plane divides the body into left and right halves. The sagittal plane divides the body into left and right halves. Visceral indicates the organs within the cavity.

3. d. Shingles is also known as herpes zoster. Alopecia is baldness. Urticaria, or hives, is an acute condition characterized by the appearance of wheals, usually due to an allergic reaction. Psoriasis is a chronic skin disease characterized by red lesions and silvery scaling thought to be caused by an immune disorder. Dermatitis is inflammation of the dermis.

4. a. A bruise is a hematoma. Impetigo is an infectious bacterial inflammation caused by *Staphylococcus* or *Streptococcus* bacteria. Verruca is warts. A furuncle is a boil or an abscess involving the hair follicle and adjacent tissue. Schleroderma is thick, densely fibrous skin, thought to be caused by an autoimmune disorder.

5. e. Hemiplegia is a spinal cord injury in which paralysis occurs on one side of the body. Multiple sclerosis is a chronic nerve disease caused by the degeneration of the myelin sheath. Encephalitis is inflammation of the brain. Quadriplegia is paralysis of all four extremities. Paraplegia is paralysis of the trunk and lower extremities.

6. c. A myocardial infarction is a heart attack. Weakness of an artery is an aneurysm. Narrowing or blockage of arteries is called arterosclerosis. Chest pain is angina. Buildup of cholesterol in the artery wall is called atherosclerosis.

7. c. Hypothyroidism is also known as myxedema (hyposecretion of thyroxine). Thyroiditis is inflammation of the thyroid. Hyperthyroidism is hypersecretion of thyroxine. Hyperparathyroidism is hypersecretion of PTH causing hypercalcemia. Hypoparathyroidism is hyposecretion of PTH causing hypocalcemia.

8. b. The sebaceous gland produces oily secretions that lubricate the skin. The pineal gland produces melatonin, which regulates the body's biological clock. The pituitary gland controls the functions of the other endocrine glands. The parathyroid gland causes bone to dissolve to increase blood calcium and phosphate levels, causes phosphate to be secreted by the kidney for excretion in urine, and activates vitamin D for increased absorption of calcium. Adrenal glands secrete several steroid hormones.

9. e. Air exchange describes a function of the respiratory system. Hormone production is a function of the endocrine system. Movement is part of the muscular system. Transportation of elements is a function of the circulatory system. Waste removal is part of the digestive system.

10. b. Homeostasis means that the body is in a state of equilibrium or balance. Homeostasis is the condition of constancy within the body's internal environment. Anabolism is the phase of metabolism in which simple substances are synthesized into the complex materials of living tissue. Metabolism refers to all the physical and chemical processes in the body that convert or use energy. Synergism may be defined as two or more agents working together to produce a result not obtainable by any of the agents independently. Catabolism is the breakdown of large molecules into small molecules.

Psychology

1. c. Behavior modification is an application of the theories of behaviorism, which focuses the attention of researchers on observable behavior. Also called behavior therapy, it attempts to modify established patterns of behavior.

2. a. Uncovering irrational beliefs, which are cognitive errors, or mistakes in how someone thinks or understands their world, is an important tool in cognitive therapy.

3. d. Anxiety is a response to a stressful situation, but it is not a defense mechanism, which is an emotional strategy used to avoid the painful feelings or thoughts arising from difficult situations.

4. b. Kübler-Ross's five stages of grief are denial, anger, bargaining, depression, and acceptance. The other choices are unacceptable because they include one choice that is not part of her model of grieving. Anxiety—included in choice **a**—may be experienced by terminally ill or grieving individuals, but it is not one of the stages of grief. Outrage—included in choice **d**—may be felt in the anger stage, but it is not a stage on its own; this choice also does not include the final stage, acceptance.

Professional Standards

1. d. Ethics is the set of values that dictates the behavior of a professional toward patients and colleagues. The medical assistant should understand ethics, know the difference between right and wrong, and behave in a fair and honest manner when treating patients and working with colleagues. Criminal law deals with cases against society such as murder or burglary. Civil law deals with the rights of private citizens and relationships between individuals, and tort law is a type of civil law that deals with wrongful acts against another person such as injury, libel, or slander. Statutes of limitation refer to the time period after an event in which a legal proceeding, such as a malpractice claim, may be filed in a court of law.

2. d. Disinterest is not an attribute that a patient looks for in a medical assistant. However, patients—as well as colleagues and other people that medical assistants come into contact with—expect a medical assistant to be dependable, courteous, and flexible and to look clean and neat.

3. c. Flexibility describes the medical assistant's ability to adjust to abrupt changes in a medical office environment. The other attributes listed in the choices are desirable in a medical assistant but don't indicate the ability to adjust to various events that take place in a medical office.

4. d. A credential does not guarantee a job. However, a credential may make the applicant a more attractive candidate for a job because the credential shows that the individual has successfully met the standards of the profession.

5. a. Knocking before entering the examination room is an example of providing privacy to a patient, because the patient may be embarrassed if the medical assistant walks into the room when the patient is in the process of undressing. Carrying on conversations in an area where others may overhear does not provide privacy.

6. b. Professions are not limited to the medical field. Law, teaching, and accounting are some nonmedical professions.

7. b. Telling the patient's physician about the abnormal test results just received from the lab is not a breach of patient confidentiality because it is proper to discuss patient information with the primary physician caring for the patient. Leaving the medical record where others may view the contents, discussing any patient information with an attorney without the patient's written consent, talking about a patient in an elevator, or allowing another patient to hear test results of a patient are all considered a breach of patient confidentiality.

8. d. Active listening consists of restating or paraphrasing what the patient has said in order to be sure that his or her comments were understood correctly by the medical assistant. Helping the patient to complete his or her thoughts can be disruptive to the patient; it can distort what he or she is really trying to say. Recording all information the patient says may make the patient reluctant to provide information because it is being taped. Writing down information while the patient is speaking may cause the medical assistant to miss much of the information provided by the patient.

9. d. When communicating with a visually impaired patient, the medical assistant should introduce himself or herself to the patient when entering the room. Since the patient is visually impaired, he or she may not be able to see the medical assistant enter the room. The medical assistant should also notify the patient when leaving the room so that the patient will not ask questions only to find out that he or she is alone in the room. Not all visually impaired patients need help with walking or finding the way to the examining room. If the patient seems to have a problem navigating the halls of the facility, the medical assistant may ask if the patient would like assistance.

10. b. All elderly patients prefer to be treated with respect, and that means avoiding terms of endearment like "Gramps" and "dear." Not all elderly patients have difficulty walking or hearing, nor do they all lose intelligence because of aging.

11. d. The medical assistant should not encourage the patient to think about happier times and forget about his or her illness. Thinking about happier times will not make a serious illness go away. The medical assistant should encourage a patient and his or her family to talk about their concerns and fears related to the patient's illness. Listening is important to help comfort patients and families because they may feel isolated. The medical assistant may be able to refer the patient and his or her family to appropriate support groups once their fears and concerns are identified.

12. a. All cultures do not use the same body gestures. Every culture has its own acceptable behaviors and body gestures. In some cultures, people do not like physical touching and hugging, others find direct eye contact rude, and still others prefer that any concerns about the patient be discussed with the oldest member of the family instead of speaking with the patient directly. It is important for the medical assistant to learn about the various cultures of the patients treated at the facility where he or she is employed in order to provide the best care for all patients.

13. b. Mentally impaired patients should be spoken to directly in simple, easy-to-understand terms. A legal contract cannot be made with a mentally impaired individual. Medical conditions are not treated by a specialist limited to mentally impaired individuals.

14. d. Trust is not a barrier to communication. Trust encourages communication, which will help the healthcare team and the medical assistant better serve the patient's needs. Closed doors, mistrust, fear, and stress are barriers that may lead to miscommunication.

15. c. When a child asks whether a procedure will hurt, the child should be answered in simple, honest terms. Delivering the information in a manner that is suitable for a child's level of understanding will do much to relieve fear and anxiety that a child may feel about the procedure. Ignoring the question, telling the child that the physician will talk to the child later, or having the parents answer the question would not be the best choices, because the parents may not know the answer and the physician may not have the time to answer the question. Ignoring the question may make the child uncooperative, while a simple explanation may relieve the child's fear and anxiety.

16. c. The verbal and nonverbal methods that may be used to convey messages such as speaking, writing, and body language are called channels. The receiver is the person to whom the message is sent. The sender is the person sending the message or information. Feedback, the final part of the communication process, is the response made back to the sender of the message.

17. b. The proper response to a patient's statement of "I can't wait until this operation is over" would be "You seem worried about the operation. Am I correct?" Feedback gives the sender the opportunity to evaluate whether the receiver understood correctly the message. Telling the patient not to worry or to forget about the operation is not helpful to the patient. The patient should be able to express his or her concerns.

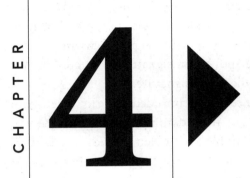

CHAPTER 4 ▶ ADMINISTRATIVE PROCEDURES

CHAPTER SUMMARY

The medical assistant is involved in many of the most important administrative practices of a medical office. These wide-ranging responsibilities can include data entry, basic communications, operation and management of equipment, maintenance of records, mail screening and processing, appointment scheduling and monitoring, efficient operation of the office, and basic functions in the practice's finances. These responsibilities are outlined on the following pages.

Data Entry

Data entry, or data processing, is the conversion of data into electronic form—that is, entering, updating, and maintaining information on a computer system, including data contained in archives. Data entry needs to be accurate and able to be understood by anyone in the office in order for the material to be reliable and usable.

Correspondence

Accurate, professionally written correspondence is a must in any medical office because these documents reflect the professionalism of the office. Correct spelling is an essential aspect of professional documents, and although the computer has a spell-check function, it does not always have the ability to check the spelling of medical terms or to highlight homophones (words that sound alike but have different meanings, such as *their*, *there*, and *they're*) that may have been used incorrectly.

Business Letters

Composing a business letter can be accomplished using four basic letter formatting styles: full-block, modified-block, indented modified-block, and simplified.

- **Full-block** is the most commonly used format for letter writing in an office because it is professional looking and easy to use. In full-block format, all lines are aligned with the left margin of the paper.
- When using **modified-block**, all lines are aligned with the left margin of the paper except the date line, complimentary closing line, and signature line, which are all centered on the page.
- **Indented modified-block** follows the directions for modified-block use, but allows the first line of each paragraph to be indented five spaces.
- The **simplified** format aligns all lines flush with the left margin of the paper and omits the salutation and the complimentary closing. Simplified style is the easiest format to use, but some medical offices feel that it is too casual for formal letter writing.

Business Letter Components

Although different formats of letter writing can be used to produce business letters, most formats have basic components in common.

- The date of the letter should be written out in full (for example, November 15, 2010 instead of 11/15/10).
- The inside address should contain the name, title, and address of the person or company receiving the letter and should be typed approximately five lines below the date line.
- The salutation, or greeting, of the letter is placed at the left margin of the letter, two lines below the inside address.
- The subject line is keyed two lines below the salutation and contains the topic of the letter.

- A complimentary closing, typed two lines below the body of the letter, ends or closes the letter using such terms as *Best regards*, *Sincerely*, or *Respectfully yours*.
- The keyed signature on a letter is typed four lines below the complimentary closing and includes the name and title of the person writing the letter. A handwritten signature is entered directly above the keyed signature.
- Reference initials, included at the lower left-hand margin of the letter, are used to indicate who is responsible for the letter. The initials of the person who composed the letter are entered in uppercase letters and the initials of the person who typed the letter are entered in lowercase letters (for example, "TK:ef"). If the person who wrote the letter also typed the letter, only one set of initials would be recorded in the reference initials section (for example, "TK").
- When other documents will be sent with the letter, enclosure notations are added to the bottom left-hand margin of letters, one to two lines below the reference initials. Examples of enclosures are laboratory reports and medical records.
- Copy notations are used when a copy of the letter will be sent to someone in addition to the addressee. A lowercase "cc" followed by a colon is entered at the lower left-hand margin of the letter, and the name of the person to whom the letter will be copied appears after the colon (for example, "cc: John Smith").
- A blind copy notation is used when the letter will be sent to other individuals without the knowledge of the person to whom the letter was written. The notation is entered at the lower left-hand margin of the letter using the initials "bcc."

Memos

A memo, or memorandum (the plural of *memorandum* is *memoranda*), is usually used for interoffice messages written and sent to other personnel to speed up the communication process. Memos can be used to notify personnel about meetings, updates, or changes in the workplace that pertain to everyone. They are written without a salutation or a complimentary closing. Many times a memo format is programmed into the computer for easier and faster use. A common memo format includes four lines, typed in capital letters and listing the date the memo was sent, the name of the person it was sent to, the name of the person sending the memo, and the subject matter of the memo.

DATE: June 8, 2011

TO: Staff of Family Health Center

FROM: Sue Jenkins, Office Manager

SUBJECT: Insurance Changes

As of January 1, 2012, the medical facility will be offering a new insurance plan to employees. Please contact Sue Jenkins at extension 2243 to set up an appointment.

Other Written Material

Transcription is the process of preparing accurate, formatted reports by converting dictated physician notes into written documents. Although medical assistants are trained in transcription, many facilities outsource patient information that needs to be transcribed because it lowers costs, allows faster turnaround times, and enables the facility to receive these documents seven days a week, which can be advantageous, especially for larger facilities. A busy medical assistant can have difficulty keeping up with the volume of transcription needed, and therefore, many facilities find that transcription is not the best use of the medical assistant's time

and skills. The medical assistant's role has changed from transcriptionist to editor and quality assurance manager, monitoring all incoming reports for accuracy.

Chart Notes (Progress Notes)

Documentation of patient care should be accurate, complete, and up-to-date. The date and time of the entry and the initials of the person making the entry should be recorded in black ink. Care should be taken to make entries into the medical record correctly, and if an error is made, then corrections should be made following the proper procedure. (See the following sections later in this chapter: "Medical Records Management," and "Making Corrections to Medical Records.")

Progress notes can be informal, but should always have correct spelling and be legibly written, using only accepted medical abbreviations. The medical record is a legal document, and therefore, information entered into it can be used in a court of law. All pertinent information should be recorded, since any treatment or procedures not charted in the medical record are considered not done. Progress notes are a permanent part of the medical record and offer guidance in providing quality care to the patient.

Proofreading

Proofreading every document carefully and checking its spelling, grammar, and punctuation helps to produce an accurate document. It is important to reread the document to be sure the message is clearly stated. Proofreader's marks include a group of symbols used to indicate changes needed in a document. Medical assistants using proofreading symbols will be able to edit and prepare accurate documents more quickly. For reference, use the *Chicago Manual of Style* chart found here: http://www.chicagomanualofstyle.org/tools_proof.html

- When setting up a computer system or moving the computer system to a new location in the office, the medical assistant must take care to place it in a well-ventilated area to prevent overheating.
- A surge protector is used to protect equipment from a sudden rise in voltage, such as an electrical storm, which could cause damage to the equipment.
- Routine maintenance should also include keeping the keyboard of the computer clean, since it harbors many types of harmful organisms. Wiping the keyboard with a disinfectant will help destroy the organisms.
- Screen savers, which appear on the computer monitor when no activity has been detected for a time, are used to protect the computer screen from burn-in, the burning of an image into the cathode ray tubes of the computer.

Equipment

Equipment used to perform routine business tasks in the medical office includes:

- calculators
- photocopiers
- computers
- fax or facsimile machine. These are commonly used in medical offices to send and receive information. Patient reports, test results, referrals to and from other physicians, prescription requests from pharmacies, consent forms, and inquiries from insurance companies are a few of the various types of fax messages sent and received by the medical office.
- scanners. Used to scan or input photos or other paper documents into the computer.
- paper shredders. Used to destroy unwanted written material, such as documents with confidential patient information that are no longer needed.

Maintenance and Repairs

Keeping the office equipment in good working condition is the responsibility of all personnel using the equipment, but it is usually the administrative medical assistant who is responsible for maintaining the equipment and arranging for repairs when needed.

Newly purchased equipment often comes with a warranty, a guarantee from the manufacturer of the equipment stating that the equipment is free of any known defects. If the equipment breaks down due to faulty parts within a specified time frame, the warranty from the manufacturer states that the defective parts will be replaced and the equipment will be repaired without charge.

An instruction manual is enclosed with newly purchased equipment to explain how the equipment operates. Agreements are similar to warranties but add extended time to the warranty for an additional price.

Warranties, instruction manuals, and agreements for equipment used in the medical office should be filed and kept in a safe place. After the expiration date, warranties and agreements can be purged from the file, but the instructional manual for each piece of equipment should be kept as long as the equipment is being used.

Routine maintenance should be performed on all equipment following the directions and suggestions listed in the instruction manual. Routine maintenance will prolong the life of the equipment and allow it to function properly. If repair services are needed for equipment, the instruction manual will usually list the names of repair services. Noting important information about each piece of equipment such as the serial number, the model number, and the name of the company that made the piece of equipment will help the medical assistant arrange for speedy repairs. General policies will help protect against damage and should be posted for all employees to see.

Telephone Techniques

The telephone is one of the most important pieces of equipment used in the medical office to provide doctors, medical assistants, and other medical personnel with vital information about patients. Most patients have their first contact with the medical office by making a first appointment or rescheduling an appointment. The telephone personality of the medical assistant should make a favorable first impression on the patient.

Telephone Personality

Telephone personality includes the tone, pitch, volume, speed of speaking, and the warmth and friendliness the medical assistant expresses when answering the phone and carrying on a conversation with a caller. It is important to listen carefully to the tone of the patient's voice, as well as to be aware of the tone of one's own voice. Stressful situations or an overly busy day in the office can affect the warm tone usually spoken by the medical assistant, which can easily be picked up by the caller. If the patient is angry, intimidated by calling the office, or feeling a lot of stress, it can often be heard in the tone of his or her voice. Listening not only to what the patient says, but also to his or her tone, provides the medical assistant with clues about the patient's feelings and emotions.

Active listening, or restating what a patient has said to be sure it was correctly understood, is one method the medical assistant can use to establish a

rapport between the patient and the medical care providers. Active listening shows that the medical assistant is genuinely interested in what a patient has to say. The medical assistant should use terms that can be easily understood by the patient; this is not the time to impress the patient with medical terminology. Even if the office is extremely busy, the medical assistant should answer the phone ideally by the first ring and definitely by the third ring. Also, if the medical assistant speaks too quickly, the patient may miss much of the conversation.

Often when phone is answered, the first words tend to be clipped off and not heard or understood completely by the patient. Buffer words help prevent the loss of important words by filling in the first portion of the conversation with nonessential words. For example, answering the phone using a greeting such as "Good morning" before identifying the name of the office, "Dr. Smith's office," will ensure that the patient will hear the complete name of the office and have no question that he or she called the correct physician's office. Before a call is ended, the medical assistant should be sure to restate the important information that was provided during the call for accuracy. The patient should be the one to end the call, so that he or she will not feel rushed or cut off. All conversations with the caller should be handled in the most courteous manner, leaving the patient with a good impression of the medical office and the medical assistant answering the phone.

Screening Incoming Calls

Medical assistants can handle many types of incoming calls and each type of call requires the medical assistant to make judgments based on learned knowledge and **patient screening**, sometimes referred to as **triaging**. Screening incoming calls means that the medical assistant tactfully inquires as to the name of the caller, the reason for the call, and the action needed. It is a method of prioritizing incoming calls, used to determine the urgency of the call and the action needed following the call. If the patient is requesting an appointment, then careful screening will help determine how soon the patient needs to be seen and the length of time needed for the appointment. Occasionally a patient may be reluctant to disclose information on the phone, because the information requested may be confidential and the patient may not feel free to discuss it with the medical assistant. Careful and tactful questioning may encourage the patient to respond to the inquiries of the medical assistant. The medical assistant should explain to the patient that a detailed description of his or her problem is not necessary. But a general idea of what the patient needs is helpful and will enable the medical assistant to determine the urgency of the patient's problem and to be sure sufficient time is allotted for the visit.

Types of Calls Answered by the Medical Assistant

The medical assistant should answer the telephone using an appropriate salutation, giving the name of the office, stating a polite offer to help, and including his or her name. The next important step is to determine whether the call is an emergency. Emergency calls need to be transferred to the physician immediately. If the call isn't an emergency, it can be directed to one of many departments, such as billing, insurance, or perhaps a registered nurse. The medical assistant can handle certain calls, such as making an appointment for a patient or taking a message from a patient requesting a prescription refill, without assistance. Specific information must be obtained from the patient in order to collect information needed to make appropriate decisions and to see that the best care is given to the patient. Depending on the size of the practice and the responsibilities relegated to the medical assistant, some incoming calls in larger offices may be transferred to other departments. In smaller offices, the medical assistant may be the person responsible for handling all nonmedical and nonemergency calls.

The following list describes the types of incoming calls that can be handled by the medical assistant, as well as the needed patient information for each type of call.

New Patient Appointments

- **Name.** The patient's legal name and date of birth are needed when making an appointment. A patient can have the exact same name as another; these patients can be easily identified by using their dates of birth in addition to their names.
- **Address.** The patient's address is needed to send patient registration forms and past medical history forms to each new patient. These forms are to be completed and brought to the first appointment.
- **Phone number.** The daytime phone number and home phone number of each patient is also needed. This information is needed in case the appointment has to be rescheduled or in case there is a question the patient must answer before he or she comes in for the appointment.
- **Insurance information.** The patient should tell the medical assistant the type of insurance and/ or policy number he or she has. (Some offices ask for both primary and secondary insurance.) Insurance information is needed to verify that the physician is participating in the patient's particular insurance plan; some offices also check whether the insurance is valid and current. If the physician does not participate in the particular type of insurance plan that the patient uses, then the office visit will not be paid by the insurance company. It will therefore be the responsibility of the patient to pay for the visit. (Many patients will opt to be treated only by a participating physician, so it is better for the patient to know whether a medical office accepts his or her insurance plan before he or she shows up for the appointment.) The patient is asked to bring his or her insurance card to the office because a

copy of the card is usually made for the medical record. Discussion of payment at the time of service through co-pays can be mentioned to the patient if it is the office policy.

- **Employment.** Employment information is often requested when a patient is making an appointment. Not all medical offices request employment information on the phone, but because the registration form often asks for employment information, it may be collected at this time by some offices.
- **Reason for the appointment.** The medical assistant should ask the patient the reason for the appointment. Knowing the reason for the appointment helps to determine the amount of time needed for the appointment and to evaluate the urgency of the appointment.

Established Patient Appointments

- **Name or address changes.** The patient should inform the medical office of any name or address changes as a result of moving, marriage, or divorce. In order to keep the medical record current, this information should be updated at every visit.
- A **patient's insurance** coverage needs frequent updating because of changes in employers, employer-offered insurance plans, or retirement. The patient may call to let the medical assistant know of such a change.
- **Reasons for appointment.** The medical assistant should ask the reason for the appointment. Knowing the reason for the appointment helps to determine the amount of time needed for the appointment and to evaluate the urgency of the appointment. If a patient needs to be rescheduled, knowing the reason for the visit will help the medical assistant meet the health needs of the patient.
- **Phone number.** A daytime phone number is needed in case the appointment needs to be changed or canceled.

Referrals from Other Physicians

- **Referring physician's name.** The medical assistant should ask the name of the physician making the referral. (The medical assistant can take the patient information. If the referring physician asks to be put through to the attending physician, then the medical assistant should transfer the call to the attending physician.)
- **Patient's name.** The medical assistant should ask the name of the patient, and then ask for the patient's address and daytime phone number.
- **Insurance information.** The medical assistant should ask for information on the patient's insurance, including the type of insurance, insurance company, and policy number.
- **Reason for and urgency of referral.** The medical assistant should ask the referring physician the purpose of the appointment and should assess the urgency of the referral. Pre-op clearance, which most insurance companies demand, needs to be made within a special time limit prior to the surgery. Many physicians will try to accommodate referrals from other physicians as soon as possible—often even on the same day.

Insurance and Billing Questions

- **Calls from insurance companies.** Insurance carriers and HMOs will call to verify patient treatment and procedures. No patient information should be given out until the caller is positively identified as the insurance company and until the medical assistant has proof that the patient has signed a release form giving the medical office permission to release the patient's information.
- **Billing questions.** If the office has a billing department, then patient inquiries about billing should be transferred to that department. Before transferring the call, the medical assistant should take down the patient's name and phone number, just in case the call is disconnected. Providing the patient with the extension number of the

requested department can be helpful if the call is terminated prematurely.

General Patient Inquiries

Patients may also call to ask about general policies of the office, to ask for directions, or to ask which insurance carriers are accepted by the facility. Patients may ask what the office's policies are concerning co-pays and methods of payment accepted, or to ask what hours the office is open. Patients may also ask about the protocol for getting medical attention during unopened hours, weekends, and holidays. The medical assistant should have access to the general policies and information about the office, which are usually located in the office policy manual. By keeping this manual within easy reach, the medical assistant can correctly answer questions about the office.

Prescription Information

Specific information is needed in order to process prescription refills or renewals. The information needed includes the full name of the patient, the patient's date of birth, the pharmacy's name and phone number, the name of the medication, the dosage, and the prescription number. A call-back number for the patient should be recorded in case there is a problem. The medical assistant should obtain this information from the patient. After the physician approves the refill, the medical assistant will call in the prescription to the pharmacy.

Test and Lab Results

Accepting normal test and lab reports is another responsibility of the medical assistant. The medical assistant can take normal reports over the phone, but most offices prefer that abnormal reports are given directly to the physician. Receiving a fax of the test or lab report is safer than receiving the result by phone because there will be a hard copy of the information, which will be more legible and accurate and take less time to obtain. Medical assistants can usually notify patients of normal lab results after the physician has read the results and given his or her approval.

Patient Progress Reports

Medical assistants also accept routine progress reports from patients. Many times, a patient leaves after an office visit with directions to call the next day and report an improvement or worsening in his or her condition. If the report from the patient is a favorable one, then the medical assistant should make a note of the patient's condition, give it to the physician, and document it in the patient's medical record. If the patient's report is not favorable and the patient is doing poorly, then a message stating that fact should be taken and given to the physician with the patient's medical record and phone number so that the physician may call the patient.

Sales Calls

In addition, medical offices receive calls from many salespeople trying to sell their items to the physician. The individual office policy manual should state how these situations are handled. Some offices may set up 15-minute appointments at certain times of the day for pharmaceutical sales representatives, while other offices will see sales representatives only if time permits; some offices may not wish to see sales representatives at all.

Deciding on What Calls to Refer to the Physician

The medical assistant needs to know which calls should be referred to the physician. Medical assistants do not give medical advice because it is not within the scope of their training. Following are examples of the types of calls that the medical assistant should refer to the physician:

- calls about abnormal lab or test reports
- calls from patients who have medical questions
- calls from other physicians

- emergency calls
- calls from the physician's family members

The office policy manual should list the various types of incoming calls, stating how they should be handled. Although the goal of the medical assistant is to be helpful to patients, medical assistants should not give out medical advice under any conditions.

Handling Special Calls

Many calls come into the medical office that will need special consideration to be handled successfully. Patience, tact, a calm attitude, and knowledge of the office policies can help diffuse tense situations, prevent frustrations for the caller, maintain patient confidentiality, and help in risk management.

Angry or Dissatisfied Patients

When an angry or dissatisfied patient calls the office, the first thing the medical assistant should do is listen. Giving the patient time to release pent-up anger may help to defuse the situation. Listening closely to what the patient is saying can help identify the problem. Do not interrupt the patient, try to offer an opinion, or try to correct the patient's view of the problem. Active listening, or restating what the patient has said, is a good way to clarify the problem. Once the problem is identified, the patient can be referred to the proper person or department. Allowing the patient to speak first and then offering to help the patient when he or she gives you a chance to respond can do much to defuse and resolve the patient's anger. If it is a problem that can be handled by the medical assistant, you may offer a solution or (if it will take time for you to resolve the problem) offer to get back to the patient. Give the patient a definite time for the return call. For example, "I will call you before the office closes today at five P.M." Be sure to call the patient back even if the problem can't be solved until the following day. The patient will become even angrier if the promised call never comes.

If the angry patient is dissatisfied with the care he or she has received, then the caller should be referred to the physician. Tell the patient that the physician will make a return call, giving an approximate time, for example, after five P.M. Many physicians make return calls after office hours so that they will have more time to talk with patients on the phone without interrupting the treatment of scheduled patients. Attach a message to the medical record, alerting the physician that the patient is dissatisfied and with what aspect of care he or she is dissatisfied.

If the patient calls and is dissatisfied about a bill, perhaps the best person to handle this problem would be either someone in the billing department or the office manager. Tell the patient you will contact the appropriate person and have this person return the patient's call. Notify the billing department or office manager of the situation, and be sure to mention that the patient is angry. Give the billing department or office manager the patient's name, phone number, and details of the call. Having the appropriate person call the patient back will give this person ample time to retrieve the record, the billing statement, or whatever data is needed in order to help clarify any incorrect information the patient may have or to resolve the problem.

The Unidentified Caller or Unidentified Information

A patient may call the office requesting to speak with the physician or requesting information that the medical assistant feels should not be given out to an unidentified caller. The medical assistant should politely ask for the caller's name and the reason for the call. If the caller requests to speak to the physician and gives you his or her name, but refuses to give you the reason for the call, take his or her name and phone number and let the physician decide what to do about the call. If the caller refuses to give his or her name and phone number, then the medical assistant can suggest that the caller send a written note to the physician regarding the message or issue he or she

HANDLING OF ROUTINE CALLS RECEIVED IN THE MEDICAL OFFICE	
CALLS HANDLED BY THE MEDICAL ASSISTANT	**CALLS REFERRED TO THE PHYSICIAN**
new patient appointments	abnormal lab or test reports
established patient appointments	patients' medical questions
referrals from other medical offices	calls from other physicians
insurance questions	emergency calls
billing questions	calls from the physician's family members
prescription renewal information	
favorable routine progress reports from patients	
calls from sales representatives	
general information about the medical office	

wishes to discuss. The medical assistant can politely state that it is the policy of the physician not to return unidentified calls. Knowing the office policies can help the medical assistant make the appropriate decision when handling difficult situations.

Hearing-Impaired Callers

Once it is identified that the patient is hearing impaired, the best approach for the medical assistant is to speak clearly, slowly, and loudly. Do not shout at the patient, as this action is disrespectful to the individual.

Non-English-Speaking Callers

Ideally, the office would have a bilingual interpreter who can speak fluently with the non-English-speaking patient. If the office doesn't have an interpreter, the medical assistant may speak a little more slowly. Speaking louder will not be useful in this situation. If the patient isn't hearing impaired, speaking louder will not help the patient interpret the message. Repeating the information and having patience will most likely get the information across to the patient. Also, the fact that a patient doesn't speak English fluently doesn't mean that he or she does not understand English well. The medical assistant can verify the patient's understanding by having the patient repeat the information.

Many times a patient will bring a family member who speaks fluent English to interpret instructions.

Personal Calls

Staff members should limit personal incoming calls to emergency situations, although you may occasionally take a quick personal call. Too many personal calls for the staff will tie up the phone lines, interfering with patient calls. Personal calls may also interrupt staff members who are caring for patients.

Personal Physician Calls

The physician decides the policy regarding calls from his or her family or friends. The medical assistant should abide by the wishes of the physician.

Callers Requesting Patient Information

Medical offices receive many incoming calls requesting information about patients. These calls may be from insurance carriers; lawyers; or patients' family members, friends, and neighbors. The medical assistant has a legal and ethical responsibility to screen these calls, giving out information only to approved persons. In-depth screening needs to be done to protect the privacy of the patient.

Calls from third parties must be carefully handled. The term **third party**, when used in the context of the medical office, usually refers to someone other than the patient who is responsible for paying the patient's bill. A third party could be an insurance carrier that is involved in the reimbursement process of an insurance claim, a lawyer hired to handle the finances of a patient, or a family member assuming responsibility for the patient's bill. Assuming financial responsibility for a patient's bill does not automatically mean that the third party is permitted access to the patient's confidential information. The patient must give written permission before any confidential information is released. A patient's concerned family member, neighbor, or friend is not entitled to any confidential patient information without proper written permission from the patient.

Concerned family members, neighbors, and even employers may try to persuade the medical assistant to disclose patient information, but it is unlawful to do so without written permission from the patient. When in doubt, don't give it out. It is easier to refuse to give out information than it is to take it back after it has been released. No information can be given to a wife, husband, or concerned adult child of a patient without the patient's written consent. A call from an attorney requesting patient information may be intimidating to the medical assistant, but the medical assistant should politely refuse to release any information until he or she has verified the patient's written consent.

Emergency Calls

It is the medical assistant's responsibility to screen all incoming calls in order to prioritize the calls so that the calls are handled in order of urgency. If a patient calls stating that it is an emergency, the medical assistant should immediately get the patient's name and phone number and ask if it is a life-threatening emergency. If the call is a life-threatening emergency, the caller should be kept on the line, and the medical assistant should call 911 using another extension. Emergency situations take precedence over all other calls. If the call is not a life-threatening emergency, then the medical assistant should ask questions to determine the urgency of the situation and to make a determination about whether the patient's problem can best be handled in the office or in the emergency room of the hospital. Good judgment is essential to handling emergencies quickly and correctly. The medical assistant must be very careful not to give the patient any advice outside of his or her training and never to give medical advice. Most offices have a list of questions used in screening calls. Information that may be requested when dealing with emergency calls includes:

- What is the name, phone number, and age of the patient?
- What happened?
- Is the patient breathing or having trouble breathing?
- Is the patient is bleeding? From what part of the body? How severe is the bleeding?
- Is the patient is conscious or unconscious?
- Does the patient feel hot? What is the patient's temperature?
- Is the patient in pain? Where is the pain? How bad is the pain?
- If the patient swallowed or ate something thought to be poisonous: What was taken? How much was taken? When was it taken? The caller should be told to bring the container of the suspected poison with the patient.

Telephone Technology, Equipment, and Services

The medical assistant should be skilled in using the various types of telephone technology, equipment, and services available for use in the medical office, including:

- automated routing units (ARU)
- multi-line telephones

- caller ID
- call forwarding
- answering services
- answering machines
- voice mail
- pagers/cellular phones
- fax machines
- email

Automated Routing Units

The medical office telephone system can be equipped to handle the many calls received throughout the day by use of an automated routing unit (ARU). The ARU allows the caller to listen to a recorded message that gives the caller the option of selecting specific departments or persons by pressing the specified number given. For example, the patient may be instructed, to "Press 1 if this call is an emergency; press 2 to reschedule an appointment; or press 3 to make an appointment." The ARU is set up to allow patients to access the medical assistant immediately in emergency situations.

Other selections on the ARU can include an extension for refilling prescriptions, canceling an appointment, speaking to the billing department, receiving test results, or leaving a message. The ARU options can be individualized to meet the needs of the practice. The ARU system was designed to decrease the waiting time for patients trying to contact the office. By directing calls to the appropriate department or person, an automated system can help decrease the number of busy signals reached by patients. However, some patients find the recorded ARU message difficult to hear and confusing to understand.

Multi-line Telephones

The multi-line telephone in the office allows the medical assistant to receive more than one call at a time. However, because only one call can be handled at a time, one of the callers must be put on hold. Specific protocol, as listed in the office policy manual, should be followed to ensure that emergency calls are not put on hold, and all other calls are answered in a prompt manner. Before placing a caller on hold, certain information should be gathered. All callers should be asked if it is an emergency call. If it is not an emergency, permission to put the caller on hold should be requested. For example, the medical assistant may ask the patient, "Would you please hold for a minute?" or "Is it all right if I put you on hold for a minute?" The caller should not wait more than a few minutes before getting through to the requested party. The medical assistant should check back on the waiting caller at least every two minutes and offer to take a phone number to return his or her call, or to put the caller through to the requested party's voice mail so that he or she may leave a message. Both of these options will prevent undue waiting time for the caller.

Whether the phone is answered by the ARU message or the medical assistant, proper telephone use is important. The telephone is an essential piece of equipment in the medical setting, and the voice answering the phone needs to be clearly understood by the caller. The medical assistant should hold the receiver of the phone approximately one inch from his or her mouth, never holding it in the crook of the neck, because this position can easily muffle the sound, making the conversation hard to understand. The patient on the phone should receive 100% of the medical assistant's concentration and attention. The medical assistant should not spend time doing other paperwork or engaging in other activities while handling a call. Better communication between the medical office personnel and the patient can contribute to a more satisfied patient. When questions are better understood by the healthcare givers and patients are answered in a friendly manner, using terms that are easy to understand, communication between the patient and the medical assistant can better meet each patient's needs.

Caller ID

Caller ID is another technology advancement used in some offices to identify the caller and phone number before answering the phone, and can be applied when the phone is in use. If the medical assistant were waiting for an important call, the caller ID would alert the medical assistant to the name and phone number of the caller.

Call Forwarding

Call forwarding gives the medical office the option of transferring or forwarding calls to another phone number, such as a cell phone. The advantage of call forwarding is that important calls and messages are not missed. If calls are forwarded to the physician's cell phone, for example, he or she will receive important messages without having to wait around in the office for the call. Please note that many physicians will not want all the calls coming into the medical office to be be forwarded to their cell phones, so this feature should be handled with great caution.

Answering Services, Answering Machines, and Voice Mail

Medical offices monitor after-hours calls in several ways. Each office selects the method that works best for notifying the physician and office of missed calls.

Because voice mail is part of the telephone system, there is no additional cost to the office to set up this option. An answering machine, on the other hand, does have an additional cost because it is a separate piece of equipment that must be purchased and attached to the telephone.

The information provided to the caller by either voice mail or an answering machine is the same. The recording will give the patient a number to call in case of an emergency situation. This type of after-hours message system is used primarily for smaller practices that rarely experience emergency situations.

Answering services—whereby an outside firm is hired by the medical office to take calls, record messages, and make contacts and referrals in case of emergencies—can also be used for after-hours calls. This service allows patients to talk to a person, as opposed to leaving a message on an answering machine or in

a voice mailbox, and may leave the patient with more confidence that the message will get through.

There are disadvantages to all these options. Many patients don't feel comfortable leaving a message on the phone, in a voice mailbox, or even with a person other than the doctor or medical assistant, whom they know and trust. Also, answering machine and voice mail messages must be retrieved often to be sure critical situations are not missed. If there are a high number of calls, then the voice mailbox or the answering machine may become full, preventing messages from being recorded. In addition, sorting a lengthy list of messages would take time, preventing patients from receiving a prompt call back from the office.

Pagers and Cell Phones

Pagers, sometimes referred to as beepers, were once carried almost exclusively by physicians to receive notice that they had a message after hours. The pager provided the physician with one-way communication, listing a number for the physician to call. Cell phones are another common and more modern device medical personnel use to receive messages when the office is closed. Cell phones are small, lightweight, and convenient to use. Because cellular connections are not secure, the use of this method to relay private information should be considered carefully in order to ensure patient privacy. Cell phones can also be used to send and receive text messages.

Facsimile (Fax) Machines

Fax machines are commonly used in medical offices to send and receive information. Patient reports, test results, referrals to and from other physicians, prescription requests from pharmacies, and consent forms and inquiries from insurance companies are a few of the various types of fax messages sent and received by the staff in a medical office. The fax machine works by sending the message from one fax machine to another (or from a modem to a fax machine) using telephone lines.

Sending information using a fax machine has several advantages over using the postal system. A fax is faster, more convenient, provides a hard copy to the office receiving the fax, and is lower in cost compared to purchasing postage stamps and waiting a few days before the information reaches the other office. Up-to-date patient information can be obtained immediately, which helps provide improved care to patients.

However, confidentiality can be a problem when sending a fax if it is sent to an unsecure location such as, for example, a mailroom. Before a fax is sent, the medical assistant should call ahead to be sure that the appropriate person will be available to receive the fax or to be sure that the fax is going to a secure location, such as a private office. A cover letter should be sent with the fax stating that the enclosed information is confidential and that it is against state and federal laws to disclose this information; however, a fax that contains sensitive or confidential information should not be sent at all, if possible. After typing in the fax number, the medical assistant should recheck the information for correctness and, after sending the fax, should call the recipient to be sure that it arrived. A fax confirmation, which is a receipt for the message successfully faxed, can be requested by pressing the appropriate button on the fax machine. The receipt should be placed in the patient's medical record for documentation.

Electronic Mail (Email)

Email sends messages in digital form over a computer network. Many medical offices use email to remind patients of their upcoming appointments or to receive notices of appointment cancellations from patients. Because email messages can be sent to a group of people at the click of a button, email is a fast, efficient, and inexpensive way to send interoffice information. Hard copies of the sent information can be printed and saved as necessary. For example, an email print-out of a patient cancellation can easily be kept in the medical record to document the cancellation. Another example would be an emailed schedule of staff in-service meetings that can be printed and placed on the bulletin board. All email messages should be written using a professional tone and accurate, concise sentences. Time-sensitive material should not be sent by email because there is no guarantee when the message will be read by the receiver.

Placing Outgoing Calls

The medical assistant also places outgoing calls. The supplies needed to make outgoing calls will depend on the nature of the call. Examples of the types of outgoing calls made by the medical assistant include:

- **Appointment reminders.** An appointment book, the patients' names and phone numbers, a calendar, and a pen or pencil are the supplies needed for appointment reminders.
- **Calls about prescriptions.** To call in approved prescription refills, the medical assistant needs the name and date of birth of the patient, the name and phone number of the pharmacy, pertinent information about the medication, the pharmacy medication number, and a phone number at which the patient may be reached in case of any questions or problems.
- **Scheduling outpatient tests and procedures.** It is beneficial to have the patient available when making calls to the needed facilities to better coordinate scheduling outpatient tests and procedures. The medical assistant should place the call from a quiet area away from activity and have a calendar available for reference, along with the patient's medical record and a copy of the requisition for the test or procedure ordered. Having the patient present to agree to the scheduled times and ask questions to clarify the preparation for the treatment or procedure will help to minimize confusion and ensure that the patient will show up on the correct date and time, properly prepared for the procedure. The medical assistant may need to call the patient's insurance company for preapproval of the test or

procedure and the facility used if the insurance company is to cover the expenses.

- **Scheduling inpatient tests and procedures.** Most scheduling for inpatient procedures and tests is confined to the departments in the hospital, and preapproval from the patient's insurance company may be needed before expenses will be covered.

- **Calling to reschedule patient appointments.** The medical assistant will need the appointment book, manual, or computer; a list of the available time slots; and patient information such as name, phone number, and the reason for the visit.

- **Collection calls for overdue patient balances.** Collection calls should be made in a private area to ensure confidentiality. The medical assistant should speak only to the person responsible for the bill. Early hour and late evening calls should be avoided, and no calls should be made to the patient's place of employment. A friendly, matter-of-fact, nonthreatening tone should be used, and the patient should be treated with respect. Often, medical offices are willing to work out a payment schedule with the patient. Check with your office manager or billing department about the policy regarding payment schedules for patients.

- **Ordering supplies and requesting equipment service.** When ordering supplies, the medical assistant should have a list of the needed supplies, the name and phone number of the supplier, and a purchase order for the needed supplies. When requesting service for equipment, the medical assistant should have the name and phone number of the repair service to be used and any relevant information about the type of office equipment to be repaired. For example, any serial numbers or information about warranties should be easily available when requesting service.

Long-Distance Calls

The medical assistant may be arranging conference calls from individuals in different time zones in the United States or making a call to the patient's family out of state. It is beneficial for the medical assistant to know the various time zones so that he or she may better coordinate calls within reasonable hours for all parties. International direct dialing is also an option when calling out of the country.

There are six time zones in the United States. The contiguous United States has four time zones: Eastern, Central, Mountain, and Pacific. Most of Alaska is located in the Alaska time zone (which is four hours before Eastern Standard Time [EST]) and the westernmost Aleutian Islands, St. Lawrence Island, and Hawaii are in the Hawaii-Aleutian time zone (which is five hours before EST). Going from east to west, time is one hour earlier for each time zone. For example, if it is nine A.M. in Boston, Massachusetts, it would be eight A.M. in Milwaukee, Wisconsin; seven A.M. in Denver, Colorado; six A.M. in Sacramento, California; five A.M. in Anchorage, Alaska; and four A.M. in Honolulu, Hawaii. This information is important because if the medical assistant has to make a call to a physician's office in California, this call should not be made at nine A.M. EST because it would be six A.M. in California, and most offices do not open that early.

Outgoing Calls Made by the Physician

Outgoing calls that should be made by the physician (rather than by the medical assistant) include calls to patients who have medical questions, patients who have poor test results, and patients who are dissatisfied with their care or treatment. The physician should also directly contact the pharmacy about questions he or she may have concerning a prescription that was written or requested. The patient's medical record, along with messages from the patient, should be given to the physician so that when the physician calls the patient, he or she will have adequate information when handling these calls.

Computer Concepts

In order to use computers effectively, the medical assistant must know computer terminology and how to use the components of the computer.

Computer Components

A computer is made up of hardware (the physical components) and software (the programs stored inside the computer that perform functions vital to medical offices), and the operating system (the fundamental software program that controls how the entire computer system operates).

Many medical offices use email to remind patients of their upcoming appointments or to receive notices from patients of appointment cancellations. Because messages can be sent to a group of people at the click of a button, email is a fast, efficient, and inexpensive way to send interoffice information. Hard copies of the sent information can be printed and saved as necessary—for example, a printed copy of an email received from a patient canceling an appointment (for documentation purposes).

Computer networks are used to share information between two or more computers, exchanging information electronically. The information exchange can occur over cables, a satellite, or a modem hooked up to telephone lines or cable lines. The Internet is an example of a computer network.

COMMON TYPES OF STORAGE DEVICES	
compact disc (CD)	unwritable disks; usually used for listening to music
CD-R	writable disk that cannot be changed once burned because entered data is permanent
CD-RW	rewritable disk used to enter data, erase data, and reenter data
flash drive	a small, removable, and rewritable storage device (also called a thumb drive or a jump drive)

COMMON TYPES OF PRINTERS	
dot matrix	least expensive; produces the lowest-quality printout
inkjet	moderately expensive; produces average-quality printout
laser	most expensive; generally produces the best-quality printout

Key Components of a Computer

TERM	DEFINITION
HARDWARE	
central processing unit (CPU)	component that allows the computer to perform basic operations
keyboard	device used to enter data into the computer
hardware	devices connected to the computer, e.g., printer, monitor, keyboard
input devices	devices used to enter data or information into the computer system
modem	device that converts electronic signals information to travel over telephone or cable lines
monitor	screen used to view activity on the computer
motherboard	circuit board allowing communication between computer parts
mouse	handheld device that controls the cursor
printer	machine that produces a hard copy or readable paper copy of data
scanner	device that converts printed images and text into digital information
storage devices	used to provide a copy of the data entered, for review or editing
touch pad	a flat, sensitive device that allows movement of the cursor by sliding one's fingers across the pad
touch screen	a screen sensitive to human touch, allowing interaction with the computer
trackball	handheld device that controls the cursor; has a rolling ball on top of the device
SOFTWARE	
computer applications	software programs designed to control the computer, helping it perform a particular task
cursor	device used to point to a specific area on the computer screen
database	software program used to arrange and sort data for easy and fast searching
graphics	computer images (pictures or artwork)
menu	list of options available to the user
screen saver	protects the computer screen from burn-in
software	computer programs that perform tasks within a computer system
spreadsheet	database used for organizing and computing numerical data into charts, graphs, and models
utility software	computer programs for virus protection
word processing	software program used to create, edit, and produce text documents
OPERATING SYSTEM	
operating system	software that controls the computer and helps it perform tasks
Random-Access Memory (RAM)	temporary memory storage that functions only while the computer is in use
Read-Only Memory (ROM)	permanent memory storage that cannot be altered

Security Measures

Security measures are essential when dealing with confidential information in a medical office. Some of the measures used to provide security and prevent unauthorized entry into the computer system include:

- **Passwords** track users entering a program. Each employee using the computer is provided with a password. Employees should be instructed not to share this password with anyone.
- **Firewalls** keep information secure on a computer by blocking outside information from entering or exiting a private network.
- **Antiviral programs** protect the computer from software programs and outside communications that aim to interfere with normal computer functioning or cause data to be deleted. Antivirus software must be updated continuously to protect the computer and data from damage.

Medical Management Software

Computers used in the medical office maintain electronic medical records (EMR) and electronic health records (EHR). An EMR is a type of computer-generated record of a patient's care from one source, such as a medical office, a hospital, or a pharmacy. An EHR documents the total care provided to a patient from all sources. For example, an EHR contains records from all the physicians in different practices who are caring for the patient. It also contains information about medical services and procedures provided by other medical providers and facilities to the patient. The EHR is a more comprehensive record of the patient's health history.

Computer software programs such as a total management system can help medical assistants to manage patient records, enter demographic data—such as birth dates—needed to complete essential forms, track and schedule appointments, complete billing statements and insurance claims, send claims electronically, post payments from patients and third-party payers, and generate needed reports.

Internet Services

A medical office uses the Internet to send insurance claims electronically; this is referred to as electronic claims transmission (ECT). Claims sent in this manner reach their destinations more quickly and with less expense than claims sent using the postal system. Payments can be made by direct deposit within a few days after transmission when an ECT system is used.

Medical Records Management

Managing medical records is one of the most important responsibilities of the medical assistant. Medical records have four uses.

1. The patient's medical record is an ongoing source of information needed to provide comprehensive and quality care to the patient. It contains past and present medical information that can influence future care. The record makes needed information available to other medical personnel involved in patient care.
2. The medical record is considered a legal document and can be used in court to protect patients or medical staff members. All entries must be accurate, complete, and written in pen.
3. Clinical information collected from the medical record can be used in research projects, such as monitoring experimental drugs or treatments used for specific diseases.
4. Information collected from medical records can be used for statistics, such as the reporting of various types of contagious diseases.

All information contained in the medical record is confidential and should be viewed only by those in need of the information. Medical record information is released only with written permission by the patient and the patient has the right to decide who can have access to the information in his or her medical record.

The **Health Insurance Portability and Accountability Act** created the government agency overseeing rules and procedures protecting medical record confidentiality. (See the "Professional Standards" section in Chapter 3.) The medical assistant must always check for written permission from the patient before releasing any patient information.

> ## MEDICAL RECORD OWNERSHIP
>
> The question often arises as to ownership of the medical record. The person or facility who created the medical record owns the actual paper record. The information within the medical record belongs to the patient. The patient has the right to see the information in the medical record, request a copy of any part of the medical record, and decide what information can be entered or left out of the medical record. Patients often express concern about keeping recorded information confidential and should be reassured that all precautions are taken to protect the material from unauthorized access.

Electronic Medical Records/ Electronic Health Records

Although the terms electronic medical record (EMR) and the electronic health record (EHR) are often used interchangeably, there is a clear distinction between the two types of records. The EMR was developed to take the place of a paper record, storing the collected clinical data about the diagnosis and treatment provided to a patient in a computer. The EHR went beyond the immediate care of the patient in a particular facility by having a broader focus. The EHR had the ability to share all the data collected by the EMR to a variety of health care providers involved in all aspects of the patient's care. The EHR allowed physician offices, hospitals, nursing care facilities, laboratories, community resources, and various specialists to participate in providing and using information from the EHR to ensure quality care to the patient regardless of where the patient was when medical treatment was needed.

EHRs have been used in some medical facilities since the 1960s. With the advancement of technology, computer software is now readily available to provide comprehensive medical information to physicians that can be used in the treatment of patients. Complex medical diagnoses have necessitated the need for prompt access to medical information on patients, a method of data management to locate important information when needed, and the ability to store the collected information for easy retrieval.

The advantages of an EHR include:

- Better patient care, due to available access to a patient's medical record. For example, if the patient's primary care physician's office is closed or if the patient is traveling when he or she becomes injured or experiences an illness, the EHR can be retrieved quickly by the treating facility. EHRs provide up-to-date treatment protocols, recommendations for lab tests, contraindications for medications being prescribed, and can even print out patient instructions, all measures which will improve patient care.
- Less chance of a lost record. Having the patient's medical record logged into a computer with a back-up system will prevent destruction and loss that can occur with a paper record.
- Multiple users at one time. With a paper record, only one health care provider can view the medical record at a time. With an EHR, the medical record information can be view by many health care providers such as the physician and the medical assistant, each entering data pertaining to the care they provided.
- Efficiency and savings. EHRs provide ease of locating data and save time since medical records are stored on a computer. Less time is spent locating EHRs than searching through rows of paper medical records that may even be misfiled. Eliminating the expense of supplies needed to maintain paper records, storage, and retrieval of active and inactive records has been an economic benefit of using EHRs.

However, there are also disadvantages to using EHRs, including:

- Cost of installing computer equipment. Technology is a big investment in a medical practice, although prices are more reasonable than in years past. The use of EHRs increases reimbursement due to coding programs which provide more accurate coding, and eliminates the need for added personnel to manage paper records and perform transcription.
- Computer downtime is always a concern since it might interfere with patient care.
- Fear of security leaks of privileged information has always been an issue as to why physicians didn't want to use computers to keep medical records. The government has worked to overcome this problem by various methods such as encryption and government regulations for password setup and maintenance.
- Expense of training time needed for all personnel involved in managing and maintaining the EHR system. Most EHR computer software programs developed are being designed to be more user-friendly and less intimidating. Templates are being set up which make using an EHR easier and more time-efficient.
- Lack of compatibility among computers in different facilities has been a problem with establishing wide use of EHRs. The barriers to incompatibility between computers have been addressed and progress has been made in this area.

EHR use will be mandatory for medical offices and hospitals by 2014, as part of the Stimulus Act of 2009. Regulations regarding the use of EHRs have been established by the National Coordinator for Health Information Technology (HIT), with the requirement that every patient must have an EHR that meets the established criteria and objectives set by the Centers for Medicare & Medicaid Services (CMS) and the Office of the National Coordinator for Health Information Technology. EHR systems have many benefits such as consistent documentation, secure patient privacy, fewer errors due to illegible handwriting, and available resources for provider use. The goal of the EHR is to provide more comprehensive care to patients regarding preventable diseases which will ultimately increase the health of the population and decrease the rising cost of healthcare.

Making Corrections to Medical Records

Even with close attention and extreme care, errors can be made when entering information in EMRs and paper medical records. The acceptable method when correcting a paper medical record error is to draw a single line through the error, write "corr." or "correction" above the error, enter the correct information, and add the date and initials of the person writing the entry. The crossed-out error should never be scribbled out completely or made unreadable.

An error in the EMR can be corrected immediately if noticed or by following the directions of the EMR system used in the office. The error is corrected using the same procedure as the paper medical record by entering "corr." or "correction," writing in the new information, and adding the date and initials of the person making the correction.

Types of Medical Records

Medical assistants must be familiar with three types of medical records.

Problem-Oriented Medical Record

The EMR or paper medical record can be organized using different methods. The problem-oriented medical record (POMR) is designed to identify, name, and number patient problems and to list them in different sections for easy access and reevaluation using a problem-solving approach. The sections of the POMR include:

1. **Patient Database**
   The patient database consists of the following items:

- patient profile: name, address, date of birth (DOB), phone numbers, emergency contacts, signed consent forms, insurance information, and other personal data about the patient needed by the medical office
- interview with patient
- information from prior medical records, if available
- family history (FH)
- physical examination with review of systems (ROS)
- laboratory and radiology reports
- medication list including prescription drugs, nonprescription drugs, and herbal supplements taken by the patient
- allergies
- previous immunizations

2. **Problem List**

The problem list keeps track of all patient health issues. The problem list can include current and past problems, active or inactive problems, and acute or chronic problems. The problems can be physiological, psychological, or socioeconomic. Once the complete problem list is developed, each problem is given a title and number. For example, the problem list could include: 1. Diabetes mellitus, 2. Hypertension, 3. Arthritis, and 4. Sore throat. As each problem is addressed by the physician, progress notes in the form of **SOAP notes** are written to record information about the problem. The acronym SOAP represents:

- **S**ubjective impression: symptoms that are experienced only by the patient and are subjective (meaning that they cannot be objectively measured), such as headache, pain, and fatigue
- **O**bjective clinical evidence: complaints or symptoms reported by the patient that can be measured or seen by others, such as bleeding, an elevated temperature, high blood pressure, or a laceration

- **A**ssessment: an evaluation of the patient's condition made using the subjective and objective information provided, including the physical exam and any diagnostic procedures performed; a diagnosis is made based on the assessment of all factors contributing to the specific patient problem
- **P**lan: management of the patient's problem by ordering further tests and procedures, by implementing treatment for the problem, or by reevaluating the patient's progress by requesting a return visit

Some facilities use SOAPER notes—adding an "E" for **E**ducation of the patient" and an "R" for "**R**esponse of the patient to the education provided"—to the SOAP notes.

Example of a SOAP Note

Patient Name: George Jones
Date: February 2, 2011
S. Complaining of severe sore throat for x3 days.
O. Throat appears red. Patient's temp 101.4° F
A. R/O strep throat.
P. Order throat culture. Will call patient in 24 to 48 hours with results and antibiotic if results are positive.

Source-Oriented Medical Record

The source-oriented medical record (SOMR) is the more traditional method of managing medical records and is still used in many medical offices. The SOMR method of record organization files patient information according to the type of source, or subject matter, generating the information. For example, all radiology reports would be filed together in one section, all laboratory reports would be filed in another section, and all physician entries would be filed in still another section. Within each section, the materials would be filed in chronological order, placing the most recent entry on top for easy viewing. Progress notes using the SOMR system do not use SOAP notes, but rather are written in paragraph style and include all pertinent information.

Strict Chronological Order

Organizing medical record information by using strict chronological order means that all incoming patient information is filed in the medical record with the most recent material on top. There are no separate sections for subject matter or lists of problems. Laboratory reports, radiology reports, progress notes, or any material needing to be added to the patient record is filed in the order it was received or written.

Patient information arranged using this system can make locating past medical information, such as the patient's last chest X-ray, time consuming. If the specific date of the patient's most recent chest X-ray is not known, then the medical assistant must search through the medical record, page by page, until the report needed is found.

Medical Record Storage Equipment

If the medical facility is using paper medical records, a storage method of records must be selected. Different types of storage units are available, each type having advantages and disadvantages to consider before a selection can be made. The type of filing cabinets used depends on the size of the storage area, the cost of the equipment, the estimated record volume, and the requirements for confidentiality.

Common types of filing cabinets often used to store medical records include vertical (or drawer) cabinets, lateral (or open-shelf) cabinets, and movable file cabinets (such as compacted cabinets or rotary cabinets).

Supplies Needed for Filing

The supplies needed for filing medical records will depend on the type of filing equipment used and the preference of the medical office.

1. **File folders:** File folders for vertical file cabinets are made with the tabs at top edge of the fold-

ers cut into different sizes. These tabs make it easier to read the labels on the folders in front to back filing. Folders used for lateral shelves are made with tabs that extend on the side of the folder, which makes it easier to read the file names. Color coding helps medical assistants easily recognize and properly file the medical records. For instance, it can help the medical assistant to recognize an active or inactive record based on the color of the sticker indicating a specific year.

2. **Outguides or outfolders:** Outguides are made of plastic (or a heavier type of material than that used in folders) and are used to keep track of medical records that are removed from the file cabinet for a length of time. Although medical records should be filed daily and remain in the medical office, occasionally the medical record may be needed by the physician to complete reports or needed for reference, preventing a timely filing. Outguides can provide information as to when the record was removed, by whom it was taken, and when it will be returned.

This information is placed in a clear plastic section of the outguide in order to help locate the medical record if it is needed before it is returned. All correspondence and information that needs to be filed for that medical record is placed in the outguide folder section, which prevents material from being lost or misplaced. When the medical record is returned, the patient information in the outguide can be placed in the medical record and the medical record file can be returned to its place in the filing system. Outguides are not used to replace medical records that are pulled daily for office visits.

3. **Labels:** Labels are used for patient identification, either by name or number. Many offices use a variety of color-coded labels designed to make retrieving and filing medical records easier and faster, to help prevent errors in filing, or to notice errors easily when they are made.

4. **Divider guides:** Divider guides are usually made of heavier material than folders so that they stand out for easy recognition. They are used to separate the files into specific sections. The divider guides have tabs that are labeled with captions identifying the major divisions of the files. For example, captions can be the letters of the alphabet, or breakdown of numbers into smaller sections, such as, tens, hundreds, or thousands. Organizing into smaller sections provides easier and faster retrieval and filing of medical records.

Filing Systems

The selection of a filing system depends on the volume of information to be filed and on the preference of the medical facility. Each type of filing system has advantages and disadvantages.

Three common filing systems include:

1. **Alphabetic filing system.** This system is simple to use, which makes it ideal for smaller facilities with limited records. Disadvantages to the alphabetic filing system include potential privacy concerns if patients' names can be viewed easily by others. Expansion of alphabetic files can sometimes be difficult because the files may need to be moved to accommodate overcrowded sections within the various letter divisions.

2. **Numeric filing system.** This system provides the advantage of additional patient confidentiality since medical records are filed by number and not by name, and it offers easy expansion (especially when using straight numbers) because each new file is added after the last file entered, avoiding the need to shift or move files. This system is used mainly in larger facilities filing large numbers of records. A disadvantage of this type of system is the extra step needed because an alphabetic record of patient names is needed to locate the numeric file.

3. **Subject filing system.** This system is used to file business information such as inventory lists, paid invoices, warranties for equipment, vendors used for purchases, repair service records, financial reports, and insurance policies. Medical offices can use subject filing for many different topics. Each topic is arranged in alphabetical order for easy retrieval and filing.

Alphabetic Filing

Alphabetic filing is probably the easiest and most common method used in medical office records management. To perform strict alphabetic filing, certain rules must be followed for separating all items into smaller indexing units—for example, using the patient's last name as your key unit. The key unit is also referred to as Unit 1. The units used in determining the alphabetic filing order include:

- Unit 1: last name
- Unit 2: legal given first name; no nicknames are used
- Unit 3: middle name or initial
- Unit 4: titles and other identifying information, such as MD, Sr., Jr., Prof., or III. If the office has patients who are couples who share the same last name, it may help to include each partner's name on the other partner's medical record as a fourth unit.

For example, Unit 1: Smith; Unit 2: Elizabeth; Unit 3: Lois; Unit 4: Mrs. Robert. This means that the record is filed first under the last name "Smith," but if there are other patients named Smith, then the next unit is the first name "Elizabeth." If there is more than one Elizabeth Smith, then the next unit is the middle name.

Basic rules have been established to standardize alphabetic filing and to maintain consistency among medical personnel responsible for managing patient records. Although there are variations for the rules used for alphabetic filing, many basic rules are used, including:

1. Complete names are filed in alphabetic sequence from last name, to first name, to middle name.
2. Hyphenated names are considered one unit, and the hyphen is removed.
3. Foreign names are considered as one unit and should be indexed as written, ignoring spaces, any capital letters, or punctuations. Some offices prefer to file names beginning with *St.* separately. The policy of the office should be followed.
4. Professional titles placed before a name or after a name can be added as Unit 4.
5. Married women use their legal first names as Unit 2. Unit 4 could be the husband's first name.
6. Seniority titles are listed in alphabetic order as Unit 4.
7. Numbers come before letters; for example, *Adam T. Brown III* would come before *Adam T. Brown Jr.*
8. Identical names with no distinguishing titles can use date of birth as Unit 4, using either the month or year for filing arrangement.
9. *Mac* and *Mc* are filed in alphabetic order, although some offices prefer to file names beginning with *Mc* separately. The policy of the office should be followed.
10. Commercial business names can be filed using indexing units, disregarding the word *the* at the beginning of a name for indexing purpose, by either putting it in parenthesis or indexing it as Unit 4.
11. Identical commercial names can be filed using the address as indexing units.

Numeric Filing

Numeric filing uses numbers instead of letters to file patient medical records. Most large offices and hospi-

tals filing thousands of medical records prefer this type of filing system (used with color coding) to manage medical records.

Numeric filing provides patient confidentiality and allows unlimited expansion of files. The different types of numeric filing include straight numeric filing, middle digit filing, and terminal digit filing. Straight numeric filing and terminal digit filing are most common.

Straight Numeric Filing

Straight numeric filing is the simplest type of numeric filing. In this system, medical records are arranged in ascending order, from the smallest number to the largest number. Examples of straight numeric filing would be 140, 141, 142, and so on, or 000123, 000124, 000125, and so on. In the example of files 140, 141, 142, and so on, the number 1 is the primary indexing unit; therefore, all records starting with a number 1 will be grouped together. Consideration is then given to the middle digits, arranging all records in sequential order, grouping all records having, for example, a number 4 as the middle unit. Finally, the items are then grouped in ascending order according to the last digits of the records. Zeros at the beginning of a group of numbers are ignored when arranged for records filing, so the file number 000123 would be arranged by using the number 1 as the primary unit, using number 2, the middle digit, as Unit 2, and finally, by using 3, the terminal digit, as Unit 3.

Terminal Digit Filing

Terminal digit filing is another common numeric system used in medical offices. In terminal digit filing, the digits, read from right to left, are separated by hyphens. The number of digits used can vary, but usually contain sections of two or three numbers.

Terminal digit filing is divided into 100 major or primary sections. Patients are given preassigned consecutive numbers when the medical record is set up, and the records are filed using the terminal digit, or last digit, in the number as Unit 1. In the number 42-65-26, the last two digits at the far right (numbers 2 and 6) are referred to as Unit 1, the middle two digits (numbers 6 and 5) are Unit 2, and the last two digits on the far left (numbers 4 and 2) are Unit 3. Using this example, all records in unit 1 (with terminal digits 26) are grouped together, then all records in Unit 2 (middle section) are arranged in ascending order, and finally, all numbers in Unit 3 are arranged in ascending order.

If color coding is used in numeric filing, then each digit—zero through nine—would be assigned a specific color. The terminal digits would have corresponding color labels attached to the tabs section of the file. This would make it easier to file records or to spot misfiled records.

Alphabetic Card System/Accession Record System

Regardless of the type of numeric system used, all numeric systems need an alphabetic card system to designate the number given to a specific patient's medical record. This card system should be locked when the office is closed, in order to protect patient privacy. Each new patient must be assigned a number for the medical record being established. Preassigned numbers are usually prepared in duplicate on labels. When a medical record is needed for a new patient, one of the preassigned numbers is removed from the label attached to the tab on the file folder, and the other label is attached to the alphabetic card. These preassigned numbers are referred to as an accession record, and are assigned and kept on file by a computer system. Using preassigned numbers helps prevent errors when setting up medical records.

Subject Filing

Subject filing can use an alphabetic system (using the letters of the alphabet, such as A, B, C, and so on) or alphanumeric systems (using a combination of letters and numbers, such as A1-1, A1-2, and so on). This type of filing system is used for correspondence, invoices, warranties, or any other general paperwork in the office that needs to be filed. A cross-reference of the material filed may be needed because an invoice for supplies could be in a file labeled "Invoices for Supplies" or in a file labeled with the name of the supply company from which the item was ordered.

Filing Procedures

Regardless of the system used to file papers or medical records, the following five specific steps should be used when filing.

1. Inspect the paper to be filed, locating the patient's name or other identifying information to be used in the filing process. All paper clips and staples should be removed before filing, and any tears in the paper should be repaired with tape. All small papers should be affixed to an 8.5 by 11 inch sheet of paper in order to prevent the small paper from being misplaced or lost when filed in the medical record.

2. Index the paper to be filed; that is, decide how the medical record or paper would be located when it will be retrieved, and use the appropriate indexing units to classify it. For example, dividing patient names into indexing units using the last name as Unit 1 is a commonly used method of indexing.

3. Code the paper or medical record, indicating how and where an item will be filed by underlining, circling, or highlighting the selected area. If there is any ambiguity or uncertainty concerning where an item should be filed, then a cross-reference card noting an alternate place that a person may look for the record in the future can be used.

4. Sort the papers or medical records by putting them in the order that they are to be filed: alphabetically, numerically, or by subject. This technique will save time.

5. Filing is the actual placement of papers in the medical record or the placement of the medical record back into the file cabinet after use.

Release Marks

It is essential that the physician has seen and read all material before any patient data can be filed in the medical record. A release mark—either in the form of a stamp or a check mark and the initials of the physician—placed in the same area on all papers to be filed is a good quality control method to safeguard against the filing of unread patient data. If patient information is filed without being read by the physician, then information about negative test results may go unnoticed and the patient may not receive the necessary care.

Special Filing Systems and Techniques

Tickler Files

Tickler files are used as a reminder system that some type of action needs to be taken, and can be used for many purposes, depending on the needs of the office. Tickler file systems can be set up by day, month, or any time frame needed by the office. They can be set up for a variety of uses. Some common uses of a tickler system can include reminders:

- to remind patients about yearly physicals
- to remind patients about monthly or quarterly blood pressure checks
- to be sure that lab results were returned for scheduled patients
- to schedule lab work or outpatient procedures for patients
- to attend monthly hospital meetings
- to follow up on insurance questions from patients

Tickler systems can be manual or computerized, depending on the preference of the staff of the medical office. When set up properly, tickler systems can increase efficiency in the medical office by keeping the staff from overlooking important information.

Cross-Referencing

Cross-referencing is used with alphabetic filing systems to aid in the retrieval of filed material. It is a notation placed in one file area listing other areas within the file system where a specific piece of information may be found.

The most important step in using a cross-referencing system is to determine the primary filing location of the record and then to decide on what the cross-reference card should include. Identifying alternative location sites (usually one or more) where the record may be filed should be helpful when searching for a file.

Locating Misplaced Records

Even with prompt and careful filing, the use of color coding, and the insertion of outguides, medical records or important papers can be misplaced or lost. Spending time searching for a misplaced record wastes valuable time. Here are some helpful steps that the medical assistant may take in locating a missing record:

- Search the entire record page by page to find the misplaced item.
- Check the records that are located in the file immediately before and immediately after the record needed.
- Check the physician's desk to see if the record is being used by the physician. An outguide may not have been prepared because the record was not removed from the office.
- Check records of patients with similar names to be sure that the item was not mistakenly filed in the incorrect record.

Active, Inactive, and Closed Files

Medical records can be divided into three categories of files.

1. **Active files** include the medical records of patients currently under the care of the physi-

cian or who were recently treated by the physician.

2. **Inactive files** include medical records of patients not recently treated. Each practice sets policies to determine when a record becomes inactive. Generally, a record is considered inactive two to three years after the patient's most recent visit. Inactive files may be removed from the easily accessible file cabinets, but must be retained by the office for a number of years, as dictated by state laws.

3. **Closed files** include medical records that are no longer needed. For example, the medical record for a patient who died or left the practice is considered a closed record.

Record Retention, Record Storage, and Purging Records

Medical offices are constantly accumulating information from various sources, such as laboratory reports and test results needed for patient care, warranties on office equipment, insurance policies, financial records, inactive and closed medical record files, and other miscellaneous data. Some types of information (such as fire insurance policies and warranties) have value for a limited time and do not need to be kept indefinitely. Other types of information such as inactive and closed patient medical records can be destroyed only after the statute of limitations expires, based on the laws of each individual state. Inactive and closed medical record files are separated from active medical record files. However, they must be available if needed and stored following the standards of preserving patient confidentiality as set forth by HIPAA. Purging is the process of appropriately disposing of files or information no longer needed. Material containing patient information or sensitive information is shredded to ensure privacy and prevent exposure of confidential information.

Mail Screening and Processing

Medical assistants are responsible for processing and screening the mail that comes to the medical office through the United States Postal Service (USPS) or via courier services such as FedEx or UPS. The medical assistant should be familiar with the various types of mail that are sent to and from a medical office.

Mail Classification

Mail delivery is classified according to weight, type, and destination of the item to be mailed. Classifications of mail that are often sent to and from the medical office include:

- **First-class mail** is used for handwritten or typed letters, bills, postcards, and personal correspondence. It is sealed and closed against inspection. Rates are based on size and weight, regardless of the distance traveled. Most of the mail sent to and from the medical office is first-class mail. The current postage rate is $0.44 per letter for letters weighing 12 ounces or less. Mail weighing 13 ounces, but not more than 70 pounds is automatically considered priority mail. First-class mail includes forwarding and return services with no additional fee. For a small additional fee, first-class mail can be upgraded to provide special services and security such as certified mail and registered mail.

- **Priority mail** is used when mail needs to get to a destination anywhere in the United States within two to three days. It includes all first-class mail weighing more than 13 ounces but not more than 70 pounds.

- **Periodical mail**, formerly known as second-class mail, is used to mail items usually prepared by printers and publishers, such as newspapers, magazines, and periodicals. Only authorized items may be sent using this class.

- **Standard mail A**, previously known as third-class mail, is used for mailing material weighing less than 16 ounces and is not eligible for first-class rates. Large amounts of printed material, such as quickly copied announcements or letters, containing nonpersonalized material and a duplicated signature may be sent by this class. This class cannot be used for personal correspondence.

- **Standard mail B**, or nonprofit mail, formerly known as fourth-class mail, includes both parcel post (that is, the mailing of packages weighing more than 16 ounces) and library rate (an economical rate intended for library use when mailing books on loan). Standard mail B is commonly used when mailing at least 200 or more identical items. The items must include a complete return address and be mailed to United States addresses only. All mail in this category needs to be separated by ZIP code and bundled with elastic bands. A business may be charged an annual fee to use this type of mailing.

- **Bulk mail** is used mainly by businesses that send large quantities of mail that meet specific criteria. An annual fee is charged for bulk mail, but the postage rates for this type of mail are discounted. Bulk mail can include a variety of mail classifications such as first-class, standard, and parcel post.

- **Media mail** is used to send books, DVDs, CDs, or any other types of media. Rates are based on weight. Delivery takes approximately one to two weeks.

- **Express mail** offers the fastest service of any type of mail offered by the USPS. Mail sent by express mail may reach its destination overnight or by the second day of mail service. Express mail is offered 365 days a year and can be delivered to most locations in the Unites States.

- **Certified mail** provides both proof of mailing and proof of delivery. Certified mail can be used to notify patients when they have been discharged from the medical practice (usually due to noncompliance with the physician's treatment advice). It can also be used to notify patients of overdue accounts.

- **Registered mail** is used to send valuable or irreplaceable items or letters. Registered mail is more expensive than certified mail, but can be delivered only to the person listed on the envelope.

- A **certificate of mailing** is used when the sender needs proof that an item was mailed, but is not necessarily concerned about when or if the item was received. For example, a certificate of mailing may be used to send a legal contract that needs to be postmarked by a certain date.

- **Special delivery mail** is charged at a special rate and ensures that the mail will be delivered as soon as it reaches the post office of its destination. The special delivery mark does not speed up the delivery between cities. Special delivery mail can include first-class, registered, or insured mail.

- **Special handling** is used to send third- and fourth-class mail by the fastest ground service. Mail labeled special handling will be delivered in about the same amount of time it would take first-class mail to reach its destination.

- **International mail** sent by offices to a location outside of the United States is classified according to weight, size, and destination. Information about rates and location sites can be obtained from the post office.

Mail may also be sent using private delivery services such as FedEx, Airborne Express, and UPS. Many of these services offer overnight delivery, operate at a competitive rate with the USPS, and have locations throughout the United States where items to be mailed may be dropped off. (In addition, some private delivery services offer pickup service.)

Postage Meter

A postage meter, used by many offices, may be purchased or leased from an office equipment dealer. A postage meter is used for faster mail delivery at the most efficient cost. Once purchased or leased, the postage meter is brought to the post office to purchase a designated amount of postage. The meter will be set for the amount of postage bought and can be refilled periodically, as needed. In the medical office, each item to be sent is weighed on an electronic scale or on a manual scale. The correct postage needed is printed out onto envelopes or onto adhesive strips that can be easily attached for mailing. Because mail that has been prepared using a postage meter does not need to be canceled or postmarked at the post office, it may reach its destination sooner. Also, using a postage meter will ensure that the exact amount of postage needed is used.

Processing Incoming Mail

The medical office receives a variety of incoming mail that needs to be processed in an efficient manner. Examples of incoming mail that may come to a medical office may include:

- laboratory reports
- certified or registered letters
- telegrams
- faxes
- payment from patients for services
- payments from third-party payers
- bills for services provided to the office
- information from pharmaceutical companies
- medical journals, magazines, and newspapers
- catalogs and advertising from office equipment suppliers
- insurance carrier updates
- correspondence and personal letters

Sorting Incoming Mail

Mail should be sorted according to importance. Telegrams, registered and certified letters, and letters marked "personal" are considered important mail and should be placed on the top of sorted mail. Once sorted, mail can be directed to the appropriate person or department.

The medical assistant should be familiar with the office policy regarding opening various types of incoming mail. Any mail addressed to the physician that is clearly marked "confidential" should not be opened by the medical assistant; rather, it should be delivered to the physician as soon as possible. Many physicians prefer that mail, even if not marked personal, sent from the Internal Revenue Service, accountants, or attorneys not be opened by the medical assistant.

Opening Mail

Opening and processing the mail should be done when the medical assistant can devote sufficient time to this duty. Each piece of mail opened should be stamped with the date it was received. Before the letter's envelope is discarded, the medical assistant should locate a return address on the letter, and the envelope should be checked to be sure it is empty. While reading the letter, the medical assistant may jot down notes in the margin of the letter noting any action that he or she needs to take. This process of annotating the mail acts as a reminder of the action needed. For example, if the patient's medical record were needed for the physician to complete an insurance form received, the medical assistant may note this in the margin, pull the record from the file, and attach the letter to the record with a paper clip so that the needed information would be easily accessible. If no action were needed, then the letter would be coded for filing.

Preparing Outgoing Mail

Envelope Selection and Letter Folding

Envelopes should be of high quality and should be heavy enough to protect the contents of the envelope from being viewed. The letter should be folded correctly so that it fits into the envelope properly and may be easily removed and read. A properly folded letter can create and impression of professional competency. Common envelope types used in a medical office include

- No. 10 envelope (measures $9\frac{1}{2}$ inches long by $4\frac{1}{8}$ inches wide). Standard size letters are folded by bringing up the bottom edge of the letter about third of the length of the paper and forming a crease. The top third of the letter is then folded down to within a quarter inch of the first crease. The letter is then placed in the envelope with the last crease going into the envelope first.
- No. $6\frac{3}{4}$ envelope (measures $6\frac{1}{2}$ inches long by $3\frac{5}{8}$ inches wide). Standard sized letters are first folded bringing up the bottom edge to within a quarter inch of the top edge. The right edge is then folded about one third of the letter width toward the center, making a crease, and the left edge is then folded toward the right edge crease to within a quarter inch. The left creased edge—the last crease made—goes into the envelope first.
- Window envelope (measures $7\frac{1}{2}$ inches long by $3\frac{7}{8}$ inches wide). Letters to be sent in this type of envelope are fan folded by folding the bottom edge of the letter up one third of the length of the paper. The letter is then turned over, and the top of the letter is folded down to the crease. The letter is then placed in the envelope so that the address shows in the window.

Addressing Envelopes

Envelopes addressed according to the standards set by the USPS can be read by an optical character reader (OCR), which is a type of scanner that electronically transforms the address information into a bar code placed at the bottom edge of the letter. Letters read by the OCR will go to the bar code sorter and will be delivered faster. Rules to be followed when addressing letters to meet the USPS standards include:

- Use all capital letters.
- Use no punctuation except for the hyphen in the ZIP code.
- Use one space between the city and state.
- Use approved abbreviations for street suffixes and locators.
- Use left justification format, using simple fonts with at least 10-point font size.
- Use dark ink on a light background.
- Use approved two-letter abbreviations for states.

Return Addresses

The medical assistant should make sure that a complete return address is placed in the upper left-hand corner of all letters mailed to ensure a prompt return if the post office is unable to deliver to the address listed on the envelope. Letters without a complete return address go to the dead letter office, where they may be opened in attempt to find the sender. If no information is provided in the opened letter regarding a return address, then the letter is destroyed.

TWO-LETTER STATE ABBREVIATIONS		TWO-LETTER STATE ABBREVIATIONS	
AL	Alabama	MT	Montana
AK	Alaska	NE	Nebraska
AZ	Arizona	NV	Nevada
AR	Arkansas	NH	New Hampshire
CA	California	NJ	New Jersey
CO	Colorado	NM	New Mexico
CT	Connecticut	NY	New York
DE	Delaware	NC	North Carolina
DC	District of Columbia	ND	North Dakota
FL	Florida	OH	Ohio
GA	Georgia	OK	Oklahoma
HI	Hawaii	OR	Oregon
ID	Idaho	PA	Pennsylvania
IL	Illinois	RI	Rhode Island
IN	Indiana	SC	South Carolina
IA	Iowa	SD	South Dakota
KS	Kansas	TN	Tennessee
KY	Kentucky	TX	Texas
LA	Louisiana	UT	Utah
ME	Maine	VT	Vermont
MD	Maryland	VA	Virginia
MA	Massachusetts	WA	Washington
MI	Michigan	WV	West Virginia
MN	Minnesota	WI	Wisconsin
MS	Mississippi	WY	Wyoming
MO	Missouri		

Envelope Notations

Notations such as "personal" or "confidential" should be typed, underlined, and aligned immediately below the return address on the left side of the envelope. Notations to the USPS should be typed in uppercase letters, immediately below the stamp on the right side of the envelope. If the letter needs an attention line, this information is typed on the line immediately above the post office box number or the street address.

ZIP Codes

Zone improvement plan (ZIP) codes are five-digit numbers used by the USPS to expedite mail delivery.

In 1983, a nine-digit ZIP code went into effect to identify geographic segments within delivery areas designated by the first five digits, such as a group of apartments, a city block, or any identity that would be helpful to speed up mail sorting and delivery. The nine-digit ZIP code is written using the first five digits separated by a hyphen and then listing the last four digits, and is referred to as a ZIP + 4 code.

Handling Special Mail

Even with careful addressing and record keeping, some mail does not get to the intended destination. Special mailing situations can include:

- **Forwarding and obtaining changed addresses.** Forwarding and obtaining changed addresses can occur when patients have moved without notifying the medical office of their new address. By writing "forwarding services requested" on the letter, the medical assistant can instruct the post office to forward the letter to the patient's new address if the move occurred within 12 months (or if the forwarding address is listed with the post office) at no expense for first-class or priority mail.

- **Address correction requested.** The notation "address correction requested" is used when the sender wants to know the patient's new address. If the letter was sent by first-class mail, then the corrected address will be noted on a sticker and returned to the sender at no additional cost.

- **Recalling mail.** Recalling mail is needed if a letter was deposited into the mailbox in error. A completed written application, accompanied by an exact duplicate of the envelope mailed, handed in to the post office, can recall the letter mailed in error. If the letter has already left the post office, a notification can be sent to the post office of the letter's destination requesting the letter's return, although no guarantee is made that the letter will be returned.

- **Tracing lost mail.** Letters mailed by certified, registered, or insured mail have a better chance of being located if the medical assistant has kept the mailing receipts until the letter has reached its destination. First-class mail is very difficult to trace. Insuring or certifying a letter is not very expensive and may be worth the expense if it is important for the letter to reach its destination.

Scheduling and Monitoring Appointments

Scheduling appointments for patient visits is one of the primary responsibilities of the administrative medical assistant. Appointments can be made by telephone or in person. Appointments can be recorded either in a manual appointment book or with a computer scheduling system. Regardless of the scheduling system used, skillful appointment scheduling can make patient flow run smoothly, which decreases waiting time and better accommodates the needs of the patient. The medical assistant must be familiar with the office policy regarding the time allotment for appointments and the preferred scheduling styles of the facility.

Appointment Book

The first step in manual scheduling is to select an appropriate appointment book. Considerations in this selection should meet the following requirements of the individual office. Appropriate time slot selection allows the office to schedule patients at specific intervals, for example, every 15 minutes or every 20 minutes. Adequate space for entering patient information should be available. Most offices record the patient's full name, daytime telephone number, the reason for the visit, a note about whether the patient is new or established, and the type of insurance.

The appointment book should also lie flat when opened (so that it is easier to use) and should be large enough to accommodate the number of physicians in the practice. Because appointments often need to be changed or cancelled, entries should be done in pencil to prevent the appointment book from becoming difficult to read. Some appointment books could include color coding for different days of the week or for different months. Also, some appointment books allow viewing of more than one day at a time. One disadvantage of the manual appointment book system is that it doesn't provide a permanent record of the day's appointments because it is written in pencil. A typed list of patients should therefore be kept for legal reference.

Computer systems for scheduling are quite popular in many offices and often come as part of the office management software package. Regardless of the type of appointment book used—either manual or computerized—problems with patient flow will occur if careful attention to the time needs of the patient, the work habits of the physician, and the best use of the facility resources and staff are not considered in the scheduling process.

Matrix

The next step after selecting the appointment book is setting up the matrix. The medical assistant should block off times that the physician is unavailable to treat patients and times the office is not open, such as during weekends, vacation, medical meetings, or holidays, so that patients are not scheduled during those times. The matrix should be done in pencil to accommodate changes.

The medical assistant must set up a matrix whether the office uses a computerized scheduling system or a manual scheduling system.

Common Scheduling Styles

There are different styles or methods of scheduling patients. Each style has its advantages and disadvantages—for both the patient and the medical staff. The facility can use any combination of the scheduling styles in order to accommodate the flow of the patients and to allow flexibility in the schedule in case of emergencies.

Stream scheduling is one of the most common types of scheduling styles used in physicians' offices. Each patient is given a specific time for the appointment and the time allowed for the appointment depends upon the reason for the visit. For example, a physical examination for a new patient would take more time than a three-month blood pressure check for an established patient would take. An advantage of this scheduling style for patients would be minimized wait time, so that the patients would not have to wait too long to receive care. An advantage for the medical staff is that the patient load would be spread out throughout the day. Certain periods in the day could be marked off to allow for emergency appointments or to allow the physician to catch up if he or she runs behind due to unforeseen problems. These marked-off times are referred to as "catch-up times."

Wave scheduling schedules three patients per hour. For example, three patients would be scheduled at ten A.M., three patients scheduled at eleven A.M., and so forth, allowing for 20-minute visits. The main idea behind this style of scheduling is to start and finish each hour on time, treating three patients per hour. All three patients would be scheduled at the same time, and the first patient to arrive would be seen first, followed by the second patient to arrive, and then the third patient to arrive. The theory behind this style is that not every patient takes the same amount of time, and most of the time the differences work out by the end of the hour. There is a disadvantage to the patient, however, with this style. If all patients arrived at the same time, one patient would have to wait approximately 40 minutes before he or she could be seen. However, most references on scheduling state that the waiting period for a patient should not exceed 15 to 20 minutes. If there will be a delay longer than 20 minutes before the patient is seen, many offices will inform the patient of the delay and offer to reschedule, or even call the patient to inform him or her that the office is running late and ask the patient to come in a bit later in order to decrease the waiting time.

Modified wave scheduling aims to address these potential issues with wait time. Only two patients are scheduled on the hour and the third patient is scheduled at half past the hour. This style allows more flexibility within the hour depending on the needs of the patient and minimizes the waiting time for patients.

Clustering, sometimes referred to as grouping, allows the facility to schedule similar procedures together in a specific time slot or day. Performing school physicals one morning or having a routine immunization clinic one morning, for instance, makes for more efficient use of time and staff members.

Open hours is a style for treating walk-in patients. No specific times are set for each appointment, but rather the hours of operation are listed and patients are seen usually on a first-come, first-served basis. With this scheduling system, patients are **triaged**, or screened, when they arrive, meaning that the most seriously injured or the sickest patient is seen first, regardless of the order of arrival. One of the advantages of this style is that the patients don't have to wait weeks or even months to get an appointment with their physician. There are disadvantages, too: patients may need to wait a long time to be seen, and the medical staff may have no patients, or too many, to treat at any given time.

Double-booking is a style that schedules two patients for the exact same time. It should be used very carefully and only if the office can accommodate more than one patient at a time. If two patients are going to be scheduled for a physical examination and both are scheduled for the same time, one patient could be taken to the lab for blood work or be seen by the physician, while the other patient is having an electrocardiogram (EKG) performed. Neither patient would be sitting and waiting for his or her appointment. Some physicians use this way of scheduling to ensure that there will not be any empty times during office hours caused by missed appointments or last-minute cancellations; however, this can result in long wait times for patients.

Practice-based scheduling refers to any method that works for the individual office. No one type of scheduling works for every facility; therefore, a practice-based style consists of scheduling techniques that are the best fit for a specific facility. For instance, a pediatrician's schedule may be set up for well-baby visits two mornings a week (clustering style) and have set appointment times the rest of the day (stream style). Another afternoon could be dedicated to immunization appointments (clustering style).

No matter what scheduling style is used, many problems with scheduling can be solved by making reminder calls to patients the day before their appointments and being sure to give each returning patient a reminder card for his or her next appointment.

Scheduling Guidelines

Scheduling guidelines include facility and staff availability, physician preferences and habits, and patient needs.

Facility and Staff Availability

In selecting an appointment style and setting up the matrix, the medical assistant should give attention to the available facilities, such as the available number of patient examining rooms. The type of practice will dictate the needs of the patients. Offices that perform minor surgical procedures may need more time with each patient, plus a recovery room to allow the patient to rest before leaving the office. More treatment rooms may need to be set up for the next surgical procedure so that the physician and patient do not have to wait. The time needed to perform procedures done by other personnel, such as blood tests, EKGs, or X-rays, needs to be considered when setting up appointment times.

Physician Preferences and Habits

The working style and habits of the physician are another consideration for time allotment in the appointment book. Physicians work differently, some preferring to be kept very busy and others preferring a slower, more relaxed environment. The scheduling style selected should fit the needs of the individual office.

Patient Needs

Regardless of the scheduling style chosen, flexibility and concern for patients are the most important factors in successful scheduling. Having some general information about the type of patients coming to the facility can be helpful in arranging the most convenient appointment times for patients. Elderly patients may need transportation. Working patients may appreciate evening or weekend appointments. Working around the individual's schedule will help ensure that appointments are kept.

New Patient Scheduling

New patients require longer appointment times. One reason for the additional time needed is that information must be gathered from the patient upon his or her arrival. Such information includes the patient's full name, phone number, reason for the visit, and type of insurance. Some offices ask for more detail before the patient even arrives, including the name of the referring physician and the patient's address, place of employment, date of birth, and insurance information, while other offices may wait to obtain this information when the new patient arrives for his or her first visit. To get started on organizing the medical record, some offices will send registration and past history forms to the patient and ask that the completed forms be returned when the patient comes in for his or her appointment. Some offices may request that new patients come in 15 minutes before the scheduled appointment to fill out paperwork. The medical assistant should remind the patient to bring his or her insurance card and co-pay, if needed, depending on office policy.

Established Patient Scheduling

Information needed from established patients requesting an appointment should include the patient's full name, a phone number where he or she may be reached during the day, the reason for the visit, and any changes in insurance information. Often the medical assistant will ask established patients to update information on file, such as addresses and insurance plan details.

Physician Referrals

Patients can be referred by the primary care physician to a specialist for evaluation or treatment of a specific disease or condition. Many types of insurances, such as health maintenance organizations (HMOs), request preauthorization before the patient can be seen by a specialist. There are three primary types of referrals:

- **Regular referrals:** requested when the primary care physician decides that the patient needs more specialized treatment; usually take about one week to ten days before being approved by the insurance company
- **Urgent referrals:** requested for more specialized, non-emergency care; can take between 24 to 48 hours for insurance company approval
- **STAT referrals:** requested for life-threatening conditions; usually faxed to insurance companies and usually approved by telephone

Referrals can be made by the physician, members of the physician's staff, or the patient needing the referral. If the patient or the staff member of the referring physician is the one calling for the appointment, the information needed for scheduling an appointment is the same as needed for scheduling a new patient. It is essential that the patient provide the reason for the appointment, so that the medical assistant may schedule an appointment for the patient as soon as possible, if needed. If the patient is referred to a medical facility for a presurgical clearance, then the appointment needs to be scheduled within a certain time frame, depending on the policy of the hospital where the surgery will be performed. Many times, if the situation is more urgent, the referring physician may call to request the appointment for the patient. If the situation is urgent, the medical assistant should make every attempt to give the patient an appointment on the day of the call or as soon as possible.

Resources for Patients

In this section, you will find resources that may be useful to patients.

Community Services

Medical facilities should be aware of the various community resources available to patients. The medical assistant should be sensitive to the needs of patients and their families when illness or disabilities occur. Many patients and their families are not aware of the resources available in the community, and these resources can be helpful in the care of the patient or in the acceptance of the medical condition.

Community resources include assistive programs or group services offered to members of the community at no cost or at affordable rates. These services or programs are designed to help the patient become as independent as is possible and to help all family members cope with medical situations. Programs such as Meals on Wheels, transportation services to and from the physician's offices, senior care, support groups for all ages and problems, and educational classes for parents are just a few of the different types of resources available in communities.

The medical assistant should keep a list of organizations and resources that would be most helpful to their patients in an easily accessible file so that they may refer patients to these programs. The specific programs on the list will depend on what services are offered in the community and on the specialty of the medical facility.

Patient Advocates

Patient advocates are liaisons between the patient and the physician or healthcare provider. Patients and their families may have difficulties understanding healthcare treatment and options. The role of the patient advocate is to help decipher the complex information presented to the patient by the physician or healthcare provider.

Clear communication between patients, family members, and healthcare providers is essential in providing quality care. An informed patient is more accepting of medical treatment, less apprehensive, and more satisfied with the care received. Patient advocates can offer support to patients and families, can assist with insurance issues and employment issues, and can help in coordinating communication and schedules with all providers involved in the patient's care.

Maintaining the Office Environment

The patient's first encounter with the medical office should make the patient feel welcome. The medical office should convey warmth and make patients feel secure and comfortable about the care they will receive. The medial assistant plays an important role in developing and maintaining this welcoming and secure environment.

Physical Environment

Safety and comfort should be the main characteristics in the physical environment of a medical office.

Entrance and Front Office

Here are some guidelines for the entrance and waiting room:

- Furniture should be comfortable, provide adequate seating, and be easy to clean.
- Seating arrangements should provide ample personal space for patients as they wait for treatment.
- Adequate lighting should be provided for reading, writing, and easy movement around the office.
- Small scatter rugs, electrical cords within walking areas, and sharp corners on furniture should be avoided.
- Nonslip mats should be placed in front of incoming doors.
- A coatrack and umbrella stand should be available.

The physical environment of the medical assistant's office is also important. Here are some important considerations:

- The office should be within sight of the entryway to allow the staff to welcome a patient upon arrival.

- A window separating the reception area from the medical assistant's office will provide privacy as the medical assistant uses the phone, although it should not be seen as a barrier between the patient and the medical staff.
- The front office should have adequate light and a sliding window to view patients arriving for appointments.

ERGONOMICS IN YOUR OFFICE

Ergonomics is the science of designing a workspace to help workers reach maximum productivity and reduce fatigue and discomfort. The furniture and equipment in the office should be designed with ergonomics in mind. Placing the computer monitor in an area that prevents glare on the screen is important in preventing eye strain. Chairs and computer keyboards should be adjusted for the height of the user, and wrist supports should be used. Properly adjusted equipment will help to prevent neck strain, back pain, and carpal tunnel syndrome.

Examination and Treatment Rooms

The arrangement and maintenance of examination and treatment rooms is critical. Here are some important guidelines:

- The rooms must be cleaned after each patient visit.
- Maintenance and repair of equipment in a timely and thorough way is essential.
- Hazardous equipment and supplies, such as surgical instruments, syringes, or caustic chemicals, should not be left within the patient's reach.
- Prescription pads should be placed in a drawer available only to the physician and other medical personnel.

- Chairs and stools that are sturdy and will not easily tip over should be used in the examination room.

Medical assistants are responsible for maintaining the examining room and treatment areas. They should have a file containing the information needed to obtain prompt and efficient repair of all equipment.

Government agencies, such as Occupational Safety and Health Administration (OSHA) and Centers for Disease Control (CDC) have developed guidelines—including what are called standard precautions—on the maintenance of medical facilities. Information about these standards can be found in Chapter 5 in the "Infection Control" section.

Americans with Disabilities Act

The **Americans with Disabilities Act**, established in 1991 and designed to protect the rights of people with physical and mental disabilities, applies to businesses with 15 or more employees. Such business, including medical offices, must comply with specific ADA guidelines for accessibility and safety. Some of these guidelines include:

- wide enough hallways or corridors to accommodate a wheelchair
- parking spaces for disabled patients, rules for which vary between states
- elevators in buildings that have more than one floor
- ramps available for easy access into the building
- door handles at wheelchair level
- bathroom with doors wide enough for a wheelchair, as well as a handicap stall with railings
- Braille text available on elevator numbers and office doors
- examining rooms arranged to accommodate wheelchairs

Fire Safety and Security Regulations

Fires can spread very quickly and easily in a medical office because of the presence of chemicals and oxygen tanks. Here are some important guidelines for preventing fires and for handling them if they occur:

- Working smoke alarms and fire alarms should be available and checked regularly.
- Fire extinguishers should be placed in an easily accessible area, and all office personnel should be trained to use the equipment properly.
- Exit doors should be clearly marked, and stairwells should be uncluttered.
- An escape plan should be placed on a wall, showing the quickest route out of the building.

The medical assistant may be the staff person designated to make a routine check of fire equipment, such as checking for frayed electrical wires and expiration dates on fire equipment.

Biohazardous waste can also create a safety issue in the medical office. Biohazardous waste consists of contaminated waste that is potentially infectious to humans or animals. Examples include:

- blood and blood products
- most bodily fluids such as amniotic fluid (from the uterus during pregnancy), synovial fluid (from the joints), pleural fluid (from the lungs) and cerebrospinal fluid (from the spinal canal)

Perspiration is not considered a biohazardous body fluid.

Protocol for standard precautions should be followed when coming into contact with or handling biohazardous substances. A spill kit can be purchased to use for cleaning up spills of chemicals and blood. Broken glass items should be placed in a hard, red plastic hazardous waste container to prevent injury.

Security is the responsibility of all employees in the medical facility. Some key factors in security are:

- Most facilities have an alarm system that should be activated each evening when the office is closed.

- All controlled substances such as narcotic drugs should be counted and double-locked for security.
- Patient records should be locked up to prevent unauthorized access to the records and safety in case of a fire.
- Any cash—for example, the cash used to make change and the cash in the petty cash account—should be locked up each evening.

Alarm system codes should never be given to anyone, and safety codes should be changed periodically.

Equipment and Supply Inventory

The medical assistant is often responsible for keeping track of inventory and ordering supplies. Inventory cards should be made for each item, listing the supplier's name, address, phone and fax number, and the cost of each item. A daily or weekly review (depending on the needs of the office) of the inventory cards will determine what supplies should be reordered.

Ordering and Managing Supplies

Ordering supplies is not as simple as it seems! Here are some pointers:

- Order supplies from reputable companies.
- Avoid changing suppliers without discussion with the office manager or the physician.
- Because many items have expiration dates, such as chemical reagents for the laboratory, take care not to over-order.
- Room to store supplies may be limited, another reason not to over-order.
- Place newly arrived supplies behind the supplies already there to ensure that the "freshest" are used last.

Office Policies and Procedures

The office policy manual usually describes general information about the medical practice and the expectation of its employees. It may include areas of appropriate dress and behavior, wages, benefits, insurance, vacation time offered, and any other information important to the employees.

A procedure policy manual is mostly concerned with the details of how to perform procedures in the office. The procedure manual may describe the proper protocol for handling volatile chemicals or may describe what instruments each physician requires for certain procedures. Administrative guidelines, such as how to handle emergency calls or how to handle supplies and inventory, may also be covered in the manual.

The advantage of written manuals is that an employee knows what is expected to meet the requirements of the job satisfactorily.

Financial Practices

Managing many of the business details of the medical practice is one of the medical assistant's responsibilities.

Bookkeeping Functions

The medical assistant may be required to perform some or all of the bookkeeper's responsibilities. These tasks may include:

- recording charges, payments, and adjustments made to patient accounts
- maintaining the business checkbook (much like a personal checkbook)
- processing payroll
- gathering necessary data for use by the practice's accountant

An outside accounting service is usually hired as the practice accountant. Accountants are responsible for the design and management of the financial systems that bookkeepers use. An accountant's responsibility is to prepare monthly financial statements and tax returns at the end of the year, and to perform other financial services that would help manage the medical office as efficiently as possible. Bookkeeping functions may be performed through the use of computer software programs or performed manually, using systems set up by the accountant in charge of the practice.

TIPS FOR ACCURATE BOOKKEEPING

- The medical assistant's bookkeeping should accurate and legible.
- Carefully forming numbers and lining up columns ensures accuracy.
- Bookkeeping tasks should be performed at a quiet time when attention will not be diverted to other issues in the office.
- Using dark blue or black ink will ensure that the numbers will be able to be easily read even over time.
- All math should be checked carefully, with the placement of the decimal points carefully checked!
- Bookkeeping should be done on a daily basis.

Manual Bookkeeping Forms

The pegboard system, also referred to as the "write-it-once" or the "one-write" system, is a manual bookkeeping system used in many offices. It consists of a day sheet, ledger cards, encounter forms, and receipts.

The pegboard has raised pegs protruding from one side of the frame that allow for easy placement of the forms. The day sheet is the basic form that is placed on the pegboard and is used to record all transaction that are posted each day.

Posting is the process of recording transactions into a bookkeeping system. Multiple no-carbon-required (NCR) forms can be placed on top of the day sheet, allowing any information entered on the top sheet to be transferred to the lower sheets easily and clearly. Writing information just once helps prevent errors.

Ledger cards, one per patient, are used to record patient transactions such as charges and payments and to keep track of the balance a patient owes. Notations can be made to signify if the claim was sent to the patient's insurance carrier.

An encounter form, also referred to as a charge slip or superbill, is an itemized account of the patient's visit, listing the procedures, diagnosis, and charges for the visit. The encounter form can serve as a patient appointment card because it has an area designed to include the date and time of the next appointment. Encounter forms are usually triple layered and can be customized for individual medical offices. The top white sheet is kept in the patient's record as documentation of the itemized services provided for the visit. The yellow middle sheet is sometimes used to submit insurance claims, and the bottom pink sheet is given to the patient as documentation of the visit services. A receipt acknowledges payment from a patient without itemizing any charges.

On a day sheet, charges are entered under the debit column and payments are entered under the credit column. The adjustment column is used to record entries such as insurance write-offs, overpayments from patients, or patient discounts or write-offs.

Petty Cash

Petty cash is money kept and used in the medical office to pay for unexpected minor expenses, such as postage due. The amount of petty cash kept in the office depends on the individual needs of each office. Small bills are kept and can be used to make change for patients, if necessary. When other minor expenses are paid using the petty cash fund, a voucher or petty cash log is filled out listing the date, the amount and reason for the expenditure, and the initials of the person taking the money. The medical assistant should balance the petty cash drawer daily. Larger bills can be exchanged for smaller bills when the medical assistant makes the bank deposit. When the petty cash funds are getting low, a check to replace the used funds can be requested.

Coding Systems

The medical office must provide a procedural code and a diagnostic code for every service provided to the patient when submitting insurance claims in order to receive reimbursement. The two main types of coding systems used to code insurance claims are current Procedural Terminology (CPT) and International Classification of Diseases, Clinical Modifications (ICD-CM).

Current Procedural Terminology

Current Procedural Terminology—developed by the American Medical Association (AMA) in 1966—is a list of terms and codes used to identify and report medical procedures and services. Written procedures are translated into a numeric code that accurately describes the procedure in uniform language. This coded information is communicated to healthcare providers and insurance carriers and is also used to collect data used for developing guidelines for medical care review. The CPT book of codes was revised for the fourth time to keep the procedural codes current, and the present issue of the book is referred to as CPT-4.

The CPT-4 edition is divided into six sections, using five digit codes to identify all medical procedures and services provided to patients receiving care in medical offices, hospitals, nursing facilities, and home care. Each section is then arranged in smaller subsections, subheadings, categories, and subcategories to provide detailed descriptions. An index section is found at the end of the book, listing every procedure and service in alphabetical order for easy reference.

- **Evaluation and Management (E/M).** Code numbers include: 99201 through 99499.

   E/M codes describe physician services based on place of service, such as office (outpatient) or hospital (inpatient); type of service, such as office visit, consult, or hospital admission; and patient status, such as new or established patient. E/M codes are also divided by patient history, physical examination, and the complexity of the decision-making process.

- **Anesthesia.** Code numbers include: 00100 through 01999.

  This section contains all codes needed for any type of anesthesia used in any procedure.
- **Surgery.** Code numbers include: 10021 through 69990.

  Surgical codes are divided by body system and are very descriptive and specific.
- **Radiology, Nuclear Medicine, and Diagnostic Ultrasound.** Code numbers include: 70010 through 79999.

  These codes are very descriptive and use detailed information when coding the procedure.
- **Pathology and Laboratory.** Code numbers include: 80047 through 89356.

  Every test and combination of test procedures can be found in this section of the CPT manual.
- **Medicine.** Code numbers include: 90281 through 99607.

  This section includes detailed codes adjusted for each procedure. This is a large section including codes for chemotherapy, immunization, and various types of injections.

Modifiers are two-digit numbers used in coding to indicate specific circumstances about the procedure or service. Modifiers can indicate, for instance, that a bilateral procedure (-50), such as a bilateral inguinal hernia repair (herniorraphy) was performed.

International Classification of Diseases, Clinical Modifications

An ICD-CM code is a standardized method used to classify diseases, conditions, symptoms, signs, and abnormal findings. Every possible health condition can be coded to translate the condition into numbers for more accurate recording and reporting. The ICD-9-CM edition will soon be replaced with ICD-10, the new revised edition. ICD-10 was set to be implemented in the United States as of October 2013; however, in April of 2012, the Department of Health and Human Services (HHS) released plans to delay the implementation of ICD-10 for one year in order to give providers more time to prepare for the necessary changes needed in their systems for the successful operation of ICD-10. The new release schedule is October 2014.

Once implemented, the ICD-10 edition will be the required coding book for reporting diagnoses used for all outpatient procedures and physician services that are performed in ambulatory care facilities and for all outpatient hospital services.

Although the ICD coding manual has been updated every year, the publishing of the new edition, ICD-10, was delayed due to substantial changes being made in this edition. ICD-9 had the ability to accurately tract and analyze various areas in health care, but due to the advancement in medical knowledge and technology, it had limitations such as outdated terminology and insufficient detailed classifications. The World Health Organization (WHO), the organization responsible for publishing ICD, recognized the need for a system that would be expandable, flexible, easy to update, and be able to collect, contain, and analyze more detailed health information. ICD-10 was developed to meet these requirements by providing greater specificity that would allow better collection of data concerning primary care risk factors, ambulatory care services, complications following surgery, and behavioral and mental disorders. There will be approximately 68,000 ICD-10 codes compared to the 14,000 ICD-9 codes. ICD-10 is designed as a one-step coding process by incorporating the V codes (Factors Influencing Health Status) and E codes (External Causes of Injury and Poisoning), directly into the coding list. The coder will be able to find an accurate code for a diagnosis without having to search through a variety of sections, reducing coding time, coding errors, and claim rejections.

To provide expandability, flexibility, and easy updating, ICD-10 codes will have up to seven alphanumeric characters per diagnosis as needed, with the sixth and seventh characters providing greater specificity needed for recording information from detailed documentation. The first character will be a letter, the second character a number, and the remaining characters either a letter or number. ICD-9 was limited to a maximum of five numeric digits, limiting expansion and updating. All the letters of the alphabet, except "U," will be used for coding existing diagnoses. The letter "U" will be used to code unnamed conditions or diseases of uncertain origin. ICD-10 will also address areas for documenting and tracking information on poisonings, injuries, threats to public health, and medical errors. The ICD-10 book will have an alphabetical and tabular listing of diseases and conditions similar to the ICD-9 book.

The research data collected by ICD-10 will be readily accessible to all health care professionals, not only to provide better communication between providers and facilities, but to provide quality care to patients by using up-to-date medical resources and research data. Educating and training office personnel and students in health care fields to use ICD-10 has already begun in order to meet the implementation date. It is imperative that the health care professionals in the United States be prepared to use the new ICD-10 edition since it will be the international standard for tracking and analyzing health data.

The ICD-9 system is published in three volumes.

- Volume I is a tabular list, listing all diagnoses in numerical order.
- Volume II is the alphabetic volume listing all disease and conditions in alphabetical order.
- Volume III contains numeric and alphabetic sections used for coding surgical procedures on inpatient hospital claims.

Supplementary health factor codes (V codes), found in Volume II, include classification of factors that influence the health status of a patient. They identify reasons for healthcare other than diseases or injuries. V codes would be used when a patient comes to the medical office for his or her annual physical (V70.0) or for a rubella screening test (V73.3).

External cause codes (E codes), also found in Volume II, classify external causes of poisoning and injuries, and identify medications. E codes are used

AN EXAMPLE OF ICD-9 CODING

Diabetes mellitus has the main ICD code 250.0. A box appears above the condition stating that a fifth code is necessary for accurate coding. For instance, for a patient with non-insulin-dependent diabetes, the fifth digit would be 0.

to provide additional information and cannot be used alone. If a patient experienced a closed fracture of the ankle when he fell into a hole, for instance, the main code for this condition would be for the fractured ankle (824.8) and an E code would be added to describe the cause of the fracture. For example, E883 states the patient fell into a hole.

Morphology codes (M codes) are five-digit codes used mainly for cancer registries. The first four digits indicate the specific histological term and the last digit indicates if the tumor is benign or malignant.

Preparing a Claim Form

The first step in coding the diagnosis is to look up the condition or disease alphabetically in Volume II. The diseases and conditions are arranged by main terms consisting of at least three digits.

Main terms are then subdivided into subterms and can even be divided further into categories and subcategories. The intent of the coding system is to define each disease or condition specifically.

Once the alphabetic code is determined, the code number is now looked up in Volume I, the tabular list of numbers. After carefully reviewing the information in the tabular section, the medical assistant can decide which ICD code to use for the patient's diagnosis or condition.

Conventions are general guidelines that help the coder determine the most specific ICD diagnostic code. Symbols, abbreviations, punctuation marks, and formatting are used to direct the coder in the right direction. A list of conventions can be found in the introduction section of the ICD-9-CM manual.

IMPORTANCE OF SPECIFICITY IN CODING

ICD-9-CM codes need to be coded at the highest level of specificity (five-digits, if needed) and CPT codes need to reflect the correct level of service. Improperly coded claims may result in a lower payment for the physician if a code indicates a diagnosis or service that is lower in complexity than actually delivered. ICD-9-CM codes missing a fourth or fifth code when needed may lead to the claim being rejected. Rejected claims slow, or even prevent, payment to the physician.

Third-Party Billing

A third party is someone other than the patient who is responsible for paying the patient's medical expenses or for a portion of the expenses. Insurance carriers are often considered third-party payers because they have entered into a contract with the patient to provide reimbursement for medical expenses that meet certain criteria.

A photocopy of both sides of the patient's insurance card should be made and kept in the patient's medical record. Some medical offices use a point-of-service (POS) device, which allows direct communication with the insurance carrier to verify the status of a patient's insurance coverage. The device is similar to a credit card machine whereby an individual swipes the card through the machine.

Many insurance carriers impose a waiting period on new subscribers. A waiting period is a specified period of time that must pass before the insurance coverage begins; the delay in coverage is usually due to a preexisting condition, such as diabetes or pregnancy.

Types of Insurance Plans

There are several types of health insurance coverage available in the United States; some insurance carriers offer more than one—or all—types of coverage.

A **capitated plan** is a form of managed care designed to provide healthcare to members for a fixed monthly cost. The capitated plan works with providers who accept a set dollar amount per patient regardless of the number of visits made to the medical office.

Major medical insurance, as its name implies, offers coverage for the most serious medical expenses or catastrophic illness. Major medical insurance usually covers inpatient and outpatient expenses after a deductible, which the patient pays out-of-pocket, is met. This type of insurance usually pays higher benefits and has a higher maximum limit on the benefits allowed.

Managed care is a general term used to indicate lower-cost healthcare coverage. Managed care plans use a variety of techniques to keep costs down, such as eliminating unnecessary medical and surgical procedures, sharing more of the healthcare costs with beneficiaries, and offering economic incentives to providers and patients to select less costly forms of treatment. A **health maintenance organization (HMO)** is a type of managed care system that offers comprehensive healthcare to an enrolled group for a fixed amount of money. The patient selects a primary care physician (PCP) from a list of providers who are under contract with the HMO. Different types of HMOs include:

- **Independent practice association (IPA):** a group of physicians in private practice who join together to treat members at a discounted fee or on a capitation basis. Patients enrolled in this type of plan must select a physician from the IPA in order to have their healthcare covered.
- **Preferred provider organization (PPO):** a managed care plan consisting of a group of physicians who agree to a predetermined pay scale for provided services. Patients are responsible for deductibles and coinsurance payments. Out-of-pocket expenses are less if the patient is treated by a physician in the PPO network.
- **Point-of-service (POS) plan:** an HMO plan that allows the member to choose a physician from

a list of physicians who have previously agreed to the discounted payment schedule. POS plans have no deductibles and small co-pays that vary depending on the type of medical treatment received. Referrals are generally necessary from the primary care physician for specialty care other than an annual gynecological exam and pediatric well-child visits. Because of the lower cost for healthcare, POS plans are popular with employers who offer healthcare benefits to their employees.

Sources or Providers of Medical Insurance

Private companies and government entities are the two main sources of health insurance coverage in the United States.

Private, or **commercial**, **insurance** companies provide individuals or groups (usually companies or associations) with healthcare coverage. Premiums are paid—by individuals, employers, or both—in exchange for various levels of coverage. The coverage offered by private companies can range across all the types of insurance previously discussed. Blue Cross Blue Shield is an example of a private insurance carrier.

Government insurance plans, including Medicare, Medicaid, Tricare, and CHAMPVA, are government-run plans that are funded by tax revenues and, in some cases, individual premiums. Coverage in these various programs can include characteristics of the types of coverage previously discussed.

Medicare, a health insurance program under Social Security, Title XVIII, was started in 1965 for individuals who are age 65 or older, or individuals who are under age 65 but are disabled and unable to work. There are four parts to the Medicare program.

- **Part A.** Medicare Part A is hospital insurance and is provided at no cost to individuals who have worked and paid Social Security taxes for at least ten years. This plan covers most medically necessary hospital care, skilled nursing facility care, home care, and hospice care. There is a yearly deductible that needs to be met before Medicare will reimburse expenses.

- **Part B.** Medicare Part B is medical insurance for which an individual must pay a monthly premium. Medicare Part B covers most medically necessary physician services, preventative care, hospital outpatient services, durable medical equipment, laboratory testing, X-rays, mental-health care, and some types of home healthcare and ambulance services.

- **Part C.** Medicare Part C allows private insurance companies to offer the same benefits that are offered by Medicare. This type of plan is referred to as a Medicare Advantage plan or a Medicare private health plan. It can be offered by HMOs, providing the same benefits but using different rules, and may have different costs and coverage.

- **Part D.** Medicare Part D provides outpatient prescription drug coverage and is available only through private insurance companies that have a contract with the government. Medicare Part D is optional and can be purchased as stand-alone insurance or in a benefit packet for individuals opting for Medicare Part C.

Medicaid, or Title XVIX, is an insurance program providing healthcare to individuals, regardless of age, whose income is insufficient to meet medical expenses. Medicaid is funded by the states and the federal government.

TRICARE, formally known as the Civilian Health and Medical Program of the Uniformed Services (CHAMPUS), is a healthcare program designed and managed by the Department of Defense that provides civilian healthcare to military personnel and their families. TRICARE offers three types of programs.

- **TRICARE Standard.** TRICARE Standard allows beneficiaries to use any civilian healthcare provider. There is an annual deductible and coinsurance to be paid out-of-pocket.

- **TRICARE Extra.** TRICARE Extra functions as a PPO, allowing the beneficiary to use a civilian healthcare provider listed in the provider's network. The discounted coinsurance is the only fee the beneficiary pays for this type of plan.

- **TRICARE Prime.** TRICARE Prime is a type of HMO that requires the beneficiary to choose a primary care physician and obtain referrals and authorizations when requesting specialty care. A small copayment is required for each visit. Military retirees and their families are charged an annual enrollment fee, which is waived for active duty military and their families.

Civilian Health and Medical Program of the Department of Veterans Affairs (CHAMPVA) is a health benefit program for veterans with 100% service-related disabilities and their family members. CHAMPVA shares the cost of the healthcare with the beneficiaries of the plan. Spouses or widow(ers), and children of a permanently disabled veteran or a veteran who died while on active duty are also eligible. The beneficiary of this plan cannot be eligible for TRICARE. CHAMPVA allows the beneficiary to select a physician and pays on a fee-for-service basis. There are deductibles and co-pays for this coverage.

Workers' compensation is a type of insurance that provides an employee who has been injured or disabled in a job-related incident with coverage for medical expenses. Most state laws mandate that employers with a certain number of employees purchase workers' compensation insurance for their employees.

RESPONSIBILITY FOR INSURANCE KNOWLEDGE

Who is responsible for knowing the ins and outs of each patient's type of healthcare insurance plan, the patient or the medical assistant? Although the medical assistant has some knowledge of healthcare plans, the patient should be encouraged to take responsibility for understanding the provisions of his or her insurance plan. Incorrectly scheduled yearly exams or treatments and procedures, for instance, may not be covered under a patient's insurance plan. The medical assistant should always take the time to verify the status of the patient's insurance coverage and the insurer's referral requirements and scheduling requirements for specific exams, as well as check whether precertification is required. By calling the insurance carrier or instructing patients to do so prior to scheduling referrals or procedures, nonpayment or other problems with reimbursement by the insurance carrier can be avoided.

Processing Claims

Processing claim forms accurately is essential in order to receive financial reimbursement for services rendered in the medical office. Most insurance carriers encourage the submission of claims electronically. There are common guidelines to follow when completing insurance claims either manually or by computer.

Claim Forms

The medical assistant should be familiar with three standardized claim forms used to report medical services to insurance carriers. The **National Uniform Claims Committee (NUCC)** is a voluntary organization that was developed to institute changes in the claim forms used in the reimbursement process. The goal was to provide standardization needed to process and send insurance claims. Two basic forms are used for insurance processing.

- **Centers for Medicare and Medicaid Services (CMS 1500)** is a standardized form used in the medical office to submit insurance claims. Previously known as the Health Care Financing Administration (HCFA 1500), the CMS 1500 is required for government programs such as Medicare and Medicaid, but may be used for most types of insurance claims.
- The **Uniform Bill 04 (UB-04)** is the standard insurance claim form used by institutions. The UB-04 form may be used for completing claims covering services such as inpatient admissions, outpatient procedures, psychiatric and alcohol clinics, and nursing facilities.

Manual and Electronic Preparation of Claims

The process of preparing manual or electronic insurance claims starts when the patient schedules an appointment. The medical assistant uses the patient registration form to gather demographic information required for the insurance claim form.

Information concerning the services rendered during a patient's visit and the related diagnosis is then entered on the claim, using the correct CPT and ICD codes. This information is obtained from the physician who includes it on an encounter form at the time of service.

The medical assistant enters the information either into a computer program or on the paper claim form and sends it to the insurance carrier. The majority of medical offices submit claims electronically because the turn-around time is quicker for reimbursements, and it is easier to trace claims if there is a problem receiving reimbursement. In fact, some insurance carriers require that claims be sent electronically. Only clean claims—that is, claims containing no errors—are accepted by the insurance carrier; dirty claims (those containing errors) will be rejected and not be paid. A rejected claim will cause a delay in reimbursement.

PRIVACY AND SECURITY OF PATIENT INFORMATION

The **Health Insurance Portability and Accountability Act of 1996** is a law administered by the U.S. Department of Health and Human Services and enforced by the Office for Civil Rights, which governs the rules and procedures that provide for the privacy and security of a patient's protected health information (PHI) (any information about the provision of healthcare, healthcare status, or payment for healthcare than can be linked to a particular person). An important part of the registration process is asking the patient to sign a consent form giving the medical office permission to release the necessary information to the insurance carrier in order to process the insurance claim. When the insurance claim is completed, a note is entered on the insurance claim form stating that the patient's signature is on file, giving permission to release information to the insurance carrier to process the claim.

Tracing Claims

A claims register, also referred to as an insurance log, is a method of keeping track of claims submitted to an insurance carrier. A claims register keeps track of information such as:

- date the original claim was submitted
- name of the primary insurance carrier
- name of the patient
- amount billed to the insurance carrier
- amount paid by the insurance carrier
- date claim sent to secondary insurance carrier
- name of secondary insurance carrier
- amount billed to secondary insurance carrier
- amount paid by secondary insurance carrier
- follow-up

A claims register can be customized to track the information needed by the individual medical office.

Sequence of Filing Primary or Secondary

Primary insurance coverage is usually provided through the insurance carrier in which an individual is enrolled. Secondary insurance coverage, usually provided as a result of being a dependent on someone else's insurance plan, applies only after the primary insurance plan has exhausted the amount of coverage provided.

Insurance carriers use primary and secondary insurance plans to coordinate benefits, allowing the maximum of 100 percent to be paid on any claim. Coordination of benefits (COB) is used by insurance carriers to avoid duplication of payments for the same service or procedure.

Even with a primary and a secondary insurance, 100% of the bill may not be covered, and some plans will require that the patient to pay the remainder or a portion of the bill. Each insurance plan has specific rules for reimbursement amounts. When both parents of a minor child have insurance coverage, the birthday rule is a method used to determine the primary insurance carrier. The birthday rule states that the parent whose birthday falls first in the year is the primary insurance carrier for the child.

Reconciling Payments

Although the claims register is helpful to keep track of the insurance claims sent to the insurance carriers, the remittance advice sent by the insurance carrier to the physician's offices summarizes all the benefits paid to the provider for the claims submitted. The remittance advice itemizes:

- charges sent to insurance carrier for a specific date of service
- amount allowed by insurance carrier
- any disallowed amount such as prearranged agreements with the physician in HMO insurance plans or capitated plans
- patient's portion, such as co-pay, co-insurance, or deductibles, if any
- amount of payment sent to the physician

An explanation of benefits (EOB) is a report sent to the patient from his or her insurance carrier itemizing the benefits paid for services provided on a specific date. Assignment of benefits is a method used by the insurance carrier to determine to whom the payment will be sent. If a patient accepts assignment, the payment will be sent to the physician's office, and the patient will receive an EOB itemizing the payment made to the physician on his or her behalf. If the patient does not accept assignment, the payment will be sent to the beneficiary, usually the patient. The medical office then bills the patient for the amount due for the services provided.

Inquiry and Appeal Process

Even with the careful collection of patient data, detailed completion of insurance claims, and proper coding, claims may not be received or may be rejected by the insurance carrier. The claims register is helpful to identify claims that are not processed in a timely manner.

Electronic claims may be paid within a week or two, while paper claims take longer to process. Each insurance carrier has a statute of limitations for payment consideration. If the medical assistant does not submit the claim within the specified time period, the insurance carrier will not honor the claim and no reimbursement will be made for that date of service. The patient cannot be billed for the charges due, and the medical office will have to write off the amount owed to the office.

If payment is denied on a submitted claim, the medical office may appeal the decision of the insurance company. The remittance advice lists a code justifying the denial, which may help in determining the problem. Many times the denial is caused by a violation of the terms of the insurance policy—for example, a yearly physical that was done too early in an annual cycle. Sometimes, a simple administrative error—such as an inaccurately recorded policy number—may be the cause.

Applying Managed Care Policies

The medical assistant is responsible for being aware of the policies of managed care health plans and should be able to apply the required policies. If referral from the primary care physician to a specialist is required, the medical assistant should facilitate the referral process for the patient.

Also, when a primary care physician refers a patient to a specialist, many insurance carriers require that the patient obtain precertification, or preauthorization, to obtain approval for the appointment. If the treatment or procedure is approved, a preauthorization number will be given as documentation that the procedure was approved. The patient must bring the preauthorization number and the completed form listing the approved treatment or procedure to his or her appointment.

Because each insurance carrier has its own policy, the medical assistant should keep a log or file listing requirements for obtaining referrals and preauthorizations from frequently used insurance carriers.

Fee Schedules

Fees, insurance coverage, and required patient payments should be discussed when a new patient calls to make an appointment. Having a clear understanding of financial responsibility can help avoid any misunderstandings in the patient-physician relationship, and many offices provide brochures discussing the financial policies of the medical facility. One of the most important steps in billing is finding out who is the guarantor, or the person responsible for paying the medical bill.

Usual, customary, and reasonable (UCR) rates are terms sometimes used in developing a fee schedule.

- The **usual** fee represents the average fee a physician charges for a service or procedure.
- The **customary** fee is the average fee charged by a provider in a specific geographical area for a specific service or procedure.
- The **reasonable** fee is the fee charged for an exceptionally difficult or complex procedure requiring more time and effort on the part of a provider.

Relative value studies create a unit value for every medical procedure in order to develop a fair and accurate fee schedule. Malpractice expenses, medical practice expenses, and the effort needed by the provider to perform each procedure are taken into consideration when developing a fair and accurate fee schedule.

Resource-based relative value scale (RBRVS) is a formula used to calculate reimbursement amounts for various procedures based on resources involved in providing services rather than on fees charged by providers in the past. Every procedure, service, and medication is given a CPT code based on the amount of time, effort, and physical and technical skill needed to perform each procedure. The RBRVS formula is adjusted for geographical areas, and an amount is calculated for payment of each procedure.

Diagnostically related groups (DRGs) are used in a **hospital inpatient prospective payment system (IPPS).** DRGs are divided into 467 illness categories, and each illness is given an ICD code. Reimbursement is based on the assumption that all patients in the same DRG category will experience the same symptoms and need the same care. In an effort to control healthcare spending, an average of the expenses incurred by the patients in a specific DRG is determined, and the inpatient facility is then reimbursed the average expense, not the actual cost of the hospitalization.

Contracted fees apply to managed care organizations in which a provider participating in an HMO agrees to provide his or her services for a fixed payment. When the HMO member visits the physician, the claim form is sent to the HMO, and reimbursement is made to the physician at the agreed-upon amount.

Payment arrangements: Because not all patients have medical insurance, and medical insurance may not cover all expenses incurred during treatment, some patients may have difficulty paying their bills.

Medical practices offer various options to help patients in these circumstances.

- **Payment plans:** If fewer than four payments are necessary, no formal document is required; if more than four payments are necessary, a formal loan arrangement between the office and the patient may be agreed upon.
- **Pre-planned monthly payments** may be accepted for prenatal care and the delivery of a baby.
- **Credit card payments** allow the patient to pay the physician and then manage the expense through his or her credit card company.
- **Special agreements:** Many physicians will agree to adjust a fee or past-due balance for a patient with limited income or for an established patient who is having a difficult time financially.

Accounting and Banking Procedures

The medical assistant may be responsible for handling some of the accounting and banking procedures performed in the medical office.

Accounts Receivable

The term *accounts receivable* refers to the amount of money owed to the medical offices for services provided. Most patients have some type of health insurance that covers a portion of an office visit. The patient may pay a co-pay at the time of service, while the remainder of the amount due is submitted to the insurance carrier for reimbursement. The amount owed on the patient account is part of accounts receivable until it is paid. Accounts receivable are tracked either with a computer program or with the manual pegboard system.

Billing Procedures

Adequate cash flow in the medical office depends on up-to-date billing practices and policies of the medical office. It is important to collect payments promptly, because the more time that has elapsed since the date of service provided, the more difficult it may be to collect payment from a patient. Billing procedures include preparing an itemized statement of all current patient charges, co-pays or payments made at the time of service, payments made by the insurance carrier, and the balance remaining for the patient to pay.

Billing statements should be sent to patients at regular intervals so that patients may budget appropriately. Many offices use a once-a-month billing system. Cycle billing, which allows the office to divide the accounts into sections and then bill each section every so many days, can allow patients to receive bills on a monthly basis, but spreads out the work involved in billing over a longer time period.

Aging of accounts identifies the length of time an account has been overdue and begins from the time the first billing statement is sent to the patient. If the bill is not paid within 30 days, it is referred to as 30 days old; if not paid within 60 days, it is considered 60 days old; and so forth. Some offices may choose to send the overdue bill to a collection agency; however, the medical office should advise the patient first of its intention to do so.

Accounts Payable

Accounts payable are the bills or amounts of money owed to others for services or supplies purchased with credit. The medical office has financial responsibilities just like any other business: supplies, maintenance of equipment, utility and telephone bills, payroll, and various types of insurance payments. The medical assistant may be responsible for managing the accounts payable. Some elements in tracking accounts payable are:

- **Purchase orders:** numbered forms to be completed for all ordered supplies; they help to keep track of items purchased, to prevent unauthorized purchasing of items, and to provide a system for payment of items received.
- **Packing slips:** detailed lists that come with delivered packages of the items shipped; they do not contain a bill or invoice. The packing slip should be compared to the original purchase order to be

sure all items listed on the packing slip match the list on the original purchase order and have been included in the delivered package.

- **Invoices**, or **bills:** A record of the charges for items or services delivered, which implies a request for payment. The invoice arrives shortly after the package arrives. When a check for the invoice is sent, the date, check number, and the amount paid should be recorded on the invoice before it is filed, making it easy to verify payment information if needed.

Banking Procedures

Banking procedures that the medical assistant may perform include receiving checks from patients and preparing deposit slips, preparing checks against accounts payable for the physician or another authorized person, to sign, and balancing the checkbook.

Receiving Checks

Patients use different types of checks when paying for services. These include:

- **Personal check:** Personal checks are the most frequently used type of check in the medical office, as most patients use personal checks to pay all their expenses.
- **Money order:** A money order is purchased for a specific amount. It is a guarantee that the amount shown on the check is available for use. Patients who do not want to send cash and do not have a checking account often use money orders for payments.
- **Traveler's check:** A traveler's check may be purchased in different denominations such as $10, $20, and $50. A signature is needed when the checks are purchased and when used. Although not too commonly used for payments to the medical office, they may be accepted.
- **Cashier's check:** A cashier's check is a bank's own check. It is prepared by the bank after receiving payment from the purchaser. Cashier's checks are guaranteed for the amount written.

- **Certified check:** A certified check is the patient's personal check that the bank has cleared or "certified." A certified check guarantees that sufficient funds are available and cannot be withdrawn for any other use.

Preparing the Deposit Slip

Deposit slips should be prepared and deposited into the bank daily. Checks received from patients should be endorsed immediately. An endorsement is a signature used to legally transfer a check to the bank in exchange for cash. A stamp marked "Pay to the order of," listing the name of the bank where the deposit will be made, followed by the physician's name, is the safest type of endorsement.

At the end of the business day, the cash and checks received are entered in the appropriate columns of the deposit slip, along with the date at the top. The deposit slip should be tallied carefully and double-checked for accuracy. Many offices use deposit slips that are duplicate so that a copy may be given to the bank and a copy may be kept for documentation of the deposit date and amount.

Guidelines for Check Writing

If the practice uses a computerized accounting system, checks should be prepared and printed on the computer; otherwise, write legibly, and follow these guidelines.

- Enter the correct date on the appropriate line.
- Be sure the numeric and written amounts match.
- Start writing the amount to be paid on the far left of the line provided. Draw a line after the written amount to cross out the unused portion of the line; this practice will prevent any unauthorized additions.
- Be sure to enter the correct name of the payee, using correct spelling.
- Be sure the check is signed before placing it in the envelope for mailing.
- Complete the check register, which is the record of all checks written, marking in the date, the check number, the name of the payee, and the amount

of the check. If the practice uses a one-write system, the information will transfer automatically to the register pages. Subtract the amount of the check from the balance amount in the checkbook.

Employee Payroll

The employee payroll can be prepared on a computer or on a manual pegboard system. If prepared manually, a separate card or page is prepared for each employee. Government regulations require the completion of certain documents and periodic reporting of earned income for each employee. These records must be kept for a minimum of four years. Information that is required includes:

- Social Security number of the employee
- gross amount of paycheck
- number of withholdings allowances claimed
- deductions for social security
- deductions for Medicare taxes, as well as state and federal taxes
- deductions for state disability insurance and state unemployment tax, where applicable

New employees must complete an Employee's Withholding Allowance Certificate (W-4), listing the number of withholding allowances claimed. Employees must complete a new form each time changes occur in their allowances, such as a marriage or a change in the number of dependants. More money will be taken out for taxes when the number of withholding claims is lower.

Employers are required to withhold income tax from the employee's earnings for payment to the IRS; the amount withheld is based on the number of claims the employee reports on his or her W-4. Employers must also withhold money from the employees' earnings for Federal Insurance Contribution Act (FICA) payments, which employers must match in an equal amount. Once paid to the government, the money is held in a trust fund and provides for the employee's Medicare coverage, retirement income, disability insurance, and benefits for survivors.

Practice Questions

1. The process of preparing documents by converting dictated physician notes into written documents is called
   a. typing.
   b. transcription.
   c. modified block.
   d. outsourcing.
   e. memoranda.

2. Which of the following would be the best salutation to use in a letter sent to a doctor?
   a. Yours truly,
   b. Dear Dr. Smith,
   c. Best regards,
   d. Sincerely,
   e. Dear Mark,

3. Which type of letter format aligns all lines flush with the left-hand margin except the dateline, complimentary closing line, and signature line?
   a. simplified
   b. full-block
   c. modified-block
   d. indented
   e. modified indented

4. Which of the following activities involves data processing?
   a. entering data
   b. updating archives
   c. maintaining data
   d. updating data
   e. all of the above

5. Which one of the following is concerned with patient confidentiality?
   a. OSHA
   b. DEA
   c. JCAHO
   d. CAAHEP
   e. HIPAA

6. Which of the following is a type of temporary memory?
   a. read-only memory
   b. random-access memory
   c. data storage memory
   d. CD-ROM
   e. monitor

7. Which printer produces the best quality printout?
   a. laser
   b. dot matrix
   c. inkjet
   d. toner
   e. default

8. Which device protects a computer from electrical damage?
   a. central processing unit
   b. modem
   c. surge protector
   d. motherboard
   e. cursor

9. All of the following are examples of hardware EXCEPT
   a. keyboard.
   b. printer.
   c. monitor.
   d. spreadsheet.
   e. central processing unit.

10. What part of the computer is responsible for allowing the computer to perform all operations?
   a. modem
   b. monitor
   c. flash drive
   d. central processing unit
   e. keyboard

11. Data storage devices include all of the following EXCEPT
   a. flash drive.
   b. CPU.
   c. CDs.
   d. CD-R.
   e. CD-RW.

12. Outguides are
   a. placeholders used to help in keeping track of medical records.
   b. used in file cabinets to separate the letters of the alphabet.
   c. completed every time the medical record is removed from the file cabinet.
   d. sources of available patient services in the community.
   e. all of the above

13. Which of the following choices is NOT a main type of filing system used in the medical office?
   a. diseases
   b. numeric
   c. alphabetic
   d. subject
   e. last name

14. The alphabetic filing system breaks down patient names into which of the following indexing units?
   a. Unit 1: first name; Unit 2: last name; Unit 3: middle name; Unit 4: title, if needed
   b. Unit 1: last name; Unit 2: first name; Unit 3: middle name; Unit 4: title, if needed
   c. Unit 1: middle name; Unit 2: first name; Unit 3: title, if needed; Unit 4: last name
   d. Unit 1: middle initial; Unit 2: last name; Unit 3: middle name; Unit 4: title, if needed
   e. Unit 1: Jr. or Sr.; Unit 2: last name; Unit 3: first name; Unit 4: middle initial

15. Which of the following is not a subjective symptom?
   a. backache
   b. dizziness
   c. stomach cramps
   d. fever
   e. chest pain

16. Who owns a patient's medical record?
   a. The patient owns the actual paper medical record and the information it contains.
   b. The information in the record is owned by the patient, but the patient does not own the paper record.
   c. The physician or facility that created the record owns the paper medical record and the information it contains.
   d. The actual paper medical record is owned by the physician or facility that created it.
   e. The patient owns information in the record, and the actual paper medical record is owned by the physician or facility that created it.

17. Medical records are used for all of the following reasons EXCEPT
   a. for research.
   b. for legal documentation.
   c. to determine patterns signaling patient needs.
   d. to keep track of patients' financial transactions.
   e. to manage patient care.

18. An advantage of electronic medical records (EMR) is that
   a. they are easy for all medical personnel to use.
   b. they are inexpensive to maintain.
   c. they are available quickly in emergency situations.
   d. their passwords do not need to be changed.
   e. they can be used by only one user at a time.

19. Which of the following is the best method for correcting an error in a paper medical record?
   a. Neatly cover the error with correction fluid so that the correct information can be entered.
   b. Draw a double line through the error in red ink.
   c. Draw a line through the error in red ink, and write "error" on the red line, covering the incorrect entry.
   d. Draw a line through the error in red ink, and sign your full name, date the entry, and write the time that the error was corrected.
   e. Draw a single line through the error with red ink, and write your initials and the date near the correction.

20. A "release" mark is made by the physician on a medical record in order to
   a. determine the indexing units of the item to be filed.
   b. indicate that the item is ready to be filed.
   c. tell the medical assistant to inspect all items before they can be filed.
   d. indicate the cross-reference information on an item to be filed.
   e. indicate that the item should not be filed.

21. Medical records are classified as
   a. closed, open, or miscellaneous.
   b. incomplete, active, or closed.
   c. closed, active, or inactive.
   d. inactive, open, or active.
   e. incomplete, inactive, or active.

22. Which type of filing system offers the most privacy for medical records?
   a. subject
   b. numeric
   c. chronological
   d. alphabetical
   e. indexed

23. Advantages of the numeric filing system include which of the following?
   a. It expands easily.
   b. It uses an alphabetic card system.
   c. No patient names are listed on the record.
   d. It is always arranged by color-coded file folders.
   e. both **a** and **c**

24. Place the following medical records in alphabetic order:

1. Scoville	Francis	J	Sr.
2. Scoville	Frances	J	
3. Scoville	Francis	J	III
4. Scoville	Francis	J	Jr.

   a. 1, 2, 3, 4
   b. 3, 1, 4, 2
   c. 4, 1, 3, 2
   d. 2, 3, 4, 1
   e. 2, 1, 3, 4

25. If a medical record were numbered 24-73-89, which group of numbers would be the primary unit when using terminal digit numeric filing?
   a. 24
   b. 89
   c. 73
   d. always the lowest number
   e. always the highest number

26. The fastest way to mail a letter using the U.S. Postal Service is
   a. first-class mail.
   b. media mail.
   c. priority mail.
   d. certified mail.
   e. express mail.

27. Notations on letters such as "special delivery" or "certified" would be typed
   a. directly below the return address.
   b. directly below the stamp.
   c. in the lower right-hand corner of the letter.
   d. in the lower left-hand corner of the letter.
   e. directly above the city and state listed in the address.

28. The correct USPS abbreviation for the state of Maine is
   a. MA.
   b. MI.
   c. M.A.
   d. M.E.
   e. ME.

29. Which of the following patient information is not essential for a medical assistant to obtain when taking a phone message?
   a. full name
   b. type of insurance
   c. daytime telephone number
   d. reason for the call
   e. action requested

30. Which of the following is an acceptable greeting for a medical assistant to use when answering the phone?
   a. "Dr. Green's office. Cindi speaking. How may I help you?"
   b. "Ellen speaking. How may I help you?"
   c. "Doctor's office."
   d. "Good morning. How may I help you?"
   e. "Who is calling, please?"

31. Telephone personality is important for all of the following reasons EXCEPT
   a. it can make a patient feel welcome to hear a friendly voice.
   b. the call the patient is making may be his or her first exposure to the office, and making a good first impression is important.
   c. it guarantees return patient visits.
   d. it will make the patient more relaxed in his or her dealings with the office.
   e. it will create a positive patient-office relationship.

32. Calls that can be handled by the medical assistant include all of the following EXCEPT
   a. favorable patient progress reports.
   b. describing general medical office information and policies.
   c. providing medical advice to patients.
   d. handling requests for appointments.
   e. providing prescription renewal information.

33. Which of the following patients should not be put on hold?
   a. a patient with a return migraine headache
   b. a patient with an elevated temperature of 100°F
   c. a patient with difficulty breathing
   d. a patient who has had an earache since yesterday, which is now causing moderate pain
   e. a patient who has a moth fluttering around in his ear

34. Annotating consists of
   a. jotting down notes in the letter margins.
   b. a reminder of an action to be taken.
   c. making a "release mark."
   d. both a and b
   e. both b and c

35. If the following patients arrived at the same time to a walk-in center, which patient should be seen first?
   a. a 35-year-old female with a sore throat for two days
   b. a 55-year-old male with a poison ivy rash on his arms
   c. a 56-year-old male with dyspnea
   d. a 14-year-old male with a swollen ankle
   e. an 82-year-old female with anorexia and confusion

36. Which type of scheduling system books three patients at the beginning of each hour?
    a. double booking
    b. stream
    c. modified wave
    d. clustering
    e. wave

37. Which of the following situations should be recorded in the patient's medical record?
    a. An established patient reschedules appointment.
    b. An established patient makes an appointment.
    c. An established patient cancels an appointment.
    d. An established patient is a "no show."
    e. both **c** and **d**

38. Which of the following entries would be included when setting up the matrix in an appointment book?
    a. entering patient names in appointment slots
    b. placing an "X" through vacation days in red ink
    c. marking off times the physician will be seeing patients
    d. placing an "X" through vacation days in pencil
    e. all of the above

39. The most important principle of scheduling is
    a. flexibility in scheduling.
    b. strict adherence to the schedule is mandatory.
    c. educating patients about the importance of being on time for appointments.
    d. emergency situations take priority.
    e. both **a** and **d**

40. Entries in the appointment book should be done in pencil because
    a. the appointment book is a legal document that can be used in court.
    b. it is easier to erase no-show appointments when the entries are in pencil.
    c. using pencil is less expensive than using ink.
    d. it is easier to change appointments when the entries are in pencil.
    e. all of the above

41. Which of the following is the method used by insurance carriers to determine the primary insurance for a dependent child of a married couple?
    a. explanation of benefits
    b. birthday rule
    c. coordination of benefits
    d. remittance advice
    e. encounter form

42. Which of the following is the insurance program that provides healthcare to individuals, regardless of age, whose income is insufficient to meet medical expenses?
    a. CHAMPUS
    b. CHAMPVA
    c. Medicare
    d. Medicaid
    e. TRICARE

43. Which of the following describes a check endorsement?
    a. the signature of the person who wrote the check
    b. the signature of the person to whom the check is written
    c. the signature from the bank that provided the check
    d. the recording of the check onto the patient's ledger card
    e. the amount of the check entered on the deposit slip

44. What is the maximum number of digits that can be used in the ICD-9-CM coding system?
   a. two digits
   b. three digits
   c. four digits
   d. five digits
   e. six digits

45. Common reasons for a Medicare-participating physician's insurance claims to be rejected include all of the following reasons EXCEPT
   a. ICD-9-CM codes are incomplete.
   b. the diagnosis and procedure codes do not match.
   c. the fee charged for the procedure is more than the insurance company will pay.
   d. the claim uses an incorrect ID number.
   e. the patient's date of birth is incorrect.

46. Which of the following is a network of physicians and hospitals that contract with insurance companies to provide discounted healthcare?
   a. group practice
   b. walk-in center
   c. POS plan
   d. PPO plan
   e. HMO plan

47. A physician who does not accept an assignment
   a. writes off the difference between the charge and the medical payment.
   b. is paid directly by Medicare.
   c. must bill the patient for the services rendered.
   d. receives 50% of the physician's charge.
   e. is not entitled to receive any payment.

48. Which of the following is insurance coverage for persons injured on the job?
   a. Medicaid
   b. TRICARE
   c. workers' compensation
   d. patient disability insurance
   e. self-insurance

49. How many major sections does the Current Procedural Terminology (CPT) book have?
   a. four
   b. five
   c. six
   d. seven
   e. eight

50. Which section of the CPT book is used to code regular office visits?
   a. medicine
   b. surgery
   c. pathology
   d. evaluation and management
   e. laboratory

51. Which section of the CPT book is used to code lacerations?
   a. medicine
   b. surgery
   c. pathology
   d. evaluation and management
   e. laboratory

52. Which form may be used to help the medical assistant keep track of insurance claims once they have been sent to the insurance carrier?
   a. a POS device
   b. a claims register
   c. a claim form
   d. an EOB
   e. a pegboard

53. Which form is sent by the insurance carrier to the physician's office, usually with a reimbursement check explaining processed claims?
   a. a POS device
   b. a remittance advice
   c. an EOB
   d. a 1490 form
   e. an assignment of benefits

54. Which of the following will result when a physician's office consistently uses a service level of coding higher than what was actually performed?
   a. The wrong diagnosis may be coded.
   b. The office may be underpaid.
   c. The office may be charged with criminal fraud.
   d. The office may be charged with libel.
   e. The medical assistant may be put into a higher tax bracket.

55. Which of the following is another name for a non-duplication of benefits clause?
   a. coordination of benefits
   b. major medical
   c. catastrophic coverage
   d. co-payment
   e. service benefit plan

56. A period of non-coverage for an illness that existed prior to the issuance of a health insurance policy is called a
   a. preexisting condition.
   b. premium.
   c. special risk rider.
   d. waiting period.
   e. prior authorization.

57. Under Medicare, a retired couple has to pay an annual deductible
   a. per illness.
   b. per every admission.
   c. for both individuals.
   d. every fifteen months.
   e. every six months.

58. Which of the following actions may be taken once a patient account has been turned over to a collection agency?
   a. Reduce the bill by the commission fee and continue billing.
   b. Reduce the bill by the commission fee and discontinue billing.
   c. Continue billing.
   d. Discontinue billing.
   e. Continue billing and add calling the patient to the attempts to collect the overdue bill.

59. Which of the following is NOT an aspect or part of a one-write bookkeeping system?
   a. day sheet
   b. ledger card
   c. explanation of benefits
   d. encounter form
   e. pegboard

60. Which of the following would be an accepted way to end the patient-physician relationship?
   a. refusing further appointments when a patient calls
   b. sending a certified letter explaining the decision to end the relationship and giving the patient ample opportunity to find another physician
   c. denying treatment to the patient and refusing his or her phone calls until the patient decides to move elsewhere for care
   d. having the medical assistant notify the patient by phone that the patient-physician relationship is over
   e. canceling arrangements with the patient's insurance carrier

61. Employee payroll deduction information that must be kept for four years includes all of the following EXCEPT
   a. employee's Social Security number.
   b. gross amount of paycheck.
   c. employee's job description.
   d. deductions for social security.
   e. deductions for Medicare taxes and state and federal taxes.

62. Safety measures in a medical office that a medical assistant may take to safeguard controlled substances include all of the following EXCEPT
   a. keeping controlled substances hidden in the back of the supply closet.
   b. keeping controlled substances under double-lock and key.
   c. keeping prescription blanks in a drawer and safely away from unauthorized individuals.
   d. keeping the key to the locked controlled substances container out of view.
   e. keeping a daily record of the controlled substance amounts at the beginning of the day and at the close of office hours.

63. All the following are part of the tools useful in tracking accounts payable EXCEPT
   a. a purchase order.
   b. a deposit slip.
   c. a packing slip.
   d. an invoice, or bill, from a vendor.
   e. payments to vendors.

Answers and Explanations

1. b. Transcription is the process of preparing accurate, formatted reports by converting physician-dictated notes into written documents. Typing is the process of using a piece of equipment such as a typewriter or computer keyboard to produce documents. Modified block is a letter-writing format. Outsourcing is a newer trend of larger medical facilities to send out paperwork to other companies that specialize in transcription.

2. b. *Dear Dr. Smith* is an appropriate salutation for a physician; first names should not be used. *Best regards*, *Yours truly*, and *Sincerely* are all examples of complimentary closings.

3. c. The modified-block format aligns all lines with the left margin of the paper, except for the date line, the complimentary closing line, and the signature line, which are centered on the page. Indented modified-block follows the style for modified-block, but with the first line of each paragraph indented five spaces. All lines are aligned with the left margin of the paper when using full-block formatting. The simplified format aligns all lines flush with the left margin of the paper and omits the salutation and the complimentary closing.

4. e. Data processing, or data entry, is the conversion of data into a form that can be used by a computer. It includes entering, updating, and maintaining information on a computer system, including data contained in archives.

5. e. The Health Insurance Portability and Accountability Act (HIPAA) is the federal legislation that regulates safeguards regarding the privacy of health information. Occupational Safety and Health Administration (OSHA) is a federal agency concerned with safety issues in the workplace. The Joint Commission on Accreditation of Healthcare Organizations (JCAHO) is an organization designed to improve healthcare in medical facilities. The Drug Enforcement Administration (DEA) oversees controlled drugs. CAAHEP stands for Commission on the Accreditation of Allied Health Education Programs.

6. b. Random-access memory is the temporary storage capacity of a computer system and is erased when the computer is turned off or if there is a power failure. A monitor is the computer screen and has nothing to do with saving data entered into the computer. Read-only memory and data storage memory are permanent types of memory. A CD-R has the ability to read data and allows data to be entered, but that data cannot then be erased or changed once the disc is burned.

7. a. The laser printer, although more expensive than the inkjet and the dot matrix, produces the best quality printout. Toner is the ink used by computers. The term *default printer* refers to the primary printer used by the computer.

8. c. A surge protector is a device used to help prevent damage caused by a sudden rise of current or increased voltage flowing into electrical equipment. The central processing unit (CPU) of a computer allows the computer to perform basic operations. The motherboard is a circuit board that allows all computer parts to communicate with one another. A modem is a device that converts electronic signals and then allows them to travel across telephone or cable lines. A cursor is a device used to point to a specific area on the computer screen.

9. d. Hardware consists of devices that are connected to the computer such as a printer, monitor, keyboard, and central processing unit. Spreadsheet software is a type of computer program that runs on the hardware.

10. d. The central processing unit (CPU) allows the computer to perform all functions. The monitor is the computer screen. The modem is used to transmit signals across telephone or cable lines. The keyboard is the unit resembling a typewriter; it allows typed information to enter the computer by sending electrical signals when the keys are pushed.

11. b. The CPU, or central processing unit, allows the computer to perform basic functions. It does not store data. The flash drive, CD, CD-R, and CD-RW are all storage devices.

12. a. Outguides are placeholders used to keep track of medical records. Although patient records should be returned to the file cabinet after use, they are sometimes removed by the physician or another team member for extended use. To help keep track of the record, an outguide temporarily replaces the record, listing the date the record was removed, by whom, and an estimated date of return. Outguides are used only when the file is removed for an extended period of time. They are not used on a daily basis. Divider guides are used to separate sections of files.

13. a. Alphabetic, numeric, and subject are filing systems commonly used in the medical office. The term *diseases* could be used as a subcategory in the subject filing system, but it is not the name of a filing system. A database is a way to organize the information, not files, in a medical office.

14. b. Alphabetic filing based on patient names uses the last name as Unit 1, followed by the patient's legal first name as Unit 2, his or her middle initial or middle name as Unit 3, and any titles such as Jr., Sr., III, Mrs. John, MD, and so on as Unit 4.

15. d. A fever is measurable by taking the patient's temperature, so it is not considered a subjective symptom. A subjective symptom is a symptom that only the patient experiences, such as a dizziness, stomach cramps, chest pain, or a backache, and that cannot be seen or measured by others.

16. e. The law states that whoever created the medical record, which is considered a piece of property, owns it. So the facility that created the medical record owns the actual paper medical record. The patient owns the information contained in the medical record and is entitled to receive a copy of any or all information in the medical record.

17. d. Financial transactions are not part of the patient's medical record. The medical record can contain a listing of the patient's employer, insurance carrier, and insurance identification number, but it does not list any charges or payments made to the office for treatment. The medical record can be used as legal documentation to provide protection to the patient and the medical staff in cases of lawsuits. It is important to have accurate and complete documentation of all missed appointments, no-shows, and all other pertinent information in the medical record. By keeping a continual record of the patient's medical care, patterns of illness, for example, can be detected and signal a need for the physician's intervention in managing the problem.

18. c. One advantage of electric medical records is that they are easily available in emergency situations. However, EMRs are expensive to establish and maintain. Also, it can takes staff members weeks or even months to feel comfortable using this system. Security issues are always a problem for computer systems and passwords for the EMR system, passwords would need to be changed frequently in order to minimize the chances of a breach in security.

19. e. Draw a single line through the error with red ink. The medical record is a legal document, and correction fluid should never be used to correct the error. The error should not be scribbled out, but remain readable. Only your initials and the date the error was corrected are needed, not your full name or the time.

20. b. A release mark (usually consisting of the physician's initials) is placed on the medical record by the physician to indicate that he or she has seen, read, and approved the item for filing. The physician's initials serve as a safety check in order to prevent any unread items, such as test results, for example, from being filed.

21. c. Medical records are classified as active, inactive, or closed. Active files include patients currently being treated in the office. Inactive files are records of patients who have not been treated in the office recently. Closed files are records that will not become active again—for example, because the patient is deceased.

22. b. Numeric filing systems offer the most privacy for patients because there are no names on the file folders, only numbers. An alphabetic file system shows the patient's name on the folder tab, which would not allow the maximum amount of privacy. Although new patient medical records are added to the numeric filing system in chronological order, meaning every new patient is added on to the last record in the system, a chronological filing system would include the patient's name and not offer maximum privacy for the patients. *Indexed* is a term that refers to a system for ordering terms or records alphabetically.

23. e. Advantages of the numeric filing system include easy expansion and the fact that there are no patient names listed on the record. Adding new records after the last record is an easy way to expand files, rather than having to move them to alleviate overcrowding in certain sections, as is often necessary with alphabetical files. Since numeric files have no names on the outside of the record, only numbers, the patient's privacy is maintained. Numeric files are not always arranged using color coding and even when they are, color-coded file folders are not commonly used. The extra step of locating the patient's name in an alphabetic card system takes time and is considered a disadvantage of the numeric system.

24. d. All the last names are the same, so Unit 2 is the next consideration when filing in alphabetic order. Frances with an "e" comes before Francis with an "i", so 2 comes first alphabetically. Numbers come before letters, which makes 3 the next to be filed. The letter "J" comes before "S," placing 4 before 1. The correct order is 2, 3, 4, 1.

25. b. If a medical record were numbered 24-73-89, then it would be filed using 89. In terminal digit filing, the last group of digits, the terminal or end digits, are considered the primary digits and are considered first when filing using this method.

26. e. Express mail will get the item mailed to its destination overnight or by the second day of mail service. First-class mail takes a few days, and certified mail is sent by first-class mail. Mail media refers to mailing films or videos and requires one to two weeks, while priority mail takes two to three days.

27. b. Notations on letters such as "special delivery" or "certified" should be typed directly below the stamp and typed in all uppercase letters. Nothing should be typed in the lower corners of the envelope because that space is left available for bar codes when the letter is read by an OCR scanner.

28. e. ME is the correct USPS abbreviation for the state of Maine. State abbreviations need to be two capital letters with no punctuation in order to be read by the OCR scanner.

29. b. Although the type of insurance would be considered essential information when scheduling an appointment, it is not needed when taking a message. The patient's full name is necessary in case any information needs to be obtained from the medical record. The daytime phone number is needed in case the office needs to change or cancel an appointment. (Because many patients are not at home during the day, the home number may not be sufficient.) The reason for the call and the action the patient requests are both essential to fulfilling the request of the patient.

30. a. The greeting should include the name of the practice or the names of the physicians in the practice, the first name of the person answering the phone, and a pleasant offer of help. Providing the name of the practice will let the patient know if the call was made to the correct office. Providing the name of the person answering the phone makes the call more personal and welcoming to the patient. It also allows the patient refer back to the medical assistant because the patient has been provided the medical assistant's name. Simply saying "Doctor's office" is too generic and does not assure the patient that the correct number was dialed.

31. c. Although a medical assistant with a pleasant telephone personality may help the patient feel more comfortable dealing with the office and the staff members, a pleasant telephone personality does not guarantee return visits. However, having a pleasant telephone personality is an important step in creating a positive office relationship.

32. c. Medical advice is not within the medical assistant's scope of knowledge. All questions about medical advice must be referred to the physician. The office policy manual in each office should list the types of calls medical assistants can handle and the types of calls that should be referred to the physician. Favorable patient progress reports; normal lab and test results; requests to schedule, reschedule, or cancel appointments; and gathering prescription refill information to be approved by the physician are some of the types of calls that may be handled by the medical assistant.

33. c. Difficulty breathing can be a life-threatening condition, and this patient should not be put on hold. After further questioning, a decision may be made to call 911 or to have the patient come into the office immediately. Certainly, further questioning would be needed in order to determine how much difficulty the patient is experiencing and how long this symptom has been present. An earache and a moth fluttering in the ear can be uncomfortable, but neither of these conditions is life threatening. Because the migraine headache is recurrent, the call needs to be attended to, but this condition is also not life threatening.

34. d. Annotating means jotting down notes in the margin of a letter as a reminder of an action needing to be done. It saves times because an annotated letter does not have to be reread in order to know what to do with it or how to follow up.

35. c. Of the patients listed as choices, the 56-year-old male with dyspnea should be seen first. Patients with breathing problems are considered to be in life-threatening situations, so they would be treated ahead of the other patients listed in this question. Although a severe poison ivy rash, if located on the face, could interfere with breathing, the poison ivy rash mentioned here is located on the patient's arms, and there is no mention of a breathing problem; although the rash may be uncomfortable, it is not life threatening. A severe sore throat could also cause swelling in the throat and, therefore, interfere with breathing, but because difficulty breathing was not given as a symptom here, this patient is not in a life-threatening situation. The swollen ankle, although uncomfortable, did not present as a compound fracture, so it is not considered life threatening. The elderly female's symptoms of anorexia and confusion, although important, do not signal an emergency.

36. e. Wave scheduling books three patients at the beginning of each hour. For example, using wave scheduling, three patients would be scheduled at ten A.M., another three patients would be scheduled at eleven A.M., and so on. Double-booking is scheduling two patients for every time slot, just in case one patient doesn't show up for his or her visit. The modified wave style gives two appointments on the hour and one appointment half past the hour. Clustering styles set aside blocks of time for patients with similar procedures or reasons for the visit, such as immunizations or a well-baby clinic.

37. e. Canceled appointments and no-show appointments need to be marked, preferably in red, in the paper appointment book or in a special section of the computer software system and should also be recorded in the patient record. It is up to the individual office whether this entry in the medical record is done in red ink, but it is essential that the date of the missed appointment is recorded. Since the medical record is a legal document, entries made in it can be used to document that a patient was noncompliant to the physician's request when he or she canceled his or her appointment without rescheduling or if he or she failed to show up for recommended medical care. If the patient decides to sue the physician because he or she did not get better, then the physician can show the court that the patient did not carry out his or her responsibility by keeping the recommended appointment. If a patient cancels an appointment but makes another appointment for a few days later, there is no need to record this information in the medical record. Also, information about scheduling an appointment is not needed in the medical record.

38. d. Setting up the matrix of an appointment book is the process of marking off, in pencil, the times the physician will not be available to see patients, the times the office will be closed, vacation days, medical meetings, or any other times when appointments should not be scheduled. Ink should not be used because the times marked off could change, and it would be difficult to remove the crossed-out sections, creating a messy, hard-to-read, appointment book.

39. e. The office must be flexible, rearranging appointments if an emergency arises to be sure acutely ill patients receive needed care. Being sensitive to the needs of others is critical in providing quality patient care.

40. d. Entries in the appointment book should be done in pencil, because it is then easier to change appointments. No-show appointments are not erased; rather, they are marked in red ink and also entered into the patient's medical record in order to serve as legal documentation that the patient was noncompliant to the physician's advice about seeking medical treatment. There is no significant cost difference between using pencil or pen.

41. b. The birthday rule is used by insurance carriers to determine the primary insurance for the dependent child of a married couple. An explanation of benefits is a form sent to the patient from his or her insurance carrier itemizing the benefits paid for services provided on a specific date. A remittance advice is sent to a healthcare provider itemizing benefits paid for patient services. Coordination of benefits is the method used by insurance carriers to avoid duplication of payments for the same service or procedure. The encounter form is generally used by physicians to itemize services provided to patients and is used to complete insurance claims.

42. d. Medicaid (Title XVIX) is the healthcare insurance program funded by state and federal government for low-income individuals, regardless of age. Champus, Champva, and Tricare are various types of government programs offering healthcare to active and retired military personnel and their families. Medicare (Title XVIII) is a government-sponsored program for individuals who are age 65 and older or who are under age 65 but disabled and unable to work.

43. b. A check endorsement is the signature of the person to whom the check was written. Before a check can be cashed by the bank, it must be endorsed.

44. d. Five digits are the maximum number that can be used when coding with the ICD-9-CM coding system. The first three digits describe the disease or illness, and the last two digits define the condition or disease, resulting in a code of the highest level of specificity.

45. c. Charging a fee higher than what the insurance company will pay for a procedure will not cause a claim to be rejected by the insurance company. The physician may charge the fee that he or she normally charges for a procedure, and Medicare will pay 80% of what they allow for the procedure. A Medicare-participating physician agrees to accept the payment that Medicare allows.

46. d. A network of physicians and hospitals that contract with insurance companies to provide discounted healthcare is called a preferred provider organization, or PPO. Patients are responsible for deductibles and coinsurance payments, and out-of-pocket expenses are less if the patient is treated by a physician in the PPO network. A group practice and a walk-in center are places for medical care, and either can operate as a PPO, if they choose. A point-of-service (POS) plan is an HMO plan that allows the member to choose a physician from a list of physicians who have previously agreed to the discounted payment schedule of the plan.

47. c. A physician who does not accept an assignment must bill the patient for the services rendered. The physician expects the patient to pay the amount charged.

48. c. Workers' compensation is federal and state insurance coverage for persons injured on the job. Medicaid is government insurance for low-income families and TRICARE is insurance for military veterans and their families. Patient disability insurance may cover short-term or long-term disability, but not those resulting from on-the-job injuries.

49. c. There are six major coding sections in the Current Procedural Terminology (CPT) book: 1. Evaluation and Management; 2. Anesthesia; 3. Surgery; 4. Radiology, Nuclear Medicine, and Diagnostic Ultrasound; 5. Pathology and Laboratory; and 6. Medicine. The last section is the index and is not counted as one of the major areas of coding.

50. d. Evaluation and management deals with office procedures, such as office visits for new and established patients. Surgery is used for surgical procedures, even those that occur outside of an inpatient setting. The medicine sections deals with procedures related to the various body systems, such as the cardiovascular, nervous, and pulmonary systems. Procedures may include an electrocardiogram for the cardiovascular system. Pathology and laboratory deals with specimen collection and processing laboratory tests performed on specimens and body fluids.

51. b. Surgery would be the section for lacerations because they would need to be sutured (stitches put in) and that procedure is considered to be surgery. The medicine sections deals with procedures related to the various body systems such as cardiovascular, nervous system, and pulmonary system. Procedures might include a pulmonary function or an electroencephalogram to measure brain waves. Pathology and laboratory deals with specimen collection and processing laboratory tests performed on specimens and body fluids.

52. b. The claims register keeps track of insurance claims sent to the insurance carrier. A point-of-service device allows direct communication between the physician's office and the insurance carrier to verify membership of a patient. The claim form is sent to the insurance carrier to request payment for medical service, and the claims register keeps track of insurance claims sent in. A point-of-service (POS) plan is an HMO plan that allows the member to choose a physician from a list of physicians who have previously agreed to the discounted payment schedule of the plan.

53. b. A remittance advice is the notification sent to the physician's offices that summarizes all the benefits paid to the provider for the claims submitted. Many times a check accompanies the remittance advice. An explanation of benefits is the report sent to the patient from his or her insurance carrier itemizing the benefits paid for services provided on a specific date. A point-of-service (POS) device allows direct communication between the physician's office and the insurance carrier, to verify membership of a patient with a particular insurance. The 1490 form is used to send in claims. Assignment of benefits is a method used by the insurance carrier to determine to whom the payment will be sent. If a patient accepts assignment, the payment will be sent to the physician's office.

54. c. Criminal fraud charges may be brought against the physician for consistently using a service level of coding higher than what was actually performed. The physician may receive more money, but it would have been obtained through illegal means. Libel is the writing of false statements, often with the effect of ruining an individual's reputation.

55. a. Coordination of benefits is another name for non-duplication of benefits. A coordination of benefits (COB) means that 100% of a medical bill will be paid by all the insurance policies that cover an individual patient. Major medical and catastrophic coverage are types of insurance policies for major illness. Co-payments are the set amounts a patient must pay at each medical visit.

56. d. A waiting period is a specified period of time that must pass before the insurance coverage may begin, usually because of pre-existing conditions. Examples of preexisting conditions include pregnancy or diabetes. Preauthorization means that the patient must have the preapproval of the insurance carrier before certain treatments or procedures may be done. Premiums are the payments made to keep the insurance active.

57. c. Under Medicare, each individual needs to pay a deductible every year before Medicare will reimburse medical care expenses.

58. d. Once a patient's account has been sent to a collection agency, billing should be discontinued because it is now up to the collection agency to collect the outstanding amount owed to the physician. Whatever amount the collection agency collects, it usually keeps about 40%–50%.

59. c. An explanation of benefits is a form sent to the patient from his or her insurance carrier itemizing the benefits paid for services provided on a specific date. It helps the patient understand what his or her insurance carrier covers for his or her medical treatment; it is not a part of the bookkeeping system of a medical office.

60. b. Sending a certified letter explaining the decision to end the relationship and giving ample opportunity to find another physician would be the proper way to end the patient-physician relationship. To deny the patient appointments or refuse to respond to phone calls from a patient may result in the charge of abandonment brought against the physician for failing to do his or her duty to provide medical care to an established patient. Notifying the patient by phone that the patient-physician relationship has been terminated will not provide the necessary documentation the physician needs to avoid an abandonment charge by the patient.

61. c. The employee's job description does not relate to payroll deductions and, therefore, does not fall under the four-year rule. The employee's gross paycheck amount and deductions for Social Security, Medicare taxes, and state and federal taxes must be kept, because that information may be needed to verify tax returns.

62. a. Keeping controlled substances hidden in the back of the supply closet is not a good security measure; they should instead be kept under double lock and key. According to the law, a record of the amounts of controlled substances must be counted before and after office hours in order to keep an accurate record of the drugs. Prescription blanks should not be left on the examination room's counter, on the physician's desk, or anywhere a patient may have access to the blanks.

63. b. A deposit slip is a record of checks deposited into the medical office's bank account. It is an important tool in keeping track of accounts receivable (payments due to come into the office), not in keeping track of accounts payable owed by the medical office.

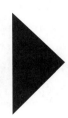

CHAPTER 5 ▶ CLINICAL PROCEDURES

CHAPTER SUMMARY

Clinical procedures are essential in a medical office. This chapter will review clinical procedures including infection control, procedures relating to the treatment area, patient preparation and assisting the physician, the patient history interview, diagnostic testing and collecting and processing specimens, preparing and administering medications, emergencies, first aid, and nutrition.

Infection Control

Infectious diseases, also called **communicable diseases**, are caused by microorganisms that may be transmitted directly or indirectly between individuals, causing infection. Infection control is an integral part of medical practice settings.

KEY PRINCIPLES OF INFECTION CONTROL

- hand washing before and after contact with patients
- separation of infected patients from the uninfected
- safe handling of needles and other sharp medical objects
- use of personal protection such as gloves
- sterilization and disinfection procedures

Infectious Disease

An infectious disease is caused by the presence of an **organism** in the body—specifically, a **pathogenic microorganism**, such as bacteria, viruses, parasites, or fungi—that grows and multiplies. **Microorganisms** are tiny living plants or animals that cannot be seen with the naked eye. Many different types of microorganisms exist in the environment; however, not all are connected to disease. **Pathogens** are microorganisms that are harmful to the body and cause disease; **nonpathogens** are harmless microorganisms and carry no risk of causing disease. Bacteria, viruses, fungi, and protozoa can act as both pathogens and nonpathogens.

Microorganisms that are considered nonpathogenic live normally on and in the human body and are known as **normal flora** or **resident flora**. A healthy balance of these microorganisms normally exists and provides protection from those microorganisms that are not part of the body's normal flora.

Normal flora exist in all places that are not sterile, including the mouth, throat, intestines, and vagina. As long as these microorganisms stay in the area of origin, they do not cause disease; they are nonpathogenic. The term *normal flora* refers to the microorganisms that are present even in the state of normal health. Such microorganisms are always present in the human body, and their number far exceeds the number of body cells. Normal flora perform many useful functions in the body, such as protection from highly pathogenic microorganisms, help in providing vitamins, and help in eliminating toxins. When normal flora are transmitted to an area of the body in which they are not normally found, they are called *transient flora*; they have become pathogens.

For example, a person may have the bacteria *Escherichia coli* growing in his or her gut. This bacteria is part of a person's necessary flora, because such bacteria provides an individual with vitamins that he or she needs to survive. But if *E. coli* gets into a person's urinary tract, then the person will end up with an infection. Women tend to get urinary tract infections more frequently than men because of the closeness of the anus to the urethra in the female body.

To grow and thrive, most pathogens require nutrients, moisture, warmth, and a suitable (usually neutral) pH environment. Some parts of the human body tend to provide a more hospitable environment for pathogenic growth than others do. Some pathogens, called **aerobic pathogens**, require oxygen for growth; those that must have an oxygen-free environment to thrive are called **anaerobic pathogens**. Eliminating the conditions required for growth is one way of reducing the transmission of the pathogens. For example, aerobic infections such as *Mycobacterium tuberculosis* require oxygen to multiply. Anaerobic infections usually happen in deep wounds; because of the decrease in capillaries, the level of oxygen is lowered in these wounds, making the environment friendly to the anaerobic pathogen.

Types of Pathogenic Microorganisms
Bacteria

Bacteria are single-celled microorganisms that reproduce via cell division, in which a mother cell divides into two identical daughter cells. Bacteria are able to live and grow outside a living host. Bacteria reproduce by cell division. Many bacteria produce spores to protect themselves under adverse conditions. A spore is a dormant type of bacteria that has formed a thick capsule around itself; it is highly resistant to heat or chemicals.

Except for spirochetes, bacterial infections are diagnosed by culture. A microbiological, or microbial, culture, allows microorganisms to reproduce in a controlled environment—a biological culture medium—in order to allow for the identification of the microbe.

Bacteria are unicellular and each type has its own characteristics. A characteristic of bacteria is that they grow into various shapes. When stained and viewed under the microscope, these shapes are used to identify the organism.

- A **coccus** is round or spherical in shape. They include staphylococci, streptococci, and diplococci. Cocci can arrange themselves in various ways such as in clusters, chains, or pairs. The prefix of the bacteria's name tells the arrangement.

  Staphylococci arrange in round clusters on skin and on mucous membranes. *Staphylococcus epidermidis* is usually nonpathogic; however, a cut, abrasion, or other break in the skin can allow invasion of the tissues by the organism, resulting in a mild infection. Species of staphylococci can cause sore throat, scarlet fever, rheumatic fever, and many types of pneumonia.

  Diplococci are round bacteria that grow in pairs. Pneumonia, gonorrhea, and meningitis are infectious diseases caused by diplococci.

- A **bacillus** is rod shaped and causes tuberculosis, tetanus, and otitis externa. Bacilli are usually aerobic, like *Bacillus anthracis* and *Yersinia pestis*. Diseases caused by bacilli include botulism, tetanus, gas gangrene, gastroenteritis produced by salmonella food poisoning, typhoid fever, pertussis, bacillary dysentery, diphtheria, tuberculosis, leprosy, and plague. *Escherichia coli* is a species of bacillus that is found among the normal flora of the large intestine.

- **Spirochetes** are long, spiral, flexible bacteria. They cause diseases such as syphilis, caused by the bacteria *Treponema pallidum*; Lyme disease, caused by the bacteria *Borrelia burgdorferi*; and cholera, caused by *Vibrio cholerae*.

- **Antibiotics** are used to fight bacterial infections; they either kill the bacteria or prevent it from reproducing.

- *Rickettsia* and **Chlamydia** are genera of bacteria known as parasites, which are organisms that must live inside another living organism in order to survive. Rickettsia spread to humans via a **vector**, which is a disease carrier that transmits a disease from an infected person to a noninfected person. Common vectors are insects such as ticks, fleas, mites, and lice. Examples of diseases transmitted by *rickettsia* are typhus and Rocky Mountain spotted fever. *Chlamydia* cause lymphogranuloma, a sexually transmitted disease.

Viruses

A **virus** is a pathogen that can grow and reproduce only after infecting a host cell. Viruses are non-living organisms consisting of either DNA or RNA, surrounded by a protein coat. Viruses reproduce by taking over cells and directing the cell to produce copies of the virus in the infected cell. A virus uses the host cells' RNA and DNA (genetic material) to reproduce. Viruses are difficult to treat because of the protein in their outer cell membrane. Antivirals are used to treat viruses by inhibiting their growth. Viruses require a living host for survival and replication. The most definitive way to determine the presence of a virus is to test the blood for antibodies to the virus. Viruses cause such diseases as the common cold, hepatitis, chicken pox (varicella), measles (rubeola), and AIDS.

Fungus

A **fungus** is a simple, single-celled organism, such as yeast, or a multicellular colony, such as mold and mushrooms. Fungi can grow outside a living host on organic material. For example, athlete's foot (tinea pedis) is caused by fungus that grows in warm, moist environments and likes to live in the outer layers of human skin. However, for short periods of time, this fungus can live in warm puddles on tile floor.

Usually fungi do not cause disease, but they can become pathogenic in certain circumstances. When the normal balance in the body's chemistry changes, through infection, disease, medication, and the like, fungi that normally live in the body may no longer be kept in check and, therefore, may become pathogenic.

Fungi are opportunistic and usually become pathogenic when the host's normal flora cannot offset the colony's growth. Examples of the diseases they cause in humans include tinea infections (such as athlete's foot and ringworm) and yeast infections (such as candidiasis).

Protozoa

Single-celled parasites are called **protozoa**, another type of pathogenic microorganism. Parasites vary from single-celled organisms to more complex creatures such as worms and insects. They commonly infect persons with low immunity. Protozoan infections are spread through the fecal-oral route, when one ingests contaminated food or water, or these infections are transmitted by mosquitoes or other insects carrying the infection. Examples of common protozoan infections are malaria, giardiasis, and a vaginal infection called trichomoniasis.

Prion

Prions, the smallest pathogens, result in damage to the tissue of the brain. The best-known infections caused by prions are bovine spongiform encephalopathy (BSE, or mad cow disease) in cows and Creutzfeldt-Jakob disease in humans. Diseases caused by prions are fatal.

HAND WASHING

Hand washing has been the backbone of infection control for more than a century. Hand washing protects the patient from cross contamination and also protects the medical assistant. Go to http://cdc.gov/handhygiene and read the fact sheet on hand hygiene.

Chain of Infection

For a pathogen to survive and produce disease, a continuous cycle, known as the chain of infection, must be followed. If the cycle is broken at any point, the pathogen dies.

The chain begins with the infectious agent, which invades the reservoir host, and is transmitted through a portal of exit from the host to a new host, through a port of entry. Infection cannot occur if the infectious microorganism is not introduced at the beginning of the cycle.

The first link of the chain of infection is the reservoir host, which is the person infected with the microorganisms. Although this person may not show signs of an infection, his or her body serves as a source of nutrients and an incubator in which the pathogen can grow and reproduce. These persons are also called carriers or reservoirs of the disease.

Reservoir Host

A reservoir host becomes infected with the pathogen and serves as a source of transfer of the pathogen. The host provides nourishment for the pathogenic organism, providing a hospitable environment in which the pathogen can grow. Living infected hosts may be **symptomatic** (having noticeable signs of the disease) or may be **asymptomatic** (free of noticeable symptoms). The reservoir host is considered contagious (a carrier of the pathogen) and can spread the disease to others.

Means of Exit

The pathogen may exit the reservoir host through contact with mucous membranes, through a break in the skin, or through the mouth, nose, throat, ears, eyes, intestinal tract, urinary tract, reproductive tract, and open wounds.

Mode of Transmission

A pathogen can be transmitted to another person by direct or indirect contact with an infected person or discharge. Modes of indirect transfer include range of situations, such as coughing and sneezing, contamination of objects touched by infected individuals, and contaminated food. Examples of direct-contact transmission include transmission through skin-to-skin contact (such as hand shaking or kissing) or the exchange of bodily fluids (such as through needle sharing or sexual contact). Pathogens can be transmitted via indirect contact with inanimate objects: when an object is capable of harboring a pathogen, it is called a **fomite**.

Means of Entry

Pathogens gain entry to the body in much the same way as they exit it, usually through contact with mucous membranes, through a break in the skin, or through the mouth, nose, throat, ears, eyes, intestinal tract, urinary tract, reproductive tract, and open wounds. Therefore, potential entry sites include the eyes, nose, mouth, throat, vagina, and rectum, as well as any wounds to the skin.

Susceptible Host

A susceptible host is capable of being infected by the pathogen. Common examples of susceptible hosts include those with poor hygiene, poor nutrition, unusual levels of stress, and other underlying diseases or disorders. Other factors causing susceptibility include some medications, age (very young and very old), and self-destructive behaviors such as tobacco use, excessive alcohol intake, and use of illicit drugs.

An infection may be **localized**, which means that it is confined to one site, and can exhibit heat, redness (erythema), swelling (edema), and pain. Or an infection can be **systemic**, which means that it involves the whole body, and the symptoms can include fever, fatigue, and headache, and so on. The susceptible host can become the reservoir host, and the infection cycle begins again.

Types of Infection

Acute infections, such as the common cold, typically have a quick onset and short duration. A clear prodromal phase, in which symptoms are generally nonspecific (examples of nonspecific symptoms include body aches, rash, and fever) may or may not occur. The duration is usually one to three weeks.

Chronic infections, such as hepatitis C, last for a long time—sometimes for years or even a lifetime. The patient may be asymptomatic, or the patient's symptoms may fluctuate.

Latent infections are those in which patients experience alternating periods of being symptomatic (relapse) and periods of being symptom-free (remission). The infecting organism, usually a virus, never leaves the body, but lies dormant between relapses. A common example of a latent infection is the herpes viruses, which can cause intermittent outbreaks of oral lesions, genital lesions, and shingles.

Principles of Asepsis

Medical asepsis, a condition free of pathogens, and infection control are crucial in preventing the spread of disease. The medical assistant should practice good medical aseptic techniques to provide a safe and healthy environment in the medical office.

The Occupational Safety and Health Administration, a federal agency responsible for the safety of all workers, issued the blood-borne pathogen standard in 1992. This standard is required by the federal government to reduce the exposure of healthcare employees to infectious diseases. The Centers for Disease Control (CDC) also recommend that standard precautions procedures be used to reduce the chance of transmitting infectious microorganism. More information on Biohazardous Material and Standard Precautions follows.

Medical Asepsis

Medical asepsis, also called clean technique, involves removing pathogens and reducing transfer of microorganisms by cleaning any body part or surface that has been exposed to them.

Hand washing is the first line of defense in the practice of medical asepsis and the single most important means of preventing the spread of infection.

Soap and the friction of rubbing the hands together loosens dirt so that it can be rinsed away with water. Standard precautions state that medical assistants and other medical professionals should clean their hands with soap and warm water or with an antiseptic agent (an agent that kills or inhibits the growth of microorganisms) prior to and immediately after any direct contact with patients and after any potential contact with pathogenic organisms. Medical assistants should avoid wearing jewelry or rings when performing procedures, because microorganisms often remain in crevices of the jewelry even after the hands are washed.

Microorganisms on the hands are classified into the following categories: resident flora and transient flora. Resident flora (also known as normal flora) normally reside and grow in the epidermis and in the deeper layers of the skin known as the dermis; they are generally harmless.

Transient flora live and grow on the superficial skin layers, or epidermis, and are transferred in a range of ways, such as through contact with contaminated equipment or infected patients. They can be pathogenic, but since they live on the surface layer of the skin, they can be killed by washing and scrubbing with an antiseptic.

Antiseptic hand washing cleans and sterilizes the hands through the physical scrubbing action and through the action of the antimicrobial soap contained in the antiseptic.

The medical assistant should wash his or her hands at the following times and under the following conditions:

- before and after every patient
- before and after breaks and lunch
- at the end of the day
- after coughing, sneezing, or blowing his or her nose
- after contact with contaminated material
- after using the restroom
- before and after wearing gloves

The medical assistant should always assume that everyone's blood and body fluids are contaminated with pathogens. Although gloves help to protect against contamination from these pathogens, wearing them does not replace hand washing, because bacteria can multiply in the moist environments inside gloves.

Medical assistants should always wear gloves whenever they risk exposure, such as when touching or handling biohazardous containers or when drawing blood or assisting in surgical procedures. Wearing gloves protects both the medical assistant and the patient from transmission of pathogens.

Levels of Asepsis

There are three levels involved in asepsis: sanitization, disinfection, and sterilization.

Sanitization

Sanitization is the removal of microorganisms using chemicals, heat, or ionizing radiation. The single most effective standard precaution that breaks the chain of infection and protects everyone is consistent, proper hand hygiene and sanitization.

To sanitize an instrument, the medical assistant will usually rinse it under cold water and scrub it with an enzymatic detergent. In some cases, the medical assistant may use an ultrasonic bath where sound waves cause vibrations to loosen debris from instruments. In addition to equipment, the medical assistant must sanitize the environment of the medical office, including surfaces such as countertops and examination tables. A solution of ten parts water to one part household bleach is inexpensive, easy to use, and effective. Regardless of the product used, the medical assistant should always take time to read the labels, follow the directions, and note the information on **material safety data sheets (MSDSs)**, which provide data about ingredients, information on how to handle or work with specific substances, and measures to take in the event of an exposure or spill.

Disinfection

Disinfection typically involves the application of a substance to equipment, surfaces, or other items to kill pathogenic microorganisms. In order to effectively disinfect an object, the medical assistant must sanitize it before the disinfection process.

Chemical disinfecting agents appropriate for instruments, surfaces, furniture, and equipment include chlorine, iodine, 70 percent isopropyl alcohol, hydrogen peroxide, or a one-to-ten solution of household bleach and water.

Sterilization

Sterilization eliminates all microorganisms from a surface or instrument through exposure to chemicals, ionizing radiation, dry heat, gas, or steam. Prior to sterilization, instruments must have been sanitized and disinfected. Some pathogens are easily destroyed; others, such as spores, are very resistant to temperature extremes and are difficult to destroy. The sterilization process, as a final stage, helps to eliminate these types of pathogens. The autoclave is used to sterilize surgical instruments and supplies. An autoclave subjects items to high-pressure steam at 121° C typically for 15 to 20 minutes, depending on the size of the load and the contents.

Surgical Asepsis

Surgical asepsis is the practice of destroying all pathogenic organisms before they enter the body. More specifically, the surgical aseptic technique is a method of performing invasive procedures so that patients are protected from pathogenic microorganisms. Examples of some procedures that require surgical asepsis include injections, urinary catheterization, wound care, tissue biopsy, and repair and suturing of lacerations.

Surgical Scrub

Surgical scrub is a style of hand washing that is much more thorough than regular hand washing and follows specific steps. Although the human skin can never be fully sterilized, the surgical scrub is designed to reduce the number of pathogenic microorganisms on the hands and forearms to the greatest extent possible.

A surgical scrub requires surgical soap, a nail file, and a sterile brush. In a surgical scrub, your hands are kept upright to avoid having the water run from the unscrubbed area of your arm onto your hands. The scrubbing process should take five minutes for each hand, covering all four sides of the fingers. Arms and

forearms should be rinsed, starting with your fingertips, wrists, then forearms, always holding the fingers upward, without touching the faucet. The faucet should be turned off with the foot, knee, or elbow and hands should be dried with a sterile towel.

Gowning and Gloving

Gowns and gloves are worn to protect the skin and prevent contamination of clothing during activities that may generate splashes or sprays of blood and other bodily fluids. Sterile gowns are worn when assisting in surgical procedures, and nonsterile gowns are worn for routine procedures.

Sterile gloves are used when assisting in surgical procedures, removing sutures or staples, or changing dressings, to prevent infectious material from entering the body.

More information on gowns and gloves is found in the Standard Precautions section on page 161.

Maintaining a Sterile Field

The instruments and supplies for surgery must be set on a **sterile field**. The medical assistant may set up the sterile tray either before or after preparing the patient's skin. The sterile tray setup must not become contaminated. If the medical assistant must turn away from the sterile tray or leave the room after setting up, a sterile towel must be placed over the tray to maintain sterility.

A common method for setting up a sterile tray is to use prepackaged sterile setups wrapped in disposable sterilization paper or muslin that are prepared by the medical office through autoclave sterilization. These packs are labeled according to use and contain most of the instruments and supplies required for the minor office surgery indicated on the label. The medical assistant opens the wrapped package on a flat surface, such as a **Mayo stand**, a broad, flat metal tray placed on a stand and used to hold sterile and nonsterile instruments and supplies. Several additional articles not contained in the prepackaged setup (such as an antiseptic, sterile gauze, disposable syringe and needle, or sutures) may need to be added to the sterile field when the package is opened.

To maintain sterility, the medical assistant should use only sterile objects to touch other sterile objects. The medical assistant should keep sterile objects in his or her field of vision. If the medical assistant cannot see an object, he or she must assume it is no longer sterile. Only the area above the waist is sterile. If a medical assistant lowers his or her hands or a sterile instrument below the waist, they are no longer sterile. The outside inch of the sterile field on all sides is considered nonsterile. The medical assistant should avoid passing nonsterile objects over the sterile field. He or she should also avoid coughing or sneezing over the sterile field. When one is wearing a sterile gown, the sterile field comprises the area above the waist, the front of gown, the gloves, and the sterile Mayo stand except the outer inch and any part that hangs below the table. The lower limit of a sterile surgical field is the waist.

If an antiseptic solution is poured into a basin on the sterile field, the medical assistant should read the label, check the expiration date, recheck the label, place the palm of his or her hand over the label, and place the cap on a flat surface with the open end up. Rinse the lip of the bottle by pouring a small amount of solution into a separate container. Pour the solution into a sterile container at a height of approximately six inches. The cap should be replaced and the label checked a third time.

Autoclave Sterilization

An **autoclave,** a sterilization device commonly used in a clinical setting, sterilizes items using steam under pressure. For sterilization to occur the temperature must reach 250°F to 270°F (120°C to 130°C) with 15 pounds of pressure for a specific amount of time, usually 15 to 20 minutes depending on the contents being sterilized. Subjecting items to steam under pressure causes the proteins in microorganisms to coagulate and the bacterial spores to be destroyed. When the chamber cools, the condensation of the steam causes the explosion of the microorganism cells, ensuring their complete destruction.

Operation of the Autoclave

Quality control methods must be maintained when operating an autoclave to ensure that proper sterilization has been achieved. Various indicators are used to check that sterilization has occurred. The two most common are color changes and culture tests.

Color change: Sterilization tape is all one color before sterilization. During sterilization, brown stripes appear. Sterilization pouches have arrows that turn from pink to brown during steam sterilization and from blue to yellow during gas sterilization.

Culture tests: Various types of culture tests for bacterial spores are also placed inside packs for quality control purposes. These strips or ampules contain bacterial spores. They are autoclaved with the equipment to be sterilized and then placed in an incubator or sent to a lab to see if any spores have survived.

Preparing Items for Autoclave

To prepare instruments for the autoclave, the medical assistant must open all hinged instruments. The medical assistant must pack items so that they do not touch each other and so that all parts of the instrument are exposed to the steam and pressure. Instruments can be placed in muslin cloth or in polypropylene autoclave bags. The medical assistant must wrap sharp instruments with gauze on the tips to prevent puncturing the bag. The medical assistant should also label packs using permanent marker with the contents, the date, and his or her initials.

Wrapping the equipment keeps it sterile after sterilization. The wrap is sterilized along with the item. After sterilization, the inside of the package remains sterile, while the outside can be touched.

Chemical Sterilization

Chemical sterilization is used when the instrument or equipment cannot withstand the high temperature of the autoclave. The medical assistant should carefully follow the instructions for mixing the solution, immersion time, rinsing, and storage of sterilized equipment. Chemical sterilization liquids like glutaraldehyde and formaldehyde are mixed according to the instructions on the bottle. The solution must be marked with the date of preparation and the expiration date. Materials must be submerged in this solution with a closed lid for eight hours or more. Items should be removed with sterile forceps and must be rinsed with sterile water to remove all traces of the chemical before the items are used on a patient.

The Medical Assistant's Role in Aseptic Surgery

Medical asepsis—critical in any medical setting—is a clean technique that aims to reduce the number and prevent the spread of microorganisms. Surgical asepsis goes several steps further: it is a sterile technique that aims to ensure that all microorganisms are eliminated from an environment in which an invasive procedure will be performed.

Assisting with minor office surgery requires a thorough knowledge of the instruments and supplies for each tray setup and the type of assistance required by the physician during the surgery. Of particular concern for the medical assistant is maintaining asepsis in the surgical environment.

Standard Precautions

The term *standard precautions* relates to a system—a set of principles and practices—used in all medical facilities to prevent the transmission of infectious materials and reduce the occurrence of **nosocomial** infections—that is, infections that develop in hospitals or healthcare settings. The system protects medical staff members who might be exposed to infectious agents when handling or coming into contact with blood, secretions, excretions, and other bodily fluid and tissues.

Standard precautions include various protective measures, such as:

- **Hand hygiene:** Following any patient contact, the medical assistant should wash his or her hands. Hand hygiene is often considered the most important means of defense against transmission of nosocomial infections.
- **Gloves:** Clean, nonsterile gloves should be worn when coming into contact with blood, body fluids, secretions, or excretions. The medical assistant should put gloves on just before coming into contact with potentially contaminated fluids, remove and discard gloves immediately after use, in order not to contaminate other items or surfaces, and then wash his or her hands.
- **Gowns:** Gowns should be worn during any activity that may result in splashing or spraying blood, bodily fluids, secretions, or excretions. The fabric should be resistant to fluids and nonsterile.
- **Mask, face shield, and eye protection:** These components protect the eyes, nose, mouth, and mucous membranes from spraying or splashing blood, body fluids, secretions, and excretions. They also protect from pathogens that are airborne.
- **Cleaning and disinfection:** All non-disposable equipment, including examination table, countertops, and chairs, should be cleaned or disinfected before treating another patient. Routine cleaning should be done after each patient has left the exam room. If a surface in the exam room appears to have been contaminated—for instance, through exposure to blood or other bodily fluids—it should be disinfected immediately, with a tuberculocidal disinfectant or diluted bleach solution.
- **Personal protective equipment (PPE):** Specialized garments, such as gowns and masks, that are critical in protecting against the transmission of infectious agents.
- **Puncture-resistant sharps containers:** These containers should be readily available in areas where wastes such as needles, syringes, or broken glass may be generated. Sharps are objects that

have acute rigid corners, edges, or projections capable of cutting or piercing and can be reasonably anticipated to penetrate the skin or any other part of the body. Placing sharps in puncture-resistant containers prevents injury and the potential spread of pathogens.

Disposing of Infectious Waste

The Environmental Protection Agency (EPA) and OSHA have created federal policies and guidelines for proper disposal of hazardous materials. Each state determines its own policy based on the federal guidelines. The policies can vary from state to state, but general guidelines include:

- Red leakproof bags are used for contaminated supplies such as gloves, gauze, bandages, gowns, and linens.
- OSHA's blood-borne pathogens standard requires that containers and appliances containing biohazardous materials be labeled with a biohazard warning label.
- The biohazard warning label must be fluorescent orange or orange-red and contain the biohazard symbol and the word *BIOHAZARD* in a contrasting color.

OSHA requires that the medical office have policies and procedures in place for preventing employee exposure to biohazardous materials. OSHA requires that all personnel who will be exposed to blood or other possible infectious material must have training in the blood-borne pathogens standard. According to OSHA, the medical office must provide hepatitis B immunization at no charge and provide healthcare workers with access to personal protective equipment, including face shields and gloves. In addition, OSHA requires medical offices to have an exposure control plan if the office has ten or more employees. This exposure control plan dictates what should happen if an employee or visitor is exposed to a biohazardous material.

Most medical offices enter into contracts with infectious waste disposal services. This service supplies the office with biowaste containers and regularly picks up the filled containers. The service disposes of the waste according to EPA and OSHA standards. The service also maintains a tracking mechanism recording the type of waste, weight, and disposal destination on a three-part manifest. The generator of the biomedical waste keeps one part of the form; the service keeps the other two parts. Once the waste has been destroyed, the service returns one part of the form to the generator as proof of disposal. The medical office maintains these records for three years.

Preparing and Maintaining the Treatment Area

The medical assistant is largely responsible for preparing and maintaining the treatment area. This section reviews the important aspects of this vital function.

Equipment and Materials

Instruments and equipment must be properly maintained, and all maintenance procedures must be documented. A maintenance log provides a complete record of all work performed on instruments or on a piece of equipment. The medical assistant must be sure to follow manufacturers' guidelines for performing instrument and equipment maintenance.

Examination Tables

Examination tables usually come with storage drawers to provide plenty of storage volume for gowns, drapes, and other items, yet are made to help organize the medical office's assortment of smaller supplies and bulk supplies. In addition, there are front drawers for easy access to items during pelvic exams. The one-piece, upholstered top of the examination table can be easily removed without tools, to allow for thorough cleaning. The footstep allows patients to feel more secure and to get on and off the table more confidently. The medical assistant should always assist the patient on and off the examination table. Retractable stirrups pull out straight and are then positioned in four lateral positions.

Autoclave/Sterilizer

Information about the use and operation of an autoclave—used to sterilize equipment—is included in the Infection Control section in this chapter.

Cast Equipment/Materials

Casts are applied to immobilize a fracture and allow the bone to heal in proper alignment. The type of cast to be used depends on the location and severity of the injury, the age and occupation of the patient, and the physician's preference. Different types of casts include:

- An **air cast** is a temporary cast that is inflated around the limb to immobilize it and can be used if some mobility is allowed. If no mobility is allowed, the patient will be fitted with a fiberglass cast, which is the most common type of cast.
- A **plaster cast** is a bandage impregnated with calcium sulfate crystals and is supplied as rolls of material in widths appropriate to a variety of sites. After water is added to the dry rolls of bandages and the wet bandages are applied to the area, a chemical reaction generates heat. This chemical reaction produces a rigid dressing when dry, in about 72 hours. The bandage molds to the area as it is applied. Plaster casts must be kept dry at all times.
- A **fiberglass cast** is applied in a manner similar to plaster casts; the polyurethane additives used in fiberglass casts harden in minutes, eliminating the extended drying time. The fabric has a more open weave than plaster, which helps maintain skin integrity.

The medical assistant must instruct the patient in proper cast care. The guidelines are as follows:

- Cover the cast when bathing.
- Keep the cast dry and exposed to air as much as possible.
- Elevate the cast to reduce swelling and pain.
- Observe the fingers and toes for changes in color, temperature, and decreased sensation.
- Call the office if there is any bad odor, loss of sensation, numbness, tingling, or bleeding around the cast.
- Clean the cast with a damp cloth.

Scales

Although many types of scales are available for measuring weight, the most common in the medical office is the balance beam scale, because of its accuracy. Some important points of operation are:

1. Weights that slide above two rows of numbered measurements indicate the weight.
   - The bottom row shows measurements in 50-pound units.
   - The top row shows measurements in 2-pound units.
2. The bottom row—which jumps in bigger increments—should first be moved to get the general range of the individual's weight.
3. The top row is then adjusted to measure the weight exactly.
4. The beam will be in balance when all weights are at set to zero and when the pointer at the end of the balance bar floats in the middle of the frame.

Oxygen

Adequate amounts of oxygen are vital to the proper functioning of the body and the health of the body's organs. If a patient's breathing is labored, supplemental oxygen may needed. Important aspects of administering oxygen are:

- Explain the procedure to patient and review safety precautions necessary when oxygen is in use.
- No Smoking signs should be placed in the appropriate areas.
- A doctor's prescription will dictate how much oxygen should be used.
- A mask should be used if the amount of oxygen to administer is between 5 and 15 liters per minute.
- A nasal cannula, that is, tubing connected to the larger oxygen delivery tubes, should be used if the amount to administer is 6 liters or less per minute.
- Humidification can be added to help keep the inside of the patient's nose from drying. Sterile water must always be used.
- The nasal prongs—which are attached at the end of the cannula leading into the nostrils—should point downward.
- The patient should be encouraged to breathe through the nose while keeping the mouth closed.

Spirometer

Spirometry is a test to measure breathing capacity. An instrument called a **spirometer** measures the air taken in by and expelled from the lungs. Several different measurements related to lung volume and capacity can be made with a spirometer. Some of these measurements are made directly by the spirometer; others are calculated.

The following procedure should be followed when performing spirometry on a patient:

- The patient should be in a sitting position with legs uncrossed and both feet on the floor.
- The patient's chin should be slightly elevated, and the patient's neck should be slightly extended.
- A nose clip should be securely placed on the patient's nose.

- The patient should take as deep a breath as possible, and the patient should blow in the mouthpiece as hard and as fast as possible.
- The patient should complete three acceptable sessions.

If the results are less than 60 percent of the predicted value, the patient may be given bronchodilators (medication used to dilate the bronchi, or air passages), and be retested to determine the impact of the inhalant on function after the bronchodilator has been administered.

Nebulizer

A **nebulizer** is a device used for patients who have symptoms of asthma, including wheezing and difficulty breathing. A bronchodilator (a medication administered to dilate the bronchi), such as albuterol, is added to the nebulizer, which causes the liquid medication to break apart into a fine spray that is inhaled by the patient through a mouthpiece or mask. Because bronchodilator medications can cause an increase in heart rate, the patient's pulse should be monitored before, during, and after the treatment.

Oximeter

An **oximeter** is a device that measures oxygen levels in the blood, as well as an individual's pulse rate. A probe is placed on a relatively translucent area of the body, such as a fingertip or earlobe; a portable fingertip unit can be placed directly on the fingertip. The oximeter then uses beams of red and infrared light to calculate the amount of oxygen the blood sample running by the probes, or unit, contains.

Thermometer

A **thermometer** is used to measure body temperature, which is one of the vital signs used to assess an individual's health status. A person's temperature can be measured at different sites in the body. Normal body temperature varies with the time of day and the site of measurement. Normal body temperature is between 96°F and 99.5°F (36.4°C to 37.3°C).

More information about body temperature can be found under "Vital Signs" on page 168.

Sphygmomanometers

The **aneroid sphygmomanometer** is an instrument used to measure blood pressure. The instrument consists of:

- an inflatable cuff
- an inflation bulb with a control valve
- a pressure gauge, with the needle pointing to a scale showing millimeters of mercury

Blood pressure cuffs come in a variety of sizes: one for adults, one for children, and one to fit around the thigh. The size of a cuff refers to its inner inflatable bladder. The cuff should fit snugly and should be applied so that the center of the inflatable bag is directly over the brachial artery to allow for complete compression of the artery. The cuff has a velcro fastener to hold the cuff in place.

The aneroid sphygmomanometer should be recalibrated at least once a year.

A **stethoscope**, for listening to the heartbeat, is also needed to measure blood pressure. The measurement is recorded in millimeters of mercury (mm Hg). It is usually given as two numbers, for example, 110 over 70 (written as 110/70).

- The top number is the **systolic** blood pressure reading. It represents the maximum pressure exerted on the artery walls when the heart contracts.
- The bottom number is the **diastolic** blood pressure reading. It represents the minimum pressure in the arteries when the heart is at rest.

More information on blood pressure can be found under "Vital Signs" on page 168.

Stethoscope

The acoustic **stethoscope** is a diagnostic device through which an examiner listens to sounds from within a patient. The parts of a stethoscope include:

- the diaphragm, which picks up high-pitched sounds and is often referred to as the chestpiece, because it is most frequently used on the chest to pick up sounds in the chest cavity.
- the bell, which is the cone-shaped side of the stethoscope chestpiece. It must be held lightly against the skin to amplify sound. The bell is best at amplifying low-pitched sounds, such as vascular and heart sounds.
- earpieces, which are connected to the chestpiece through tubing. When the earpieces are placed in the examiner's ears, the acoustic waves coming from inside the patient can be heard.

Electrocardiograph

The **electrocardiogram** (ECG or EKG) is the written record of electrical current as it moves through the heart. The **electrocardiograph** machine is connected to the patient with wires and electrodes that are sensitive to the electrical impulses generated by the patient's heart. This electrical activity is transmitted to the main unit of the electrocardiograph machine and is represented on electrocardiograph paper through specific waveforms, which are then reviewed and analyzed by the physician.

The waves of electrical impulses responsible for cardiac cycle produce a series of waves and lines on an electrocardiogram, which is the tracing made by an electrocardiograph. These peaks and valleys, called waves or deflections, are labeled with the letters P, Q, R, S, T, and U. Each letter represents a specific part of the pattern.

The information obtained aids in the diagnosis and treatment of cardiac problems (such as ischemia or arrhythmias); abnormalities in the size of the waves or the various time intervals indicate certain types of heart problems. ECGs are also commonly done prior to major surgical procedures in order to establish baseline health information about a patient and to identify potential cardiac disorders.

The Stylus and Paper

The horizontal axis of the paper represents time and the vertical axis represents amplitude. The stylus marks the ECG paper as it moves horizontally at a rate of 25 mm/sec.

The voltage, or strength, of the heartbeat is also recorded on the paper. Voltage can be displayed as either a positive or a negative deflection. One millivolt (mV) of electrical activity moves the stylus upward over 10 mm.

All ECG machines are **standardized** so that an ECG can be interpreted in the same manner, regardless what part of the world a patient is in. Standardization needs to be checked each time the ECG machine is used; the manufacturer's manual explains exactly how the standardization process works.

Leads and Electrodes

Ten sensors called **electrodes** are placed on the patient's arms, legs, and chest to pick up the electrical activity of the heart. Each of the electrodes is connected to color-coded lead wires by a metal clip. The lead wires transmit data about cardiac electrical activity to the ECG machine. Each **lead** records the electrical impulse through the heart from different angles. The ECG machine amplifies the electrical waveforms created by deflection of the stylus.

The standard ECG consists of 12 separate leads, or recordings, of the electrical activity of the heart from different angles. The 12-lead ECG produces a three-dimensional record of the impulse wave.

Lead I to lead III: The first three leads recorded are called the standard, or bipolar, leads because each of these leads uses two limb electrodes to record the heart's electrical activity. The right arm electrode is the negative pole, and the left leg or left arm electrodes are the positive poles. Roman numerals I, II, and III are used to identify the leads. These leads are also known

as Einthoven leads, and they show a frontal view of the heart's activity from side to side.

Augmented leads: The augmented leads are designated voltage right arm (aVR), augmented voltage left arm (aVL), and augmented voltage left leg (aVF). The electrical activity recorded by these leads is small, so the ECG machine amplifies or augments the electrical potential when recorded. These are all unipolar leads with a single positive electrode that uses the right leg for grounding.

Precordial leads: The precordial, or chest, leads are unipolar and provide a transverse-plane view of the heart. They are identified as V1, V2, V3, V4, V5, and V6. The *V* means "chest," and each of the numbers represents a specific location on the chest. Precordial leads measure the electrical activity among six specific points on the chest wall and a point within the heart.

ECG Artifacts

Artifacts are caused by improper technique, poor conduction, outside interference, or improper handling of a tracing.

Because electrocardiograph machines are sensitive to electrical activity, they sometimes record electrical activity from sources other than the patient's heart. Examples include electricity from nearby equipment or even the patient's own noncardiac muscle movement. When the ECG stylus moves in response to this interfering electrical activity, it records markings on the ECG strip known as artifacts, which are distracting and irrelevant.

Microscopes

The **microscope**, an optical instrument consisting of one or more lenses used to magnify objects, is used in the medical office to examine microorganisms and to count cells. The compound microscope is the most common type used in the medical office.

Binocular microscopes minimize eyestrain and have adjustments to allow for variations in spacing between the user's eyes.

Parts of a Microscope

- The **eyepiece** has three or four objective lenses and rotates to bring the objective into working position. The grip should be used to rotate the lenses.
- The **objective lenses** determine the magnification power of the microscope. The magnification power is marked on each objective. The longer, or higher power, objective magnifies × 40 (for closer observation). With the use of oil, the third objective, sometimes called the oil immersion lens, magnifies × 100.
- The **stage of the microscope** is a flat surface that holds the slide for viewing. An opening in the solid surface allows illumination of the slide from below.
- The **condenser** concentrates the focus of the light rays on the slide. The condenser is adjustable. In the lower position, the light focus is reduced; in the higher position, it is increased.
- The **diaphragm**, located in the condenser, consists of interlocking plates that adjust into variable-sized openings, or irises, thus controlling the amount of light from the source in conjunction with the condenser. The greater the need for light, the more highly magnified the slide must be.
- The **light source** is housed in the base of the microscope.

Several precautions should be used when handling the microscope.

- The microscope should be lifted with one hand holding the arm and the other hand under the base.
- The microscope should be operated on a sturdy surface.
- The lenses of the eyepieces or of any of the objectives should not be touched.
- Lenses should be cleaned with lens paper dipped in lens cleaner.

- The stage and other metal parts should be kept free of excess oil.

Ophthalmoscope

The **ophthalmoscope** is a lighted instrument used to examine the interior of the eye. It consists of:

- the base, or handle
- the concave mirror
- a light source
- rotating disks of lenses, operating by dials, which allows a patient's eyes to be viewed at various depths and magnifications

The examiner can view specific landmarks on the patient's fundus, such as the **optic nerve**, which transmits visual information from the eye to the brain, and the **macula**, an oval-shaped part of the eye that absorbs excess blue and ultraviolet light.

Otoscope

An **otoscope** is a device used to look into the ear. The head of the otoscope houses a light source and a lens that magnifies at a low power. An ear speculum, used to open up the ear canal, is placed at the front end.

To examine the ears of an adult, the ear canal must be straightened by pulling on the **pinna** (the projecting part of the ear lying outside of the head), and then the ear **speculum** is inserted in the external ear canal. When examining children's ears, the examiner should pull the top of the child's ear up and out to straighten the ear canal.

Endoscopes

An **endoscope** is an instrument used to see inside a hollow part of the body. It is made up of a flexible or rigid tube (or shaft), an eyepiece with a light source, an opening for inserting instruments, and a system of lenses that transmits images of what is being viewed.

There are a variety of types of endoscopes, depending on which part of the body is being examined, including:

- gastrointestinal tract: gastroscope, colonoscope, sigmoidoscope
- air passageways: bronchoscope, nasopharyngo-scope
- urological system: cystoscope, ureteroscope

The medical assistant may be called upon to assist in endoscopic examinations. His or her primary role is to assist the patient into the correct position and to drape the patient properly.

Mobility Assistive Devices

Patients who require assistance to maintain mobility may use crutches, a cane, a walker, or a wheelchair. Medical assistants often are responsible for teaching patients how to use these ambulatory aids safely.

Crutches

One crutch or a pair of **crutches** can be used to assist an individual with his or her gait, or way of walking. Crutches can be made of aluminum or wood. Axillary crutches are fitted to the patient's armpit height. The axillary bars, the padded parts at the top of the crutches, should fit two inches below the patient's axillae, or armpits.

Canes

A **cane** is used when a patient needs extra support and stability, but requires only a small measure of assistance. The tripod (three legs) or quad (four legs) cane is useful when the patient needs stability. The tripod cane stands alone when the patient needs to use his or her hands or have other support. To measure for proper cane length, have the patient stand erect. The cane should be level with the patient's hips and the patient's elbow should be bent at a 30° angle.

Walkers

A walker is a lightweight aluminum frame on which a patient can lean for stability while walking. The walker frame should be level with the patient's hip, and the patient's elbow should be bent at about a 30° angle.

Wheelchair

A **wheelchair** is a mobility device to assist people who have difficulty walking or are unable to walk because of illness, injury, or disability. The wheelchair dimensions—such as seat height, width, and depth—are important in allowing for a proper fit. It depends not only on an individual's size, but also on his or her needs. For instance, the height of the seat is important if individual needs to use the wheelchair at an office desk.

Preparing the Patient and Assisting the Physician

Vital Signs

Taking a patient's vital signs is one of the most important tasks a medical assistant will perform in the course of the day. These measurements provide valuable information about a patient's health status.

Vital signs, sometimes called cardinal signs, include:

- temperature (T)
- pulse (P)
- respiration (R)
- blood pressure (BP)

Vital signs measurements fall within certain average ranges (called normal values) when a person is in good health. Measurements recorded at a person's first visit provide a baseline for comparing measurements taken during subsequent visits. A baseline is a known, or initial, value to which later measurements can be compared.

Height and weight are also important for accurate diagnosis. Weight fluctuations can be a sign of disease, and the height-to-weight ratio gives information about a person's nutritional status.

EXAM ROOM PREP

Preparing and maintaining the treatment area provides a comfortable and healthy environment for the patient. To prepare the examination rooms, use the following guidelines:

1. Clean and disinfect exam tables, countertops, and faucets daily.

2. Change the exam table paper after each patient by unrolling a fresh length of paper.

3. Check the supply of gowns and drapes.

4. Remove dust and dirt from furniture and towel dispenser.

5. Replace biohazard containers as needed.

6. Empty waste containers frequently.

7. Check the exam room frequently to ensure that there are ample supplies and that equipment is properly cleaned.

8. Verify that each piece of equipment is in proper working order.

Temperature

A number of physiologic factors can affect temperature. Body temperature increases temporarily in response to infection, dehydration, hormonal fluctuations, and exposure to a warm environment. Normal body temperature—between 96° F and 99.5°F (36.4°C to 37.3°C)—varies with certain factors:

- time of day
- site of measurement
- gender
- temperature of the surrounding environment
- elderly persons may have an average temperature as low as 96.8°F
- diurnal rhythm, which causes body temperature to be lower in the morning and higher in the late afternoon

The body creates heat energy as a byproduct of metabolism and exercise. Three main factors affect the production and conservation of heat:

- **Metabolism:** Chemical processes in the body, such as digestion, respiration, and ovulation, produce heat.
- **Muscle movement:** Action of the muscles produces energy, which in turn creates heat; muscle activity can be both voluntary—as in exercise—and involuntary—such as shivering.
- **Constriction of superficial blood vessels:** Superficial blood vessels run close to the body's surface; their constriction helps to keep the body's internal heat constant.

The body loses heat in three ways: perspiration, elimination, and the dilation of the superficial blood vessels. Nearly 85% of the body's heat is lost through the skin as a result of perspiration. The rest is lost through the lungs and the excretions of bowel and bladder.

Taking a Patient's Temperature

Temperatures can be measured at different sites in the body:

- **Oral temperatures** are measured by placing the thermometer under the tongue. The patient should hold the thermometer with lips closed.
- **Tympanic temperatures** are measured by pulling the ear up and back for adults, and down and back for children, to straighten the ear canal. Press the button, and the results will be displayed.
- **Rectal temperatures** are measured by positioning the patient on his or her side. The left side is the preferred position because the rectum is angled in this direction. The rectal temperature is usually 1° higher than those taken through other routes because of the highly vascular, closed cavity of the rectum.

- **Axillary temperatures** are measured by placing the tip of the thermometer in the middle of the axilla. The patient's upper arm should be crossed over the stomach to hold the thermometer in place. Axillary temperatures are usually 1° lower than those taken through other routes because this area is not a closed cavity.

Electronic and disposable are the two types of thermometers most commonly in use in medical facilities.

- **Electronic**, or **digital**, **thermometers** are battery operated and portable and can obtain a temperature in one minute or less. A disposable cover fits over the probe for sanitary use. A digital thermometer can be used orally (in the mouth), axillarily (under the arm), or rectally (in the rectum).
- **Disposable thermometers** are single-use thermometers, usually made of thin strips of plastic with specially threaded dot or strip indicators. The indicators change color according to the temperature. This type is used for oral, axillary, or skin temperatures.

Abnormal Temperature Fluctuations

In the response to infection or injury, the hypothalamus may raise the body's core temperature. An individual who has a fever is said to be febrile or pyrexic. One who does not have a fever is afebrile. Shivering or chills produce heat, which is retained by the constriction of surface blood vessels, causing a higher temperature.

The higher temperature is believed to improve the body's ability to fight off infection, but temperatures above 101°F to 102°F (39.3°C to 39.9°C) are usually treated.

Hyperpyrexia. A fever higher than 105°F, hyperpyrexia is a serious condition that may cause convulsions, brain damage, and even death. Hyperpyrexia or hyperthermia (excessive body heat) may occur in infants and young children with a fever because of infection or in people of any age who exercise vigorously in hot, humid weather, especially if they do not replace the fluids lost by sweating. The skin may be hot, flushed, and dry, the pulse rapid, and the person may experience a headache, dizziness, confusion, and visual disturbances.

Fevers can be characterized according to their duration and timing:

- A **continuous** fever stays at about the same elevation all the time or returns to the same level about four hours after being treated with medication.
- An **intermittent** fever rises (spikes) and returns to normal in a regular pattern.
- A **remittent** fever rises and falls, but always remains above normal.
- A **relapsing** fever appears to go away and then returns. This may happen once or several times.

Hypothermia. A lowering of the core body temperature below 95°F (35°C), hypothermia is usually the result of long exposure to cold temperatures and occurs more quickly when a person is wearing wet clothing.

Early signs and symptoms of hypothermia include shivering, blue skin, mental confusion, numbness, and slurred speech.

Pulse

A **pulse** is the beat of the heart represented through the pulsating flow of blood through superficial arteries, that is, arteries close to the skin. The pulse rate, a calculation of the number of heartbeats in a set period of time, usually a minute, measures the two-phase action of the heart:

- **Contraction:** The heart contracts, pushing the blood through the arteries; this outward action is felt as outward pressure on the arteries.

- **Relaxation:** The heart momentarily rests, causing the artery walls to resume their original state.

The pulse is palpable, or able to be felt, in sites on the body where arteries can be compressed against bone. The most common methods for obtaining a pulse rate are:

- **radial pulse:** the most common site, located on the inside of the wrist, on the thumb side, about one inch from the thumb's base
- **carotid pulse:** commonly used in emergencies, located on the throat, in the grooves between the larynx (Adam's apple) and the long muscle on the front side of the neck (called the sternocleidomastoid muscle)
- **brachial pulse:** used typically for blood pressure measurement, located inside the elbow (a location called the antecubital space)

Other, less common methods for measuring the pulse rate are:

- **temporal pulse:** located at the temple, on the side of the head, in front of the ear
- **femoral pulse:** located in the groin; used to monitor circulation in the leg
- **popliteal pulse:** located at the back of the knee; also used to monitor circulation in the leg
- **dorsalis pedis pulse:** located on the top of the foot, between the first and second metatarsal; used to gauge lower limb circulation.
- **apical pulse:** located at the apex of the heart; used on cardiac patients; requires a stethoscope.

Respirations

Respiration involves the movement of air into and out of the lungs so that gas exchange can occur in the alveoli, which are the tiny air sacs in the lungs. A cycle of action and reaction takes place during respiration:

1. The buildup of carbon dioxide causes the pH level in the blood to drop.
2. As the pH level decreases, a message is sent to the medulla oblongata in the brain, which then sends out a message to the body to increase the rate and depth of respiration.
3. As a result, more carbon dioxide is eliminated from the body.
4. Blood pH rises back to a more normal level.
5. When pH levels rise too high, messages to and from the medulla oblongata stimulate a decrease in the rate and depth of respiration.
6. This allows the body to retain more carbon dioxide, lowering the pH level to normal.

Inspiration and Expiration

Two actions make up the respiration cycle.

- **Inspiration,** or the act of breathing in, occurs when the diaphragm and other muscles contract, pulling the thorax upward and outward. At the same time, the lungs expand, causing the air to be pulled in through the mouth and nose.
- **Expiration,** or the act of breathing out, is usually passive. The diaphragm and other muscles simply relax, allowing the rib cage to return inward and downward as air is expelled from the lungs.

Measuring Respiration

Respirations can be measured simultaneously with the pulse measurement. The medical assistant should continue holding the patient's wrist while observing the patient's chest. This will prevent the patient from altering the respirations.

The respirations have three characteristics: rate, rhythm, and depth.

Rate: The rate is the number of respirations per minute. The normal respiration rate for adults is 12 to 20 breaths per minute.

- **Bradypnea** is the term used for abnormally slow breathing.

- **Apnea** is the term used for absence of breathing.
- **Tachypnea** is the term used to describe rapid breathing. Tachypnea may be caused by asthma or emphysema.

Rhythm: The rhythm of respirations is normally described as even and regular. Abnormal variations of rhythm occur with injury or disease. Dyspnea is a condition of rapid respirations, and the expiratory phase becomes prolonged because the patient has to work harder to breathe out. This may be caused by lung disease and asthma or chronic obstructive pulmonary disease (COPD).

Depth: The depth of respiration may be described as normal, deep, or shallow. Respirations depth may be altered because of injury or disease. Respirations become deeper with physical exertion and become more shallow at rest.

Blood Pressure

Blood pressure reflects the pressure exerted against the arterial walls by blood and is recorded as a fraction. It is measured with the use of a stethoscope and a sphygmomanometer, which consists of an inflatable cuff, an inflation bulb with a control valve, and a pressure gauge, with a needle pointing to a scale showing millimeters of mercury (mm Hg).

- **Systolic pressure**, the top number, indicates the highest pressure exerted against the arterial walls during ventricular contraction.
- **Diastolic pressure**, the lower number, represents the lowest pressure exerted against the arterial walls when the heart is at rest between contractions.
- The difference between the two is the pulse pressure.

The sounds heard during blood pressure measurement are Korotkoff sounds. The Korotkoff sounds have five distinct phases.

- Phase I begins with the first sound heard when deflating the cuff. It is a sharp tapping sound. Note this first sound, as this will be the systolic reading of the blood pressure.
- Phase II is the result of more blood passing through the vessels as the cuff is deflated. The sound is that of a soft swishing.
- Phase III occurs when blood continues to travel through the vessels as the cuff is deflated. A tapping rhythmic sound can be heard.
- Phase IV is when blood is passing through the vessels fairly easily as the cuff is deflated. The sounds heard will be muffling and fading of the tapping sounds.
- Phase V is when the blood is flowing freely and all sounds have disappeared. This disappearance of sounds is noted and recorded as the diastolic pressure.

The blood pressure is recorded on the patient chart in a fraction format. The position of the patient (sitting or lying down) and which arm was used should be documented.

Normal blood pressure values are:

- systolic: less than 120 (millimeters of mercury)
- diastolic: less than 80 (millimeters of mercury)

Blood Pressure Abnormalities

There are two possible blood pressure abnormalities: hypertension, blood pressure that is consistently above normal, and hypotension, blood pressure that is consistently below normal.

Hypertension: The most commonly seen form of hypertension is primary, or essential. This type of hypertension has no apparent cause or cure, but is treatable.

Secondary hypertension is the result of some underlying condition such as renal disease, pregnancy, endocrine imbalances, obesity, arteriosclerosis, or atherosclerosis. Once the underlying condition has been removed, the blood pressure returns to normal. Secondary hypertension can be treated.

Hypertension that progresses slowly is referred to as **benign**—that is, the development of the disease takes a long time to cause serious problems.

Malignant hypertension, on the other hand, follows a quick line of progression and will cause serious cardiovascular damage.

Hypotension: Hypotension is blood pressure persistently below normal, usually below 90/60. Hypotension is defined as a blood pressure so low that the patient is unable to function normally. It is usually a result of various conditions such as hemorrhage, traumatic or emotional shock, central nervous system disorders, or chronic wasting disease. With treatment for the underlying problems, the blood pressure usually will return to the range of normal readings.

Orthostatic, or postural, hypotension occurs in several circumstances:

- when a person rapidly changes position from supine to standing
- when standing in one position for too long
- as a side effect of certain medications

Orthostatic hypotension happens when the blood pressure has momentarily dropped; the person will feel dizzy and may have blurred vision. Care should be taken when helping patients change to an upright position, as orthostatic hypotension can lead to syncope, or fainting.

Weight and Height

Height and weight are also important tools for diagnosis and treatment of patients, as both—and changes in either—can indicate alterations in health status.

Measuring Weight

In most acute and long-term care settings patients are weighed in kilograms. In ambulatory care settings, such as medical offices, patients may be weighed in pounds or kilograms, depending on office policy.

However, the trend is changing toward using metrics across the board. Therefore, medical assistants must become familiar with the metric system and learn the formulas required for conversion.

In many cases, the patient's weight is measured with each office visit. Accuracy in measuring and recording a patient's weight is very important, because medications and procedures are commonly based on a patient's weight. Any significant weight change since the last visit should be brought to the physician's attention because it may indicate a health problem. Special attention should be paid to specific types of patients:

- A child's weight is plotted on a growth chart along with his or her height to determine whether growth patterns are normal.
- A pregnant woman's weight is carefully noted on each visit as part of the data needed to monitor the pregnancy.
- A patient on a weight-loss program must also have his or her weight closely monitored to determine the effectiveness of the program.

Measuring Height

Methods for measuring height vary, depending on the age and size of the patient.

- Infants are measured during each visit so that their growth can be plotted on growth charts. They are measured lying down, and the measurement is recorded as length in centimeters.
- When the child reaches toddler age and is capable of standing, a standing measurement may be taken.

Adult height is typically measured in feet and inches and is done on the first visit and then only as needed—for example, when there is concern about osteoporosis, or degenerative changes of the vertebrae. A slight decrease in the height of an elderly patient is not unusual, but may indicate a problem.

Body Mass Index

Body mass index is another method used to interpret body weight. The BMI expresses the correlation of an individual's weight to his or her height, providing an indication of the risk of developing chronic health conditions associated with obesity. Many healthcare providers believe that the BMI is a more accurate standard for interpreting body weight than height and weight tables.

The BMI can be calculated, but charts are available—and are standard "equipment" in a medical office—that show the results of the calculations. The charts show height on one axis and weight on another axis; the numbers at the intersection of the appropriate height and weight measurement indicate the BMI.

Physical Examinations

The physical examination provides much information about a patient's health status. A medical assistant will be called upon to assist the physician or other healthcare providers during the examination. Knowing the basic components of the examination is important for deciding what equipment and supplies should be on hand, what position the patient should be in, and how the patient should be draped.

Techniques Used in a Physical Examination

The following describes the techniques used in an examination.

Inspection involves gathering information about the patient through observation. The physician will look at the patient's general appearance and behaviors, including how the patient walks, talks, and makes eye contact.

Palpation involves the examination of the patient's external body through touch with the hands and pads of the fingers. Palpation can include:

- skin, revealing information about temperature, moisture, and texture

- organs, feeling the size, shape, symmetry, and firmness of organs and to detect the presence of masses

Percussion involves tapping on body structures with the fingers or a small hammer to note the sound. The nature of the sound reveals information about the structures beneath. For example, the abdomen will usually have a more high-pitched, vibrating sound caused by greater air content; the area over the liver usually sounds duller because of its denser, vascular structure.

- **Direct percussion** involves tapping directly on the patient's skin.
- **Indirect percussion** involves laying the non-dominant hand or finger on the patient's skin and then tapping it with the fingers on the dominant hand.

Auscultation involves listening to the sounds of the body with a stethoscope (see "Stethoscope" on page 165). Sites and uses of auscultation are:

- lungs, to determine whether they sound clear or have abnormal sounds caused by narrowed airways or the presence of fluid
- abdomen, to assess bowel sounds. Normal sounds include stomach gurgling caused by intestinal peristalsis, the progressive, wavelike involuntary movement that propels the contents forward.
- vascular system (blood vessels), noting the rhythm as well as the presence of abnormal sounds, such as murmurs

Mensuration involves various body measurements, such as:

- height or length
- circumference of the head, chest, abdomen, and sometimes other extremities

- joint motion, to determine the degree of flexion and extension

Manipulation uses hands-on techniques to assess joint symmetry and to note passive range of motion, which is the distance and direction a joint can move to its full potential. It may also be used to employ therapeutic force to increase joint mobility and realign dislocated joints.

The medical assistant's presence may not be required for every examination or treatment. However, in cases where the physician and patient are the opposite gender—especially when the procedure involves areas of the body usually considered private—the medical assistant should remain in the same room.

Components of the Physical Examination

The standard physical examination is organized according to body system and, to some extent, follows a head-to-toe order. However, the physician may vary the examination depending on many factors, including the patient's age, primary complaint, and purpose for the visit.

The physical examination generally includes the following components in this order:

- general appearance
- skin
- arms and hands
- head and neck
- eyes
- ears
- nose
- mouth and pharynx
- chest and lungs
- cardiovascular function
- breasts
- abdomen
- genitalia and rectum
- legs and feet
- mental status

The physician will examine each component for normal and abnormal findings.

Body Positions

The medical assistant helps during the examination by instructing and assisting the patient in assuming various positions. The purpose of each position is to allow the physician better access to and visibility of the body part being examined. To help promote patient privacy and comfort, the medical assistant should provide careful draping.

Sitting Position

The sitting position is commonly used for examination of the upper body, including the head, eyes, ears, nose, throat, neck, chest, lungs, arms, and hands.

Common uses: Upper respiratory symptoms (such as sore throat, sinus pressure, cough, and earache) and painful or inflamed joints of the arms, hands, and fingers.

Supine Position

Also called the horizontal recumbent, the supine position is commonly used for examination of the breasts, anterior chest, heart, abdomen, and lower extremities. This is a position in which the patient is laying flat, face-up toward the ceiling.

Common uses: Breast cancer screening, heart problems, pain in the abdomen, lower leg, or foot.

Dorsal Recumbent

The dorsal recumbent position is sometimes used for rectal and vaginal examinations, particularly if the patient cannot tolerate lying on her back with her feet in stirrups. In the dorsal recumbent position, the patient is lying flat or nearly flat with legs apart, knees bent, and feet near the side edges of the examination table. It may also be used for patients with back or abdominal pain, because bending the knees relieves stress on the lower back and facilitates relaxation of abdominal muscles.

Common uses: Routine examinations and for those with vaginal or rectal pain, burning, or unusual discharge; also useful for those complaining of abdominal, pelvic, or back pain.

Lateral, or Sims, Position

In the lateral position, also called the Sims or side-lying position, the patient lies on his or her side with the upper arm forward on the table, lower arm behind, lower leg flexed slightly, and upper leg flexed deeply with his knee resting in front on the examining table.

Common uses: Anal and rectal examinations, some vaginal examinations, and such procedures as administering rectal suppositories and enemas; facilitates a better view of the patient's urethral opening.

Fowler Position

The Fowler position is similar to the upright sitting position, except that the head of the examination table is elevated as close to 90° as possible to provide support for the patient to lean against it and to allow the legs to rest outstretched on the examination table. It is used for the same reasons as the sitting position and is particularly useful for patients who are feeling short of breath, because the upright position facilitates maximal lung expansion.

Common uses: Similar to the sitting positions; also for patients who are short of breath, as the upright position helps the patient expand his or her lungs to the maximum.

Semi-Fowler Position

The semi-Fowler position is similar to the Fowler position with the head of the examination table at only 45°. The patient reclines with legs outstretched on the examination table.

Common uses: Many purposes, including to examine the chest and heart; provides comfort for patients who need extra rest and relaxation.

Lithotomy Position

The lithotomy position is used for vaginal examinations and particularly useful when a speculum is required to examine the cervix and collect a specimen for a Papanicolaou (Pap) smear. In this position, the patient reclines face-up, with legs apart and feet placed in stirrups.

Common uses: Routine vaginal exams, the collection of cervical tissue sample for Papanicolaou (Pap) smears, for women who have complaints of pelvic pain or unusual vaginal pain, burning, or discharge.

Trendelenburg Position

In the Trendelenburg position, the patient lies with his or her head approximately 30° lower than his or her outstretched legs and feet. Many patients do not tolerate this position well or for long because it makes breathing more difficult. Therefore, the medical assistant should consult with the physician before assisting a patient into this position.

Common uses: Not typically used in the medical office; helpful for patients in shock or with extremely low blood pressure; also for abdominal surgery because gravitational force causes abdominal contents to shift toward the chest.

Knee-Chest Position

In the knee-chest position, the patient sits on his or her knees with the chest and face resting forward on a pillow, arms lying to either side of the head, and buttocks in the air. This position may be awkward, embarrassing, and difficult for many patients to assume. Therefore, the medical assistant must help the patient with positioning and remain with him or her for the entire time to provide stability and emotional support.

Common uses: For rectal and sigmoid colon examinations and, rarely, for vaginal examinations.

Instruments and Supplies Needed During the Physical Exam

The medical assistant helps with the examination process by keeping the examination room clean, disinfected, and restocked as needed between patients. The medical assistant should check the schedule ahead of time and note the purpose of each patient's visit in order to anticipate the equipment and supplies that will most likely be needed, to prepare the patient for examination, and to assist the physician as needed. Having all items ready and close at hand saves time and earns the respect and appreciation of the physician and patient. The patient will also appreciate attention paid to his or her comfort and privacy needs.

Instruments used in the physical examination assist the physician to see, hear, or feel areas of the body. The instruments, supplies, and equipment are kept in a convenient location in each examination room. Supplies include a tape measure, gloves, tongue depressors, and cotton-tipped applicators. Instruments include the following:

- **Laryngeal and pharyngeal mirrors** are stainless steel instruments with long, slender handles and small, round mirrors. They are used to examine the pharynx and larynx.
- **Nasal speculum** is a stainless steel instrument that is inserted into the nostril to help in the visual inspection of the nasal lining, membranes, and septum. The tip of the instrument is inserted into the nose, and the handles are squeezed, which opens the end and allows for maximum inspection inside the nostril.
- An **otoscope** is used to visualize the ear canal and the **tympanic membrane,** i.e., the eardrum. More information on the otoscope can be found on page 167.
- The **tuning fork** is used to test for hearing. It is a stainless steel instrument with a handle at one end and two prongs at the other end. The examiner strikes the prongs against his or her hand, causing them to vibrate and produce a humming sound. When the tuning fork is vibrating, the handle is placed against a bony area of the skull near one of the ears to test for hearing.
- An **audioscope** is also used to test hearing, specifically to screen patients for hearing loss. It is composed of a range of indicators and selection buttons, which are used to adjust the tones. The examiner places the tip of the instrument into the patient's ear, produces various tones, and asks the patient to respond to questions about each of the tones.
- An **ophthalmoscope** is used to examine the interior components of the eye. More information on the ophthalmoscope can be found on page 167.
- A **penlight** or **flashlight** provides additional light to a specific area during the examination. The penlight or flashlight is used to examine the pupils and provide additional light for examination of the throat or other body parts.
- A **reflex hammer** or **percussion hammer** is used to test neurologic reflexes. It has a stainless steel handle and a hard rubber head. The head is used to test the reflexes by striking the tendons of the ankle, knee, wrist, and elbow. The tip of the handle may be used to stroke the sole of the foot to assess the Babinski reflex (a reflex noted by extension of the great toe and abduction of the other toes).
- A **stethoscope** has a bell or diaphragm at one end that is placed on the patient's body. More information on the stethoscope can be found on page 165.
- A **vaginal speculum** is inserted into the vagina to expand the opening to visually examine internal female reproductive structures and to collect samples of cells for Pap smears or discharge for diagnostic testing. To obtain the cervical cells, a spatula, cervical scraper, or histobrush is used.

The medical assistant must also keep the following smaller supplies stocked:

- alcohol pads, used to clean the skin prior to an injection or to clean medical equipment between patients
- gauze pads, used to dress a wound, stop bleeding, or apply medication

- cotton-tipped applicators, used to apply mediation or collect a specimen
- lubricant, used to reduce anticipated discomfort from rectal examinations
- tongue depressor, used to depress the tongue for easier examination of the throat

The following safety and hygiene supplies should also be monitored and maintained:

- antibacterial soap or cleanser
- paper towels
- examination gloves
- biohazard waste containers
- sharps containers
- gowns
- masks

The patient who must wait for a few minutes will also appreciate the medical assistant who provides reading material. Such material should include educational pamphlets as well as an assortment of current magazines.

Physical Therapy Modalities

Physical therapy **modalities**, or treatment methods, are often used in orthopedic, chiropractic, and physical therapy offices to treat orthopedic conditions.

Cold Application

The application of moderate cold to a localized area constricts blood vessels as the body attempts to prevent heat loss. This constriction leads to decreased blood supply to the area. The application of moderate cold for a short time is used to prevent edema, or swelling. Through the constriction of peripheral blood vessels, bleeding can be controlled. Cold also slows the movement of blood and tissue fluids in the affected area, resulting in less pressure against pain receptors and, therefore, less pain. In the early stages of an infection, the local application of cold inhibits the activity of microorganisms. In this way, suppuration, or discharge, is decreased and inflammation is reduced.

Cold application should always be placed in a protective covering, because applying cold directly to the skin could result in skin burn. The cold application should be administered in cycles limited to 20 minutes on and 20 minutes off.

Common uses: Immediately after direct trauma such as a bruise, minor burn, sprain, strain, joint injury, or fracture.

Heat Application

The application of moderate heat to a localized area of the body for a short period of time (15 to 20 minutes) produces dilation, or an increase in diameter, of the superficial blood vessels in the area as the body tries to rid itself of excess heat. This results in an increased blood supply to the area, accompanied by erythema, a reddening of the skin, along with an increase in tissue metabolism. Nutrients and oxygen are provided to the cells at a faster rate; wastes and toxins are carried away faster.

Heat promotes muscle relaxation and is often used for the relief of pain caused by excessive contraction of muscle fibers. Heat modalities can be either wet or dry. Edema, or swelling, in the tissue can be reduced through the application of heat because the increased blood supply functions to increase the absorption of fluid from the tissues through the lymphatic system.

Common uses: Reducing muscle spasms.

Ultrasound

An **ultrasound** is a treatment modality using high or low frequency sound waves transmitted to surrounding tissue. The sound waves penetrate the muscles to cause deep tissue or muscle warming and are used to treat muscle tightness and spasms. The warming effect also causes **vasodilation** (an increase in diameter of a blood vessel) and increased circulation to the area to assist in healing.

Common uses: Treatment of sprains, strains, and other acute ailments.

Transcutaneous Electrical Nerve Stimulation

Transcutaneous electrical nerve stimulation (TENS) is a machine that uses electricity, with electrodes applied to the affected area. The electrical signal disrupts the pain signal being sent from the affected area so that the patient experiences less pain.

TENS uses an electrical current to cause a single muscle or a group of muscles to contract. By placing the electrical current on the appropriate muscle fibers, the medical assistant can force a gentle muscle contraction, allowing the muscle to increase in strength. The contraction of the muscle also promotes blood supply, causing increased healing.

Common uses: Treatment of a pulled back muscle.

Paraffin Bath

A **paraffin bath** is useful in treating chronic joint inflammation. A mixture of seven parts paraffin and one part mineral oil is heated to approximately 125°F (52°C). The body part is placed in the paraffin and then removed, leaving a thin coating of paraffin on the skin. This is repeated several times until the body part is coated. It is then wrapped in plastic and a towel to allow the heat to penetrate into the tissue. The paraffin is kept on for 30 minutes before being peeled off.

Common uses: Reduction of pain, muscle spasms, and stiffness in patients with arthritis.

Patient Education

Patient education is performed under the direction of the physician. The amount and types of education the medical assistant will be expected to provide will vary. To educate patients, the medical assistant will need to help them accept their illness, involve them in the process of gaining knowledge, and provide positive reinforcement.

Changes in the nature of medical care are increasing the importance of patient education. More than ever before, patient education is now being conducted in office-based medical practices.

Health Maintenance and Disease Prevention

The roles a medical assistant takes in patient education include:

- giving all patients information about healthy habits and encouraging them to make lifestyle choices that will improve their general health
- providing information or answering questions about procedures, diagnostic tests, and follow-up care for acute illness or injury
- providing intensive one-on-one education for self-care and self-management of chronic illnesses such as asthma, diabetes, or hypertension

New information can be presented to patients in a range of ways: discussion and talk, information sheets and pamphlets, videos and websites, and so on. Therefore, the medical assistant should help the medical practice be prepared to provide instruction to patients in ways that are most useful to the individual patient. Preparing lists of approved websites or maintaining a file of approved information sheets on various conditions and treatments, for instance, will help the medical facility fulfill its role in educating patients about their health.

Preparation for Procedures

Before a diagnostic procedure, the patient must be instructed as to what the procedure is, where it will be performed, how long it will take, how to prepare for the test, and what will happen after the test. The medical assistant needs to become familiar with preparation for frequently ordered tests, but should check with the testing facility if he or she is unsure about that facility's particular preparation protocols.

- Preparation for X-rays often requires dietary or bowel preparation, especially when they involve the gastrointestinal or urinary tract. The patient needs to understand what diet to follow and how to prepare the bowel, including what supplies are needed and where to purchase them.

- Preparation for blood tests may require that the patient fast. For example, a lipid profile usually requires an 18-hour-long fast, and an overnight fast is standard for a fasting blood sugar test. Other blood tests are repeated at regular intervals; for example, a prothrombin time is repeated monthly for patients taking the anticoagulant warfarin.

- Instructions for imaging tests vary. For a pelvic ultrasound, the bladder needs to be full. For an MRI (magnetic resonance imaging) or mammogram, the patient needs to be reminded not to wear any metal products. For mammograms, the woman should not use any antiperspirant on the underarm or under her breasts.

- Some tests require that the patient stop any medications or avoid certain foods in the days before the test, and patients need specific instructions when these tests are scheduled.

Patient Administered Medications

Although the doctor or other primary care provider instructs the patient about medications, the medical assistant may need to reinforce these instructions, such as:

- continuing to take the entire prescription even after feeling better, as is the case with antibiotics
- taking the prescription with food, as is the case with some antibiotics and most nonsteroidal anti-inflammatory drugs (NSAIDs)
- eating foods high in potassium, as is necessary when taking diuretics

Some medical offices and other facilities have instruction sheets for their medical assistants to use with specific medications. These sheets, prepared by a licensed healthcare professional, include specific points for instruction, including the patient's understanding of the medication's proper use, the medication's actions, coping with the side effects, adverse reactions to report to the office, and how to assure understanding of following up lab work that may be necessary.

Pharmacies also often give instruction sheets to patients when a prescription is filled. The medial assistant should encourage patients to read these instruction sheets.

Patient History and Interview

The medical history includes all of the information a patient can give about previous healthcare, medical problems and potential medical problems, and previous and current treatment. This history becomes part of the patient's medical record.

This information is necessary for the physician to evaluate the patient's current condition and determine how to treat him or her.

Personal Data

Every patient fills out a patient information sheet at the first visit, with demographic, billing, insurance, and health information.

The demographic information includes name, address, telephone number, Social Security number, marital status, sex, age, date of birth, employer, employer address and phone number, and emergency contact information.

Chief Complaint

The chief complaint is the main problem that brought a patient to the medical office. If the patient has come for a routine physical examination, there may be no chief complaint. Important information to be recorded about the patient's chief complaint include:

- **Symptom:** A change in the body that indicates altered function or disease and that the patient experiences through his or her senses or sensation. These changes are called **subjective** complaints, because they cannot be measured or validated.

- **Sign:** A change that can be observed and measured, such as weight gain. These changes are called **objective** complaints, which means they can be observed and measured.

Additional information to describe the chief complaint include:

- location: where the symptoms are located
- quality: how one would characterize the symptoms
- severity: quantitative aspects of the illness, that is, intense, moderate or mild pain
- chronology: when the illness began and how long it lasted
- source: what the patient was doing when the complaint began or was first noticed
- what makes it better or worse: what the patient has done to relieve symptoms or make them worse
- associated symptoms: what other symptoms the patient is having

Past, Present, Family, and Social History

A new patient will fill out a questionnaire about his or her past medical history, or the medical assistant will fill out the questionnaire by asking the patient questions regarding his or her medical history. There are three elements of past health history:

- family history: taken to understand the general health of family members and the diseases that run in families
- previous hospitalizations, surgeries, and injuries: including the date and reason for hospitalization or the date and type of injury; for women, also include hospitalization for childbirth and type of delivery
- illness or medical problems: should be as complete as possible, because something overlooked by the patient may be important in a current or future diagnosis

The present history includes:

- ongoing medical problems: should be as complete as possible
- current medications: including over-the-counter as well as physician-prescribed medications
- allergies: including all allergies, such as medication, food, materials (such as latex), and so on
- social history: including appetite, sleeping, diet, exercise, caffeine, smoking, alcohol, street drugs, and occupational history

If the patient fills out a questionnaire, the medical assistant will review the questionnaire with the patient and fill in any missing sections or clarify answers.

Review of Systems

A review of systems (ROS) is a systematic review of each body system to detect any symptoms that have not yet been revealed. The physician completes the review of symptoms by asking a series of questions related to each body system; the result is a preliminary assessment of the type and extent of physical examination required. The review of systems includes:

- head and neck
- eyes
- ears
- mouth
- nose and throat
- respiratory
- cardiovascular
- digestive
- urinary
- male genitals
- female genitals
- obstetric history
- musculoskeletal
- skin
- neurological

Laboratory Testing and Collecting and Processing Specimens

Collecting and processing specimens for testing is an important duty of the medical assistant. The timing of the collection, the processing, and the method used are all geared toward giving the physician accurate results.

Blood Samples

Venipuncture, also known as phlebotomy, is the removal of a sample of blood, usually from a superficial vein. The procedure is performed to obtain a blood sample for analysis, or as a source for blood donation. A dermal puncture is a removal of blood from the capillaries. This collection procedure is used when a small quantity of blood is needed or when the patient's vein is too small or fragile for a venipuncture.

A venipuncture is most frequently performed using the veins in the antecubital space of the forearms and the inside of the elbow. Another site that can be used is the back of the hand.

Blood may be drawn from a vein using one of two methods. Blood may be drawn directly into an evacuated tube, a glass or plastic tube sealed with a rubber stopper, using a multi-sample needle. Alternately, blood may be drawn using a needle and syringe, which is a tube attached to the needle. In the evacuated-tube method, the vacuum inside the tube provides the pressure to pull blood out of the vein. In the syringe method, manual pressure on the plunger pulls blood from the vein.

Venipuncture Equipment

Having the proper equipment and supplies at hand is one of the keys to being able to perform a fast and easy blood draw. The most common method of drawing blood is using evacuated tubes. The following equipment is necessary for an evacuated tube blood draw:

- **Needles:** A needle for drawing blood must have a large enough opening to prevent damage to the red blood cells, or hemolysis. Different needles are used for a single sample or for multiple samples; a multiple-sample needle has a rubber sheath that fits over the end of the needle and penetrates the rubber stopper of the evacuated tube so that blood does not leak out while the tubes are being changed. The medical assistant should choose the needle length that is easiest to control, using a combination of personal preference and an evaluation of the stability of the vein.

- **Winged infusion set:** A winged infusion set, or butterfly needle, can be used on pediatric patients, the elderly, and patients with small or difficult veins. It can be attached either directly to a syringe or to an adapter that screws into a plastic holder for use with evacuated tubes. This allows more tubes to be drawn.

- **Needle holder:** A needle holder is a cylinder that the needle is screwed into. Needle holders come in different sizes to accommodate the size of the collection tube.

- **Tourniquet:** A tourniquet is a thin strip of non-latex rubber used to tie around the arm to help locate a vein. The tourniquet is tied three to four inches above the elbow and should not be left on for more than one minute because of the risk of hemoconcentration, or a decrease in the fluid components of the blood.

- **Alcohol:** An alcohol swab is used to clean the site before the venipuncture to prevent infection.

- **Gauze and tape:** Gauze is used to absorb blood after the venipuncture and to aid in applying pressure to the site. Adhesive tape is used to secure coverage to the venipuncture site.

- **Evacuated tube:** A tube with air evacuated from it to create a vacuum. When using the evacuated-tube method, a plastic holder holds the needle in place and supports the evacuated tube(s). The vacuum in the tube draws the blood into the tube. Each tube fills with blood until the vacuum is exhausted.

Some tubes contain one or more additives, depending on the test that will be done on that sample. The stopper color identifies the additive in the tube. Different brands of evacuated tubes (called systems) have a different color coding. The medical assistant must learn and remember the color-coding for the particular system used in any office in which he or she works. Blood drawn by the syringe method is usually put into an evacuated tube for transport to the lab.

Tubes with no additives are used to allow a clot to form. These are used to perform tests on chemicals in the serum (the liquid portion of the blood after all of the cells and clotting elements have settled and formed a clot). These include blood chemistry analyses such as tests for the presence of glucose, cholesterol, electrolytes, therapeutic drugs, alcohol and street drugs, hormone measures, and serology.

BLOOD COLLECTION TUBES		
COLOR	**ADDITIVE**	**TESTS**
yellow	sodium polyanethol sulfonate	blood or body fluid cultures
light blue	sodium citrate	coagulation
red	none	chemistry, serologic, toxicology
gold or tiger	silica particles to enhance clot formation	chemistry, serologic
green	heparin	chemistry
lavender	ethylenediaminetet-raacetic acid (EDTA)	hematology
gray	potassium oxalate or sodium fluoride	chemistry

This chart is an example of a system of color coding for evacuated tubes.

If blood analysis cannot be done immediately, a tube with a silica gel (called a serum separator tube, or SST) is used. This tube must be centrifuged as soon as possible after clot formation. After centrifuging, the gel separates the serum from the cells. Separating the serum from the blood cells prevents the cells from altering the chemistry of the serum.

Order of Draw

The order of draw refers to the order in which tubes are filled when multiple tubes are collected for multiple blood studies. The following order is recommended to minimize problems if small amounts of additives from a previous tube get into tubes drawn later.

1. Sterile tubes for blood culture
2. Tubes without additives
3. SSTs—tubes that contain silica gel
4. Tubes for coagulation studies. If only coagulation studies are ordered, a tube without additives should be drawn first (and discarded) to prevent tissue thromboplastin from entering the tube for coagulation studies.
5. Other tubes containing anticoagulants
6. Other tubes with additives

Sites to Avoid

Evacuated tube method: The evacuated tube method is appropriate for medium and large veins. The best veins are the median cephalic or lateral basilic veins the antecubital area. Do not use scarred, sclerosed, or injured veins, or veins in areas with a rash, bruise, tattoo, or other skin lesion, or an **arteriovenous fistula** for renal dialysis.

If a patient has had a mastectomy (removal of the breast), do not draw from the arm on the side of the removed breast. Do not draw from an edematous area (an area of swelling due to fluid collection). Do not draw from the arm in which an intravenous drip (IV) is in place.

To avoid needle-stick injuries, the medical assistant should never recap a needle. An available sharps container or one of the safety devices designed for blood drawing should always be used. These include holders that slides down to enclose the needle after use or needles that blunt while still in the vein. A hemolyzed blood specimen or one taken from an atypical area, such as a hematoma or the area above or below an intravenous drip, shows marked differences in many tests.

Syringe method: The syringe method is appropriate for small and delicate veins. The syringe method should be used on the veins of the antecubital area. A 22G or 23G, 1" to $1\frac{1}{2}$" needle should be used. Only about 10 mL of blood can be obtained using this method.

The blood must be transferred from the syringe to evacuated tubes before it clots. For safety, use a blood transfer device. Attach the transfer device to the syringe. Insert an evacuated blood collection tube into the transfer device/syringe assembly. Next, allow the blood to transfer from the syringe to the tube using the tube's vacuum. Do not depress the plunger of the syringe. When the appropriate number of tubes is filled, dispose of the syringe and transfer device as one unit according to your institution's policies.

Dermal Puncture

A dermal, or skin puncture, is performed to obtain capillary blood. **Capillaries** are the small blood vessels that carry blood to and from the small arterioles to the tissues and return blood to the small venules. Common sites used for dermal puncture include the ring or middle finger (called a finger stick) and the plantar surface (underside) of the heel. The finger stick is most common.

Any blood test can be performed with blood from a capillary specimen, but not enough blood is obtained for multiple tests or for repeating a test to confirm results. Capillary specimens may be taken on infants and children when small amounts of blood are needed or when it is difficult to perform venipuncture because of inaccessible or collapsed veins.

Equipment and Supplies

To obtain a capillary blood specimen, the following equipment and supplies may be used:

1. Lancet, to pierce the skin. Manual lancets are single blades for making small incisions—disposable lancets are used for adults and a disposable automatic lancet is used for an infant. A disposable lancet is placed in a plastic holder and the system's platform is placed on the patient's finger. A plunger is depressed and the spring causes the lancet to puncture the skin. The advantage of such a system is that it standardizes the depth of puncture.
2. Blood collection device. Microhematocrit or capillary tubes are either plastic or glass-coated with a plastic sheathing to minimize the risk of shattering. Capillary tubes can be either plain or heparinized to avoid blood clotting. They are closed by pressing one end in sealing clay. Microcollection containers are small plastic tubes with removable, color-coded caps. The tip is shaped like a scoop, to direct the blood flow off the side and down the tube. The color of the cap may indicate the type of additive, if any, in the tube. For instance, a lavender-colored top indicates there is EDTA in the tube, as in evacuated tubes.
3. Alcohol pads and gauze pads
4. Sealing clay

Finger sticks are usually performed on the middle or ring finger of the nondominant hand. There is good capillary flow in this area and enough subcutaneous tissue to prevent accidental puncture of the bone (as might occur on the little finger). A finger stick should not puncture deeper than 3.1 mm on an adult or 2.4 mm on an infant or child.

Urine Specimens

Urine specimens are used for a variety of tests and collected in a variety of ways, the most common of which are discussed here.

Routine or Random Specimen

Random urine specimens can be used for a variety of tests, including urine pregnancy tests and urinalysis. Random specimens are not recommended when a UTI is suspected.

To collect a random urine sample, the patient should be instructed to void into the specimen cup, filling the cup with approximately 50 mL to 100 mL of urine. After the specimen is collected, the container must be tightly capped to avoid leaking. If the patient is unable to void, he or she should be instructed to drink water and try to eliminate later, perhaps after the physical examination.

Clean-Catch Midstream Specimen

Collection of clean-catch midstream urine is the method of choice for most healthcare providers. This type of specimen, if properly collected, provides an excellent sample for most urine tests. A clean-catch midstream specimen can be used for routine urinalysis, urine cultures, urine pregnancy testing, and microscopic examination, as well as for culture and sensitivity testing. It may be helpful to post instructions for clean-catch specimens in appropriate urine collection sites.

First Morning Specimen

When a concentrated urine specimen is needed, as in pregnancy testing, the first morning sample is the specimen of choice. Formed elements and urine chemicals such as nitrites are best studied at that time. Unless the patient is hospitalized, first morning specimens must often be collected by the patient at home. Label the specimen cup with the patient's name and give it to the patient with explicit instructions and any necessary supplies before the patient leaves the office.

The patient should be instructed to deliver the specimen as soon as possible, no more than four hours after the urine is collected. If the specimen cannot be transported immediately to the testing facility, it should be refrigerated.

24-Hour Urine Specimen

The 24-hour urine collection can be used for a number of tests. One of the most important factors affecting the specimen collection is determining the specific container in which the specimen will be collected. A laboratory test reference guide should be consulted whenever a 24-hour urine test is ordered. Some 24-hour procedures require the addition of a preservative into the container before the specimen is collected; other tests use no preservative but require that the specimen be refrigerated between voids.

If a preservative is added to the 24-hour specimen container, the container must be labeled as to the type and amount of preservative added. Most tests require that urine specimens be protected from light. Also, the total volume or weight must be carefully measured and recorded.

Containers

Three different types of containers are used for collecting urine specimens. Urine cups for single samples can be either sterile (for culturing urine) or nonsterile (for random specimens to conduct general urinalysis). Urine containers for 24-hour collection are larger and may contain preservatives, such as boric acid or hydrochloric acid. The medical assistant should always check the procedure manual to determine which preservative to add before giving the collection bottle to the patient.

Stool Specimens

A stool, or fecal, specimen is collected to test for bacteria and/or parasites if a patient's chief complaint is persistent diarrhea that does not respond to the usual treatment. It can also be collected for an occult blood test, to see if there is hidden blood in a patient's stool.

Fecal collection can be accomplished either by using a rectal swab or by collecting a portion of a bowel movement. The methods for collecting a specimen from a bowel movement are discussed here.

- **Adults:** For adults who are capable of using a toilet, the method of collection is fairly straightforward. The toilet should be covered with a large sheet of plastic wrap. A depression in the middle of the plastic wrap should be made to allow for collection. Following the bowel movement, part of the stool should be collected using the collection spoon.
- **Infants:** Collecting a specimen from a diaper is also straightforward. The diaper should be lined with plastic wrap. Once the stool specimen has been provided, use the collection spoon to add sufficient stool to the collection vials.

In both cases, a specimen spoon is used to collect the specimen, and enough stool should be collected so that, when inserted into the specimen vial, it will bring the liquid level to the fill line.

If a large volume of specimen is collected, such as a 24-hour fecal fat specimen, the total volume or weight must be accurately measured and recorded.

Sputum Samples

A sputum sample may be necessary to diagnose tuberculosis, pneumonia, or other infectious disease of the lungs and lower respiratory tract.

Expectoration is the coughing up of mucus from the lungs and throat. This is the least uncomfortable method of sputum collection for the patient and is used when the patient is able to produce sputum by coughing. If the expectoration method is to be used, the patient should be instructed to drink plenty of liquid the night before, not to brush his or her teeth or use mouthwash in the morning, and to give the specimen before eating. The patient should be instructed to take a deep breath and cough vigorously to obtain the lower respiratory secretions. The patient should never simply spit into the specimen cup, as saliva is not composed of lower respiratory secretions and is not appropriate for a sputum specimen.

Suctioning equipment can also be used to collect a sputum sample. The medical assistant will require special training for the use of this equipment.

Throat Culture Specimens

To obtain a throat culture, a tongue depressor is used to hold the tongue down and a sterile swab. The specimen is obtained with a sterile swab from the back of the throat; care must be taken not to touch the tongue or teeth after the specimen is obtained.

The test is performed either by growing a culture in an incubator or by using a rapid strep test kit, which will be discussed in detail further in the chapter. If the rapid strep test is negative, a culture is recommended. To cause the least discomfort to the patient, a medical assistant should take specimens on two swabs simultaneously, rather than having to swab the throat twice.

Vaginal Specimens

A vaginal culture is collected using a swab. The sterile polyester tipped swab contains a preservative (buffer) to maintain the integrity of the specimen. The laboratory will test the specimen for bacteria, viruses, or fungal infections.

During a speculum examination by the physician, and prior to any examination or manipulation of the cervix or vaginal tract, the swab is lightly rotated across the posterior fornix of the vagina for approximately ten seconds to absorb cervicovaginal secretions. The swab is then removed and placed into the plastic sleeve.

Wound Specimens

A wound specimen is a specimen from a cut or surgical incision that has become infected. A wound may contain aerobic or anaerobic bacteria. Aerobic bacteria require oxygen to survive, whereas anaerobic bacteria thrive under conditions without oxygen. Deep wounds are especially likely to contain anaerobic bacteria. It is important that specimens be collected to perform aerobic and anaerobic cultures. Gram stains should also be performed on all wound specimens.

Use a sterile swab to collect a specimen from a wound that appears to be infected when directed to do so by the doctor. The specimen collected must be a true representative sample. A swab for a wound culture collected from the surface of the wound generally does not yield the same results as one taken from the depths of the wound.

Processing Specimens

Processing the specimen is as important as the collection. If the specimen is not processed properly it could lead to inaccurate results and unnecessary risk to the patient.

CDC Guidelines

Infection with biohazardous material can occur during specimen collection, handling, transporting, or testing. Potentially infective specimens include blood, body tissue biopsy specimens, urine, exudates, and bacterial cultures and smears. Infection can occur through aspiration of a pathogen, accidental inoculation by a needle stick, aerosols created by uncapping specimen tubes, centrifuge accidents, and entry of pathogens through cuts and scratches.

The CDC recommends safety precautions regarding handling of all patient specimens. These precautions include an infection control plan, engineering and work practice controls, personal protective clothing and equipment, sufficient training and education, provision of hepatitis B vaccination, and medical intervention after exposure incidents.

The Clinical and Laboratory Standards Institute (CLSI) also has guidelines for the laboratory worker with regard to protection from blood-borne illness caused by contact with patient specimens. The CAP offers a voluntary accreditation program for clinical laboratories that includes biosafety measures. One important precaution that can be taken is labeling of potentially biohazardous material.

Washing the hands is undoubtedly the most effective means of preventing infection. Information on proper hand washing technique can be found at the beginning of this chapter under "Medical Asepsis" (page 157).

Specimen Handling and Preservation

It has been said that the results of laboratory testing are only as good as the specimen sent for testing. Specimens that are handled improperly after collection may provide erroneous results, causing unnecessary compromise to the patient's health.

The following are reasons why a specimen might be rejected by a lab:

- quantity not sufficient (QNS)
- hemolyzed specimen
- specimen collected in the wrong container
- unlabeled specimen
- contaminated specimen
- delay in transport

All microbiology specimens should be transported as soon as possible to the laboratory. Transport media, such as CO_2 ampules or capsules for anaerobic bacteria, should be activated. For instance, culture tubes are activated by squeezing the sides of the culture tube to release the holding fluid.

Urine specimens must be refrigerated if they cannot be transported immediately.

Proper Labeling

Proper labeling and transport protocols are important for accurate microbiology testing results. A label must include:

- patient's correct name
- patient identification number, or a bar code
- site of the specimen collection
- type of culture ordered (e.g., throat culture for beta strep, vaginal culture for gonorrhea)
- date and time of the specimen
- doctor's name
- initials of the person performing the specimen collection

Quality Control

Quality assurance (QA) is a comprehensive set of policies and procedures utilized to assess the reproducibility of a test result. Quality control (QC) is a process to ensure the validity or accuracy of test results.

Every POL, or physician office laboratory, needs to establish a quality assurance, quality control, and clinical standards program to monitor its performance and improve in areas in which it determines it is deficient.

QC Testing

Quality control is a method of ensuring that all factors involved in the testing procedure at a POL are performing as expected. The factors assessed include:

- personnel
- manufactured test kits or reagents
- instruments
- supplies

Manufacturers prepare a sample of a tested substance that has a known value, or a positive or negative outcome; this is known as a control reagent. If the medical assistant is responsible for performing QC procedures in the POL, he or she will run the control sample as if it were a patient's specimen and compare the results with the expected values provided by the manufacturer of the control reagents. A positive control should yield a positive result and a negative control should produce a negative result. Some controls such as glucose controls have numerical values. The expected value is provided as a range. As long as the control falls within the range, the testing procedure can be used for patients.

Possible reasons for faulty test results include:

- Human error. If the test is run manually, human error can cause incorrect results.
- A problem with the chemicals or reagents being used. Chemicals and reagents should always be checked to see if they have expired or are other-

wise bad. Reagents may get contaminated with bacterial growth from improper use.
- A problem with the laboratory equipment. In situations where automated testing equipment is used, control samples are sometimes run along with the patient samples; other times, the samples are run first and results checked to see if they are within the acceptable range.

For many pieces of automated testing equipment, QC tests are performed first thing in the morning, before running patient specimens, and at regular intervals throughout the day or after a certain number of tests have been run. Results of QC tests are recorded in the QC log. Instruments should be cleaned daily and preventive maintenance should be performed according to the manufacturer's recommendation.

Performing Selected Tests

Once a specimen is collected, the tests performed on it reveal a whole range of factors relating to health status and disease. This section describes the tests that are performed with specimens collected, and the purpose of those tests.

Urinalysis

A physiologic change in the body caused by disease can create a disturbance in one or more of the functions of the kidney. Detection of such a disturbance can be made with the examination of urine and other body fluids.

Physical Urinalysis

The physical examination of urine includes determination of the color, appearance, and specific gravity. The color and appearance of the urine specimen may be evaluated during preparation for another testing procedure, such as the chemical testing of the urine or before centrifugation of the specimen in preparation for microscopic analysis.

Color: The following list describes aspects of the color of urine that should be noted.

- The normal color of urine ranges from almost colorless to dark yellow.
- Dilute urine tends to be a lighter yellow in color while concentrated urine is a darker yellow.
- The color of the urine is the result of the presence of a yellow pigment known as **urochrome**, which is produced by the breakdown of hemoglobin.
- Classifications that are used to describe the color of urine include light yellow, yellow, dark yellow, light amber, amber, and dark amber.
- Abnormal colors may be caused by the presence of hemoglobin or blood, bile pigments, and fat droplets.
- Some foods and medications can also cause the urine to change color.

Transparency: The transparency or clarity of urine is usually examined at the same time as the color evaluation. Fresh urine is usually clear, or transparent, but becomes cloudy as time goes by. Cloudiness in a urine sample may be the result of the presence of bacteria, pus, blood, fat, yeast, sperm, mucous threads, or fecal contamination. Classifications used to describe the appearance of urine include clear, slightly cloudy, cloudy, and very cloudy.

Specific gravity of urine measures the weight of the urine compared with the weight of an equal volume of distilled water. Specific gravity indicates the amount of dissolved substances present in the urine, providing information on the ability of the kidneys to dilute or concentrate the urine. Acceptable values are:

- normal range: from 1.003 to 1.030
- usual range: from 1.010 to 1.025

The reagent strip method is the most common method used to measure specific gravity. It involves a color comparison determination using a reagent strip that contains a reagent for specific gravity. The reagent strip is dipped into the urine specimen and the results are compared with a color chart.

Chemical Examination of Urine

Substances present in excess amounts in the blood are usually removed by the urine. The chemical testing of urine is an indirect means, therefore, of detecting abnormal amounts of chemicals in the body. The chemical examination of urine can also be used to detect the presence of blood and nitrite.

Chemical tests that are routinely performed during a urinalysis include testing for pH, glucose, protein, and ketones. Other chemical tests that may be performed include testing for blood, bilirubin, urobilinogen, nitrite, and leukocytes.

Urine analysis is broken down into two general categories:

- Qualitative analysis of urine indicates whether a substance is present in the urine and also provides an approximate indication of the amount of the substance present. The interpretation of qualitative tests usually involves the use of a color chart, with results recorded in terms of trace, 1+, 2+, or 3+; trace, small, moderate, or large; or negative or positive.
- Quantitative analysis of urine indicates the exact amount of a chemical substance that is present in the body; the results are reported in measurable units.

The most important tests performed on urine examine the following elements:

- **pH:** The pH level indicates the acidity or alkalinity of a solution. The pH scale ranges from 0.0 to 14.0. The lower the number, the greater the acidity; the higher the number, the greater the alkalinity. A pH reading of 7.0 is neutral; a reading below 7.0 indicates acidity; and a reading above 7.0 indicates alkalinity.
- **Glucose:** No glucose should be detected in urine. Glucose in the blood is filtered through the nephrons and is reabsorbed into the body. If the glucose concentration is the blood becomes

too high, the kidney is unable to reabsorb all of it back into the blood, the **renal threshold** is exceeded, and glucose is spilled into the urine; this is called **glycosuria**.

■ **Protein:** Protein in urine (**proteinuria**) usually indicates a pathological condition if found in several samples over time. Some of the conditions that may cause proteinura include glomerular filtration problems, renal disease, or bacterial infection.

■ **Ketones:** Ketones are the normal products of fat metabolism and can be used by muscle tissue as a source of energy. When large amounts of fat are metabolized by the body, the muscles cannot handle all of the ketones that result. Large amounts of ketones accumulate in the tissues and body fluids; this condition is called **ketosis**. The body rids itself of these excess ketones in the urine. This is called **ketonuria**. Conditions that may lead to ketonuria include uncontrolled diabetes mellitus, starvation, and a diet composed almost entirely of fat.

■ **Bilirubin:** Bilirubin is the breakdown of hemoglobin. Bilirubin is normally transported to the liver and excreted into the bile; eventually, it leaves the body through the intestines in the feces. Certain liver conditions, such as gallstones, hepatitis, and cirrhosis, may result in the presence of bilirubin in the urine. This is called **bilirubinuria**.

■ **Urobilinogen:** Urobilinogen is normally excreted by the liver into the intestinal tract. Bacteria present in the intestines convert it to urobilinogen. Most urobilinogen is excreted in the feces. Conditions such as excessive hemolysis of red blood cells, infectious hepatitis, cirrhosis, congestive heart failure, and infectious mononucleosis may increase the urobilinogen levels in urine.

■ **Blood:** Blood is not normally found in urine (unless it is present as a contaminant during menstruation). Blood in urine is called **hematuria**.

Hematuria may be the result of an injury or disorder such as cystitis, tumors of the bladder, urethritis, kidney stones, and certain kidney disorders.

■ **Leukocytes:** Leukocytes found in urine is known as **leukocyturia**. Leukocytes found in the urine indicate an inflammation of the kidneys and the lower urinary tract.

■ **Nitrate:** Nitrate is a compound of nitrogen and oxygen found in many food items. Some pathogenic bacteria posses the ability to convert nitrate to nitrite. Nitrite in the urine suggests the presence of these pathogenic bacteria and indicates a possible urinary tract infection.

Reagent strips are commonly used to test the urine in the medical office. The number and type of reagent areas included on the reagent strip depend on the particular brand of reagent strips. For instance, Multistix 10 SG strips contain ten reagent areas for testing pH, protein, glucose, ketones, bilirubin, blood, urobilinogen, nitrite, specific gravity, and leukocytes.

The chemical testing of the reagent strip can be performed manually by placing the reagent strip in the urine and, at a certain time period, comparing the color on the reagent strip to the values on the container. A urine analyzer is used to perform an automatic chemical examination of urine with reagent strip. The reagent strip is fed into the machine and prints out the results.

Microscopic Urinalysis

The microscopic exam is a method used to confirm the results of the physical and chemical urine evaluation. The medical assistant can prepare the urine for microscopic examination, but a physician or other qualified healthcare professional must read and record the results.

Substances that may be found in the microscopic urine include RBCs, WBCs, epithelial cells, crystals, bacteria, and other substances.

Hematology

Hematology is the study of blood, including the morphologic appearance and function of blood cells and diseases of the blood and blood-forming tissues. Laboratory analysis in hematology examines blood for the purpose of detecting pathologic conditions. Hematology testing also includes blood cell counts, evaluating the clotting ability of the blood, and identifying cell types.

The most frequently performed hematology test is the complete blood count (CBC). The tests included in the CBC are:

- red blood cell count (RBC)
- white blood cell count (WBC)
- platelet count
- hemoglobin (Hgb)
- hematocrit (Hct)
- differential WBC count (diff)
- RBC indices

Hematologic laboratory tests can now be performed in the medical office, due to advances in automated blood analyzers designed for use in the medical office. Automated blood analyzers provide accurate test results in a short time.

Red Blood Cell

Red blood cells, the most common type of cell in the blood, are responsible for delivering oxygen to the body. The RBC count is a measurement of the number of RBCs in whole blood.

ACCEPTABLE RANGES FOR RBC COUNT		
CATEGORY	NORMAL RANGE	NORMAL AS EXPRESSED ON LAB REPORTS
healthy woman	4 to 5.5 million/ cubic mm of blood	4 to 5.5 (x10⁶/mm³)
healthy man	4.5 to 6.2 million RBCs/cubic mm of blood	4.5 to 6.2 (x10⁶/mm³)

Abnormal levels in RBC count can result from several factors or conditions.

- decrease in the RBC count: anemia, Hodgkin's disease, and leukemia
- increase of RBCs: polycythemia, dehydration, and pulmonary fibrosis

White Blood Cell

White blood cells play a major role in the immune system. There are five types of white blood cells (or leukocytes), each having a certain size, shape, appearance, and function:

- neutrophils
- eosinophils
- basophils
- lymphocytes
- monocytes

The purpose of the differential cell count is to identify and count the five types of WBCs in a representative blood sample. An increase or decrease in one or more types may occur in pathologic conditions, which may assist the physician in making a diagnosis.

The differential cell count can be performed automatically or manually. The automatic method is faster and more convenient.

Automatic method: This procedure involves the use of a blood cell counter, such as the Coulter cell counter. Specimen requirements: an ethylenediaminetetraacetic acid (EDTA) anticoagulated blood specimen, which is obtained through venipuncture. The blood cell counter automatically performs the differential count and the results are printed on a laboratory report.

Manual method: This procedure requires that the medical assistant make two blood smears. Some pointers on preparing the blood smears follow.

- Blood smears should be made within two hours of the specimen collection.

- After preparing the blood smear, the medical assistant places the slides in a protective container for transport to an outside laboratory.
- Because WBCs are clear and colorless, they must be stained first with an appropriate dye (usually Wright's stain) before a differential count is performed. The nucleus, cytoplasm, and any granules in the cytoplasm take on the characteristic color of their cell type, which aids in proper identification.
- A minimum of 100 WBCs is identified on the blood smear and each is identified as one of the five types of leukocytes and the number of each type is translated into a percentage. This then reflects the overall distribution of WBCs in the patient's bloodstream.

The normal range for each type of WBC making up the total number of leukocytes is:

- neutrophils: 50% to 70%
- eosinophils: 1% to 4%
- basophils: 0% to 1%
- lymphocytes: 20% to 35%
- monocytes: 3% to 8%

Platelets: Platelets are colorless cell fragments that play a vital role in blod clotting. The platelet count, also part of the CBC, assists in evaluation of bleeding disorders that occur with liver disease, thrombocytopenia, uremia, and anticoagulant therapy.

Normal ranges for platelet counts are: 150,000 to 400,000 per cubic millimeter.

Hematocrit

A hematocrit test involves separating the components of the blood. The solid or cellular elements are separated from the plasma in a blood specimen that has been prepped with an anticoagulant and put through a centrifuge.

- bottom layer: heavier RBCs packed together

- top layer: clearer, lighter plasma, which is straw-colored
- middle layer: yellowish gray layer that holds the platelets and WBCs; called the buffy coat

The purpose of the test is to determine the percentage volume of RBCs in whole blood. The normal hematocrit ranges are 37% to 47% for women and 40% to 54% for men.

A low hematocrit reading may indicate anemia and a high reading may indicate polycythemia.

The microhematocrit method is used most often in the medical office to perform a hematocrit. Capillary blood is drawn directly from a skin puncture into a capillary tube lined with an anticoagulant agent. After collecting the specimen, one end of the capillary tube is sealed and the tube is placed in a microhematocrit centrifuge. The centrifuge spins the blood at an extremely high speed. Within one to three minutes, the RBCs are packed and the results can be read.

Hemoglobin

Hemoglobin is a major component of RBCs. It carries oxygen to the tissue cells of the body and is responsible for the color of the RBCs. It therefore can be used to measure the oxygen-carrying capacity of the blood. The normal ranges are 12 to 16 g/dL for an adult female and 14 to 18 g/dL for an adult male.

A hemoglobin determination is performed as an individual test or part of the CBC, with either capillary or venous blood.

A decreased hemoglobin level can indicate several conditions, including:

- anemia
- hyperthyroidism
- cirrhosis
- severe hemorrhaging
- hemolytic reactions
- certain systemic disease such as leukemia and Hodgkin's disease

Increased levels of hemoglobin can indicate several conditions, including polycythemia, chrronic obstructive pulmonary disease, and congestive heart failure.

The most accurate and dependable technique for measuring hemoglobin levels involves the use of a blood analyzer.

Erythrocyte Sedimentation Rate (ESR)

The erythrocyte sedimentation rate is a screening tool to analyze inflammatory processes. An increased ESR can indicate a range of conditions: It can be a sign of a simple bacterial infection, or a sign of an autoimmune disease such as systemic lupus erythematosus, rheumatoid arthritis, or Crohn's disease.

The ESR test consists of placing a well-mixed anticoagulated blood sample in a tube for one hour to measure how fast the RBC settle to the bottom. Normal RBC are biconcave-shaped and settle at a steady rate. Conditions in which the RBC are abnormal in shape, such as sickle-cell anemia, or conditions that affect the amount of fibrinogen in the plasma, such as hypofibrinogenemia, can change the sedimentation rate.

There are automated tools for performing ESR testing; however, the test is usually performed manually using either the Westergren method or Wintrobe method.

Westergren method: A sample of venous blood is mixed with a 3.8 percent sodium citrate solution (an anticoagulant agent) and left to stand vertically for an hour. The ESR is measured in millimeters of sediment that forms in one hour (mm/hr).

Normal ranges ESR using the Westergren method are:

- Males: 0–9 mm/hr
- Females: 0–20 mm/hr
- Children: 0–13 mm/hr

Potential sources for error using the Westergren method are incorrectly mixing the solution, disrupting the tube during the test, or not placing the stand level.

Wintrobe method. A sample of venous blood is thoroughly mixed with EDTA anticoagulant and then transferred to a Wintrobe tube. The tube is filled with 1 mL of blood and set vertically in a rack and left to stand for one hour.

Normal ranges for ESR using the Wintrobe method are:

- Males under 50: 0–15 mm/hr
- Males over 50: 0–20 mm/hr
- Females under 50: 0–20 mm/hr
- Females over 50: 0–30 mm/hr

The potential sources of error in the Wintrobe method include a dirty Wintrobe tube, disturbances during the test, the rack and tube not being level, and a blood specimen that was not mixed well.

Coagulation

Coagulation studies measure the ability of blood to clot. A prolonged coagulation time makes a person less likely to develop blood clots, especially after heart bypass surgery, heart valve replacement surgery, or any other procedure that disrupts the normal smooth lining of the arterial wall lining of the heart.

All patients on anticoagulant medication therapy need to have the blood monitored regularly for its clotting ability. The aim of anticoagulation therapy is to prolong the amount of time it will take for blood to clot, without making that time so long that the person has excessive bleeding. The goal is to make the length of time it takes to clot three times longer than normal.

Anticoagulation therapy is also used on a person who has a history of blood clots, such as thrombophlebitis, and to prevent heart attack or stroke in individuals with significant risk factors.

There are 12 coagulation factors in human plasma that are involved in clot formation. Formation of a clot has been further subdivided into two pathways.

- Extrinsic system: The clotting factors involved in this system are dependent on vitamin K for their production.

- Intrinsic system: The clotting factors involved in this system are NOT dependent on vitamin K for their production.

The two coagulation studies performed most frequently are:

- prothrombin time (PT), which measures extrinsic pathway factors; it is a measure of the clotting ability of the blood and can help diagnose problems with bleeding.
- partial thromboplastin time (PTT), which measures intrinsic pathways.

Prothrombin time (PT): Used to monitor patients receiving warfarin (Coumadin) therapy. Because prothrombin is produced in the liver, liver disease can also cause an increase in PT, which puts the patient at risk for bleeding episodes.

The normal PT for patients not taking warfarin is between 11 and 14 seconds. The range for individual patients taking warfarin should be established by the physician.

Partial thromboplastin time (PTT): The screening test for hemophiliacs (people whose blood does not clot or clots slowly) who are deficient in factor VIII (hemophilia A) or factor IX (Christmas disease). The PTT is also the most common coagulation test for assessment of heparin therapy. Normal ranges should be established for each laboratory, but they are usually between 30 and 45 seconds.

The PTT is a two-stage test, requiring two reagents: contact factor and phospholipid. The procedure for using each brand of analyzer is different. The medical assistant should be sure to follow the manufacturer's directions.

Blood Chemistry

Blood chemistry involves quantitative measurements of all chemical substances in the circulating blood and other body fluids. Common chemistry blood tests include glucose, hormones, lipids, drugs, and antibodies.

Chemistry testing can be done on an analyzer or individual test kits.

Glucose

When carbohydrates are digested, simple sugars such as glucose are generated. Glucose travels from the bloodstream to provide energy to the body's cells and tissues. The body produces two hormones that aid in the regulation of blood glucose levels: insulin and glucagon. Glucagon converts the stored glucose levels into glucose when blood glucose levels become low. The pancreas releases insulin to facilitate the transport of glucose from the bloodstream to the tissues and cells, thus lowering blood glucose levels.

A fasting glucose is the term applied to testing for glucose levels when a patient has been fasting (nothing ingested except for water) for 12 hours. The fasting glucose normal values are 70–100 mg/dL.

Glucose monitoring can easily be done in the medical office. Many glucose monitors are available to patients to monitor their glucose at home.

Kidney Function Tests

BUN—or blood urea nitrogen—is a test of how well the kidneys are functioning.

Urea nitrogen is produced as a waste product in the process of metabolizing proteins. It forms in the liver and travels via the bloodstream to the kidneys to be excreted. Since the kidneys are involved in the elimination of urea from the body, testing the level of urea nitrogen is one way to understand how well the kidneys are functioning.

One potential problem in using BUN as a test for kidney function, however, is that other causes, such as problems with the liver, can lead to changes in the levels of urea nitrogen.

Liver Function Tests

The liver is a multipurpose organ whose many functions include detoxification, protein synthesis, and production of bile, which aids in digestion. The tests associated with liver function measure proteins or enzymes in the blood that are involved in the operation of the liver. The levels of these substances, therefore, are a window into liver function. Standard liver function tests (LFTs) include:

- **Bilirubin:** This test measures how bilirubin, which is a waste product of the hemoglobin in the blood, is cleared from the blood by the liver.
- **Albumin:** This test measures the level of albumin, which is a protein manufactured by the liver.
- **ALT and AST:** These two indicators—alanine aminotransferase (ALT) and aspartate aminotransferase (AST)—are enzymes associated with liver cells; the level of both enzymes are raised when the liver is damaged; since AST elevations may be caused by diseased organs other than the liver, ALT is used a more targeted indicator for inflammation of the liver.
- **ALP and GGT:** These two indicators—alkaline phosphatase (alk. phos.) and gamma-glutamyl transpeptidase (GGT)—are also enzymes, in this case associated with the liver, in particular the bile ducts, or channels within or outside the liver; elevated levels can indicate obstruction in the bile ducts.

Lipid Profile

Lipids are fats or fatlike substances that do not dissolve water. Lipids provide an alternative energy source. Blood lipids that are responsible for cardiovascular disease are classified as lipoproteins. Lipoproteins are complex molecules made of fats attached to proteins. Two important types of blood lipids are cholesterol and triglycerides.

Cholesterol: An important component of cell membranes, cholesterol is used in the production of hormones and bile. Most of the cholesterol circulating in the body is manufactured by the liver. A portion of cholesterol—known as dietary cholesterol—comes from an individual's diet.

High cholesterol means that there is excessive amount of cholesterol in the blood called **hyper-cholesterolemia**. High cholesterol may cause fatty deposits, or plaque, to build up on the walls of the arteries, a condition known as atherosclerosis. As the atherosclerosis progresses, the arteries become more occluded, or blocked, which can eventually lead to a heart attack or stroke.

Cholesterol is transported in the blood as a complex molecule known as a lipoprotein. Two types of lipoproteins contain cholesterol:

- **Low-density lipoprotein (LDL)**—known as "bad cholesterol" since an excess amount of it in the blood can cause plaque to build up on the arterial walls. LDL comes from ingested fats and from the liver. It is delivered to the blood and to the muscles where it is deposited on the cells.
- **High-density lipoprotein (HDL)**—known as the "good cholesterol" since HDL removes excess cholesterol from the cells and carries it to the liver to be excreted. A high HDL has been shown to reduce the risk of heart disease. A low HDL is a risk factor for coronary heart disease.

Triglycerides. The most common form of fat in the body and food, they are a major source of energy in the body. When calories are ingested, but not used immediately, the body converts the excess to triglycerides, which are then stored in fat cells. Through the action of hormones, triglycerides are released from fat tissue to provide energy to the body between meals.

Hypertriglyceridemia, a condition marked by excess levels of triglycerides in the blood, can cause coronary artery disease through a buildup of lipoprotein at the artery walls, as in conditions of high cholesterol. Other conditions, however, such as diabetes mellitus, can result in increased levels of triglycerides; therefore, care must be taken in a diagnosis. A lipid profile includes:

- total cholesterol
- HDL cholesterol
- LDL cholesterol
- triglycerides

Because triglyceride levels are affected by the consumption of food, the patient must be instructed to fast for at least 12 hours before collection of the blood specimen.

Hemoglobin A1c

Hemoglobin is part of the red blood cells; it transports oxygen in the body and helps to process glucose and monitor diabetes.

When an individual consumes food containing glucose, the circulatory system absorbs the glucose from the digestive tract. Glucose tends to bind to protein, including a protein that makes up hemoglobin. When glucose attaches, or is glycosylated, to this protein, it forms hemoglobin A1c.

Therefore, when a diabetic patient's blood sugar is too high, the hemoglobin A1c rises: It builds up and combines with hemoglobin—that is, it becomes glycated, producing increased amounts of A1c. By measuring a patient's homoglobin A1c level, then, the medical assistant—and the patient—will be able to monitor the blood sugar level and therefore the status of the patient's diabetes.

Immunology

Immunology is the study of the immune system. It deals with antigen and antibody reactions.

- **Antigen**—a substance that is capable of stimulating the formation of antibodies in an individual. Antigens may consist of protein, glycoprotein, complex polysaccharides, or nucleic acid. Some examples of antigens include bacteria and viruses, bacterial toxins, allergens, and blood antigens.
- **Antibody**—produced by the body in response to it being invaded by an antigen. Antibodies are capable of combining with antigens, resulting in antigen-antibody reactions.

Laboratory testing in immunology deals with the study of antigen-antibody reactions to assess the presence of a substance or to assist in the diagnosis of a disease.

Mononucleosis Test

Mononucleosis is an acute infectious disease commonly seen in children and young adults. It is caused by the **Epstein-Barr virus (EBV)**. Its symptoms include:

- sore throat
- fatigue
- lymphadenopathy
- splenomegaly

A patient with symptoms of mononucleosis will have a mono test, as well as other clinical testing including a CBC and liver enzymes.

The rapid mono test is usually be performed in a medical office. Most mononucleosis tests do not look for EBV, but rather test for **heterophile antibodies**, which are sometimes present when a patient is infected with EBV.

Strep Test

The most common streptococcal condition is streptococcal sore throat, or streptococcal pharyngitis, which usually affects children and young adults and is caused by a Group A beta-hemolytic streptococcus known as *Streptococcus pyogenes*. Streptococcal pharyngitis is a potentially serious condition because some patients develop a **sequela** condition. A sequela is a morbid secondary condition that occurs as a result of a less serious primary infection. A sequela of streptococcal infection is **rheumatic fever**.

Rapid streptococcus tests directly for group A streptococcus from a throat swab in a very short time. Most tests only take about four to ten minutes. The most frequent streptococcus test is the direct antigen identification test, which confirms the presence of group A streptococcus through an antigen-antibody reaction. The test works by combining particles sensitized to the streptococcus antibody with the throat specimen. If group A streptococcal antigen is in the specimen, it combines with the antibody-sensitized particles to produce a color change that can be observed. Rapid streptococcus test kits also include a control that determines whether the test results are accurate.

C-Reactive Protein (CRP)

During inflammation and tissue destruction, an abnormal protein called C-reactive protein (CRP) appears in the blood. Patients with inflammatory conditions or disorders accompanied by tissue destruction have positive results to this test.

CRP rises during systemic inflammation and is used in testing for such illnesses as rheumatoid arthritis and lupus. It also may be an additional method of evaluating a patient's risk for cardiovascular disease.

Pregnancy Testing

Pregnancy testing, which is based on immunological principles, relies on the detection of the **human chorionic gonadotropin (HCG) hormone**, which is secreted by a fertilized egg. HCG levels can be detected from urine or serum.

The serum **radioimmunoassay** test for HCG is used to detect HCG in blood serum. This test can detect pregnancy earlier and with more accuracy than a urine pregnancy test. A serum pregnancy test can usually detect pregnancy at approximately the eighth day after fertilization.

Immunoassay tests provide for the rapid, qualitative detection of HCG in urine and blood. The immunoassay testing takes about five minutes to perform. The results are observed by a color change if the results are positive. If the the antibody in the sample contains the antigen, then a color change will appear in the kit, indicating a positive result.

Microbiology

Microbiology is the scientific study of microorganisms and their activities. Microorganisms are tiny living plants and animals that cannot be seen by the naked eye, but can be viewed under a microscope.

An infectious disease is one in which a microorganism is transmitted directly or indirectly between individuals, causing infection. Sources of human infection include other humans, animals, and sometimes the soil.

Bacteria

Bacteria are microscopic unicellular organisms that do not have a nuclear membrane enclosing their genetic material. Bacteria are classified into three basic groups based on their shape: cocci (round), bacilli (rod-like), and spiral bacteria. More information about bacteria can be found in the first section of this chapter, under Types of Pathogenic Microorganisms (page 154).

The Gram Stain Method of Classifying Bacteria

The Gram stain, named for the Danish scientist who developed the technique, is the most basic method for, and usually the first step in, identifying bacteria. Testing the chemical and physical qualities of the bacteria's cell walls, the Gram stain classifies bacteria into two groups: gram-positive or gram-negative.

A bacterium tests as gram-negative or gram-positive according to the ability of its cell wall to either retain or lose color through decolorization. This identification of gram-negative or gram-positive aids in identification of an organism.

Bacteria that are Gram-stained are observed for their characteristic shape and fall into one of the following categories: gram-positive rods, gram-negative rods, gram-positive cocci, or gram-negative cocci.

GRAM-POSITIVE DISEASES	GRAM-NEGATIVE DISEASES
streptococcal sore throat	whooping cough
scarlet fever	gonorrhea
rheumatic fever	meningitis
diphtheria	bacillary dysentery
lobar pneumonia	cholera
tetanus	typhoid fever
	plague

The Gram stain technique is a four-step process:

1. First, a primary stain—crystal violet—is used. This stains the culture purple.
2. Iodine then is applied to "hold" the stain.
3. This is then followed by the application of a decolorizer, alcohol-acetone, which removes the purple color.
4. Finally, a counterstain, usually safranine, is applied.

When stained according to the manufacturer's directions, the gram-positive bacteria stain purple and the gram-negative stain pink/red.

Parasites

Parasitology includes the study of all parasitic organisms that live on or in the human body. In parasitic relationships, the host is harmed as the parasite thrives. Parasites are transmitted by ingestion during the infective stage, direct penetration of the ingestion during the infective stage, direct penetration of skin by infective larvae, or inoculation by an arthropod vector. It is not possible to identify a parasite accurately on the basis of a single test or specimen. Most parasites are identified in urine, sputum, tissue fluids, or tissue biopsy samples.

Helminths. Helminths are parasitic worms. They live on or within another living organism and nourish themselves at the expense of the host organism. They can live in animals or humans and are usually transmitted through the soil, by infected clothing, or through contaminated food or water. Helminths go through the same life cycle as other worms. The adult worm lays eggs (ova). The ova develop into larvae. Larvae grow into adult worms, which lay eggs, and the cycle begins again. Diagnosis is usually based on microscopic examination of feces for ova and parasite and the patient's signs and symptoms.

Other Microorganisms

Other pathogenic microorganisms include virus, fungus, and protozoa. Information on these microorganisms can be found in the first section of this chapter, under Types of Pathogenic Microorganisms (page 154).

Tuberculosis Testing

The Mantoux test is used to test for tuberculosis. The Mantoux test is administered through an intradermal injection using a tuberculin syringe. It is important that the medical assistant draw up the proper amount of tuberculin solution.

- Injecting too much of the solution might trigger a reaction not caused by a tuberculous infection.
- Injecting too little of the solution results in insufficient solution being injected into the skin to cause a reaction. This will invalidate the test because if no reaction occurs, it cannot be accepted as a negative reaction.

The medical assistant must inject the solution properly:

- The injection must be made into the intradermal layers of the skin to form a wheal.
- If the injection is made into the subcutaneous layer, a wheal does not form.
- If the injection is too shallow, the injection may cease leakage of the tuberculin solution onto the skin.

Once the test has been administered, the results must be read within 48 to 72 hours. The medical assistant should use inspection and palpation to read the test results. If **induration**, or hardening, is present, the medical assistant should rub his or her fingers lightly from the area of normal skin to the indurated area to assess its size. The area of induration should be measured in millimeters.

The extent of induration is the only criterion used to determine a positive reaction. If erythema, or redness, is present without induration, the result is negative. The diameter of induration should be measured horizontally to the long axis of the forearm, and the results should be recorded in millimeters. If no induration is present, 0 mm should be recorded.

The following reactions might indicate tuberculous infection:

- The formation of vesicles, or fluid-containing lesions of the skin. If vesicles are present, the test is interpreted as strongly positive and warrants further diagnostic procedures to determine whether active TB is present.
- Induration of 10 mm or more constitutes a positive reaction and warrants further diagnostic procedures to determine active TB is present.
- Induration of 5 mm should be interpreted as a positive reaction for an individual who lives in close contact with a person with infectious TB, an HIV infected individual, or an individual at risk for HIV but whose HIV status is unknown.
- A doubtful reaction is an induration measuring 5 mm to 9 mm. Retesting is recommended using a different site of injection.
- A negative reaction is an induration less than 5 mm.

Guaiac (Occult Blood) Testing

The guaiac (occult blood) test screens patients for the presence of occult blood, which is blood present in the feces but not visible to the eye. Blood in the stool can indicate a number of conditions, including hemorrhoids, diverticulosis, polyps, colitis, upper gastrointestinal ulcers, and colorectal cancer, which is one of the most common cancers in people above the age of 40.

The test assesses the presence of blood in stool specimens collected from bowel movements on three different days. The purpose of using three specimens is to provide for the detection of blood from gastrointestinal lesions that exhibit **intermittent** bleeding. The patient must collect the specimens at home and return the prepared slides to the medical office for developing. The medical assistant is responsible for providing the patient with instructions on collection

and proper care and storage of the slides until the slides are returned to the medical office.

The patient must follow a special high-fiber, meatless diet beginning three days before the guaiac slide test and continuing until all three slides have been prepared. Meat contains animal blood that could lead to a false-positive test result, and a diet high in fiber encourages bleeding from lesions that may bleed only occasionally. In addition, fiber adds bulk, which promotes bowel movement.

The medical assistant should perform a quality control procedure after the patient's slide test has been developed, read, and interpreted.

Although the primary use of the guaiac slide test is to screen for colorectal cancer, other important uses of this test include screening for an upper GI ulcer or for disorders casing gastric and intestinal irritation. A positive test results on the guaiac slide test indicates blood in the stool, although the cause of the bleeding still must be determined.

Medical Imaging

While a medical assistant cannot take X-rays, he or she must be capable of preparing a patient for a medical imaging exam and must be informed of the safety procedures associated with this X-ray technology.

Safety Measures

Both the person performing the X-ray procedure and the patient need protection against excessive radiation or radiation reaching parts of the body to which radiation is a danger, such as the reproductive organs and thyroid.

Some of the protective equipment needed includes:

- gloves
- lead apron that reaches below the waist to protect the internal organs of the trunk and the reproductive organs of both women and men
- goggles
- leaded neck protector to shield the thyroid

The X-ray technician also stays as far away from the X-rays as possible, stepping out of the room or behind a lead-lined barrier while the X-ray machine takes the image. The technician is also responsible for the proper working of the X-ray machine to ensure that it does not emit excess radiation.

Patient Preparation and Instruction

Patient preparation for routine radiography involves several instructions and precautions:

- The outer clothing that covers the radiographed are should be removed; a gown should be provided if appropriate.
- No metal objects should be included in the radiation field because these items will appear as artifacts on the images. This includes jewelry, zippers, snaps, and other clothing fasteners; underwire bras; and the contents of pockets.
- Nonmetal objects that are thick or heavy should also be removed. Buttons and the heavy seams in jeans are examples of other clothing items that can cause artifacts on radiographs if they are in the imaging field.

The patient must remain still while the exposure is made. If more than one exposure is needed, the film is changed, the patient is repositioned, and the steps are repeated until the examination is complete.

Preparing and Administering Medications

Medical assistants are expected to have a basic knowledge of medications. This includes knowledge of prescription drugs and over-the-counter drugs. To understand the important functions of these drugs, the medical assistant must understand pharmacological principles, be able to translate prescriptions, and be prepared to answer basic patient questions.

Pharmacology

Pharmacology is the study of drugs, including their properties and effects on living organisms. Drugs—substances that can modify one or more functions of a living organism—are used to treat, prevent, diagnose, and cure disease.

A healthcare provider will prescribe, or indicate, a drug to be administered or given to a patient. The **prescription** indicates the drug's **dosage**, and the number of times the drug should be taken (such as twice per day or once per week). The medical assistant is responsible for understanding the various drugs that can be prescribed as well as the drug dispensing laws in the state where he or she works. The medical assistant must also have the skills to prepare and administer medications to patients safely.

Qualified medical practitioners who prescribe, dispense, or administer drugs must comply with federal and state laws. The laws govern the manufacture, sale, possession, administration, dispensing, and prescribing of drugs. All drugs available for legal use are controlled by the Food and Drug Administration (FDA).

Drugs that have the potential for abuse or addiction are regulated by the Controlled Substance Act of 1970. This act controls the manufacture, importation, compounding, selling, dealing in, and giving away of drugs that have the potential for abuse. These drugs are known as controlled substances and include heroin and cocaine and their derivatives and narcotics, stimulants, and depressants. The Drug Enforcement Agency of the U.S. Justice Department monitors and enforces the act. Under federal law, physicians who prescribe, administer, or dispense controlled substances must register with the DEA and renew their registration as required by state law.

Classes of Drugs

Drugs can be classified in a number of ways:

- drugs used to treat or prevent disease (e.g., hormones or vaccines)

- drugs that have a principal action on the body (e.g., analgesics and anti-inflammatory drugs)
- drugs that act on specific body systems or organs (e.g., respiratory and cardiovascular)

Drug Forms

There are two basic forms of drugs: solids and liquids, categorized based on how easily the medication dissolves.

- Solids include tablets, capsules, sustained-release capsules, caplets, lozenges, creams, ointments, suppositories, and **transdermal** patches. Some forms are actually semisolid but are placed in the solids category.
- Liquids include elixirs, emulsions, liniments, lotions, solutions, spirits, sprays, suspensions, aerosol suspensions, syrups, and tinctures. **Tinctures** and elixirs are preparations that contain alcohol; individuals recovering from substance abuse should be cautioned that such preparations contain alcohol and that an alternate preparation may be needed.

Drug Actions

A drug's action is the ability of the drug to act on body processes at the cellular level. Drugs can stimulate (speed up) or depress (slow down) cellular function. Some drugs can destroy cells or replace substance. However, drugs cannot make a cell function in a new or different way. It is important for medical assistants to understand the action of a drug from the time it enters the patient's body until the time it is excreted. A drug's action and use can be broken down into three main categories: pharmacokinetics, pharmacodynamics, and pharmacotherapeutics.

Pharmacokinetics

Pharmacokinetics is the study of the action of drugs as they move through the body. These actions include absorption, distribution, metabolism, and excretion.

Absorption is the passage of medication through some surface or opening of the body at the site of administration of the drug into the body's bloodstream. Key factors that affect absorption include:

- Type of drug. For example, adequate absorption of the beta-blocker propranolol depends on normal blood circulation through the liver. Thus, absorption of propranolol in patients with liver disease will be decreased, while absorption of other drugs in such patients will not be impaired.
- Amount of drug. For example, a physician will commonly prescribe a "loading" dose, or large initial dose, of penicillin for a patient with an infection in order to establish therapeutic penicillin levels more quickly in the bloodstream.
- Route of administration. For example, the body will absorb more slowly a medication given by mouth than one injected because a medication given by mouth must go through the digestive system before it is absorbed into the bloodstream.
- Bioavailability of the drug, or a percentage that expresses the amount of the drug that reaches the bloodstream and the length of time needed for it to do so. For example, fluoxetine hydrochloride (Prozac) has a high bioavailability of 72% with a peak concentration in the bloodstream within six to eight hours of administration.

Distribution: After absorption of the drug into the bloodstream, the circulatory system distributes it into the body fluids, tissues, and cells, carrying it to the intended site of action. Distribution of the drug may be slow or fast, depending on the patient's size and the amount of the drug given. Circulation impairment can also affect the ability of the medication to be distributed to the intended site.

Metabolism: After the body uses the drug, it must inactivate it (or break it down chemically) in order to eliminate it. This process is called **metabolism** or biotransformation. Chemical reactions break down the drug into different substances that the body can easily use and excrete. If these substances are harmful to the body, the body must also detoxify the substances before elimination. The liver is the major organ involved in drug metabolism. Several factors can affect metabolism, including age, the presence of liver disease, and characteristics of the drug.

Excretion is how the body eliminates a drug. Similar to food, after the body has used the drug, it must be eliminated. Most drugs are excreted in urine; thus, the kidneys are the major organs involved in drug excretion. However, the body may also excrete drugs through feces, hair, lungs, breast milk, and skin.

Pharmacodynamics

Pharmacodynamics is the study of the body's biochemical and physiological response to a drug. In other words, pharmacodynamics studies what the drug does to a person's body and how that effect is achieved. Many factors affect pharmacodynamics, or the drug's action in a person's body, including the patient's size, age, and genetic makeup.

Pharmacotherapeutics

Pharmacotherapeutics is the study of the use and effect of drugs in the treatment and prevention of disease. The medical reasons physicians and other health professionals prescribe drugs are:

- to cure disease
- to treat symptoms of a disease
- to diagnose disorders and diseases
- to replace a deficiency
- to prevent disease

DRUG CLASSIFICATIONS

DRUG CLASSIFICATION	COMMON USE	EXAMPLE
analgesic	relieves pain	ibuprofen; acetaminophen
anesthetic	decreases sensation	lidocaine (Xylocaine)
antacid	neutralizes acid	Tums; Mylanta
antibiotic	inhibits or eradicates the growth of microbes	penicillin; augmentin
anticoagulant	prevents clotting	heparin; coumadin
anticonvulsant	prevents seizures	Dilantin; Tegretol
antidepressant	decreases or inhibits depression	Prozac; Elavil
antidiarrheal	decreases or inhibits diarrhea	Lomotil; Kaopectate
antiemetic	decreases or inhibits nausea	Compazine; Dramamine
antihistamine	controls symptoms of allergies	Benadryl; Claritin
antihypertensive	controls high blood pressure	Lopressor; Aldomet
anti-inflammatory	controls inflammation	ibuprofen; Celebrex
antipyretic	decreases fever	acetaminophen; ibuprofen
antiarrhythemic	controls arrhythmia	Norpace; digoxin
cathartics	accelerates defecations	Castor oil; Epsom salts
diuretic	decreases body fluid by increasing urination	Lasix
fungicides	decreases fungal infections	nystatin

This list of drug classifications includes both common uses and examples of each drug type. Some drugs listed in the table are prescribed for off-label use—that is, purposes other than those approved by the FDA.

Drug Uses

A drug's use is the therapeutic effect it has on a person's body.

Drugs that cure: Some drugs can cure disease. For example, a bacterial throat infection known as strep throat can be cured by taking an antibiotic, such as penicillin. Also, the fungal infection ringworm can be cured after a full course of an antifungal drug.

Drugs for palliative care: Drugs used to treat a disease without curing it seek to relieve or alleviate symptoms of that disease. This type of treatment is sometimes called **palliative care**. For example, at present, there is no cure for arthritis. However, the physician may prescribe an anti-inflammatory drug to reduce the inflammation caused by arthritis, thereby decreasing pain. Although the patient's pain decreases, she still has arthritis. Similarly, an antihistamine will not cure allergies but will reduce and relieve some symptoms associated with allergies.

Drugs for prevention: Drugs can help prevent conditions and diseases. Such drugs are commonly called **prophylactic drugs**. For example, oral contraceptives help prevent pregnancy and vaccinations prevent tetanus, diphtheria, measles, mumps, rubella, hepatitis B, and chicken pox.

Drugs as supplements: Drugs can replace a deficient substance in the body. For example, a diabetic patient, whose pancreas lacks the ability to produce adequate insulin, may take replacement insulin by injection. Calcium supplements help achieve adequate levels of calcium when the patient's diet does not contain a sufficient amount. Patients with hypothyroidism (low thyroid hormone production) can take levothyroxine (Synthroid), a synthetic form of thyroid hormone.

Drugs for diagnostic purposes: Drugs can help diagnose a disease or disorder. For example, a **radiopaque dye**, also called a contrast medium, is injected into patients for certain tests. The dye aids visualization of glands and organs, helping the physician make a diagnosis.

Drugs used in an emergency: Emergency pharmaceutical supplies should include certain basic drugs. Details on these drugs are covered in this chapter in the section called "Common Emergency and First-Aid Supplies and Equipment" (page 214).

Side Effects and Adverse Reactions

Unfortunately, even if a prescribed drug provides the desired therapeutic effect, it can also produce effects other than the therapeutic or desired effect.

An adverse reaction is an unexpected, usually dangerous, response to a drug. Adverse reactions can occur as a result of a patient's health status, the number of drugs the patient is taking, or the length of time the patient has been taking the drugs. Such reactions can be classified as an allergic reaction, idiosyncratic effect, cumulative effect, toxic effect, or tolerance.

- Allergic reaction. An **allergic reaction** is an immune response to a drug that results in inflammation and organ dysfunction. Reactions can occur immediately or even days after drug use. Reactions range from itching, sneezing, or a mild rash to life-threatening symptoms.
- Idiosyncratic effect. An **idiosyncratic effect** is an abnormal drug response in a patient with a peculiar defect in his body chemistry. Because of the defect, administration of the drug causes effects that are totally unrelated to the drug's normal pharmacological action.
- Toxic effect. Sometimes the body cannot metabolize and properly excrete a drug, causing a cumulative drug action. The drug stays in the body and when the patient takes subsequent doses, the drug level in the blood rises, becoming unsafe for the patient and causing symptoms of overdose. This can cause a **toxic effect** that is harmful to the patient. Some drugs are inherently toxic, such as chemotherapeutic drugs, which cause the death of healthy tissue and may cause heart attack and brain inflammation.

- Tolerance. When a patient has taken a drug for an extended period of time, the desired effect may lessen or will not occur at all. This effect is called **tolerance**. Because the body of a patient who has developed a tolerance is accustomed to the drug, the physician may have to increase the dose to achieve the desired effect or change the drug completely.

Drug Interactions

A drug interaction happens when the combination of a drug with food or other drugs creates an effect in the body. When patients take more than one drug, the combination of drugs can affect the actions of the drugs in harmful or beneficial ways. The combination of two or more drugs can cause three difference effects: synergism, antagonism, and potentation.

- **Synergism**, or a synergistic drug effect, occurs when two drugs have a greater therapeutic effect together than the expected effects of each drug alone.
- **Antagonism**, or an antagonistic drug effect, happens when drugs work in opposition to one another. For example, antibiotics negate the effects of most oral contraceptives. When the physician prescribes antibiotics to a patient taking oral contraceptives, the patient should be advised to use an alternative form of birth control during the course of antibiotic therapy.
- **Potentiation** is an interaction between two drugs that enhances the effect of either drug, producing a heightened response similar to an overdose. Unlike synergism, in potentiation, the two drugs are taken for different conditions. For example, a patient taking the anticoagulant warfarin (Coumadin) may wish to take aspirin for a headache. However, the asprin will heighten the patient's response to the anticoagulant and this may be harmful to the patient.

Substance Abuse

Drug abuse, also called substance abuse, is the misuse of alcohol and other drugs. Abuse of drugs may involve legal or illegal medications and can occur suddenly or develop over time. Psychological dependence (when a person merely thinks he or she needs the drug) can turn into physical dependence (when a person's body needs the drug to prevent adverse effects, including death). Commonly abused drugs include:

- alcohol
- marijuana
- nicotine
- central nervous system stimulants (such as methylphenidate)
- central nervous system depressants (such as opiates)

The medical assistant can direct a patient who abuses drugs to a treatment facility or a support group, such as Alcoholics Anonymous or Narcotics Anonymous.

Prescriptions

A prescription is a physician's order authorizing the dispensing of a drug by a pharmacist. Prescriptions can be authorized in different forms, including handwritten, computer-generated, and telephoned or faxed to a pharmacy.

A prescription is written on a specially designed form, supplies for which must be kept in a safe place, that includes directions to the pharmacist for filling the prescription and instructions to the patient for taking the medication. The specific information must include:

- Date. A pharmacist cannot fill a prescription unless the date the prescription was issued is indicated on the form. The reason for this is that a prescription expires after a certain length of time. In most states, a prescription for a drug (except controlled drugs) expires one year from the date of issue.

- Physician's name, address, telephone number, and fax number. This information is preprinted on the prescription form. It identifies the physician issuing the prescription and provides the necessary information should the pharmacist have a question and need to contact the medical office.
- Patient's name and address. This information is important for insurance billing and for properly dispensing the medication.
- Patient's age. The patient's age is important to the pharmacists when they are double checking the physician's order to ensure the proper dosage is being dispensed.
- Superscription. The superscription consists of the abbreviation Rx, which comes from the Latin word *recipe* and means "take."
- Inscription. The inscription states the name of the drug and the dose.
- Subscription. The subscription gives directions to the pharmacist. This generally is used to designate the number of doses to be dispensed. It is recommended that numbers and letters be used to indicate the quantity to be dispensed.
- Signatura. The signatura (abbreviated Sig.) is a Latin term that means "write" or "label" and indicates the information to be included on the medication label. It consists of directions to the patient for taking the medication. The name of the medication is also included on the label.
- Refill. This part of the prescription indicates the number of times the prescription may be refilled.
- Physician's signature. A prescription cannot be filled unless it is signed by the physician.
- DEA number. The number assigned to the physician by the DEA must appear on the prescription for a controlled drug.

Common prescription abbreviations include:

- q: every
- bid: twice a day
- tid: three times per day
- qid: four times per day
- qh: every hour
- po: by mouth

Preparing and Administering Medications

Before a medical assistant can administer a drug, he or she may need to calculate the dose prescribed by the physician. To do so, the medical assistant must understand various systems of measurement and ways to convert from one system to another.

Calculation of Dosage

When a physician orders dosages, the medical assistant must administer the correct amount of medication. Because the dosage ordered will not always match the available doses, the medical assistant must calculate the proper dosage for the patient.

Systems of Measurement

In order to accurately calculate dosages, the medical assistant must have an understanding of the metric, household, and apothecary systems of measurement. No matter what system is used, medications dispensed to patients are measured in quantities of liquid (volume) or solid (weight).

Metric system: The metric system is a system of weights and measures based on the units of ten. For instance, the basic unit of length—the meter—can be divided into 10 or 1,000 units, to arrive at smaller units called decimeters or millimeters; or can be multiplied by 10 or 1,000, to arrive at larger units called decameters or kilometers.

The metric system is the most commonly used system for drug dosages, using the basic unit of mass, or weight—the gram—and the basic unit of volume—the liter.

- solid medication: measured by mass, or weight; common unit is milligram (mg)

- liquid medication: measured by volume; common unit is the milliliter (mL), sometimes called the cubic centimeter (cc)

Apothecary and household systems: Although the metric units of milligrams and milliliters are most common in medication dosages, the apothecary and household systems are sometimes used.

- The apothecary system. The units of weight in this system include grain and ounce. Volume measures in the apothecary system include minim, fluidram, pint, and quart.
- The household system. The measures for liquids are drop, teaspoon, tablespoon, fluid ounce, pint, cup, and quart. Household measures for weight are ounce and pound.

CHART OF COMMON CONVERSIONS

METRIC MEASURE	APOTHECARY OR HOUSEHOLD MEASURE
1 gram (g, gm)	15 grains (gr) or 1,000 milligrams (mg)
60 milligrams (mg)	1 grain (gr)
1 kilogram (kg)	2.2 pounds (lb) or 1,000 grams (g, gm)
1 milliliter (mL, ml)	15 drops (gtt)
5 milliliters (mL)	1 teaspoon (tsp) or 60 drops (gtt)

Some of the units of measure for apothecary and household units are the same, which can cause confusion. In addition, teaspoon and tablespoon containers are commonly poorly calibrated; thus, the patient may get too much or too little of the medication. These units of measure also are used to measure both liquid and dry ingredients, adding more confusion. In addition, household measures do not provide precise measurement of smaller quantities of prescribed drugs. For example, 60 mg of a drug would equal less than one-fourth of a teaspoon, the smallest unit in the household system. For these reasons, medications are most commonly ordered in metric doses and should be calculated in metric doses.

Calculation Methods

To administer the correct amount of medication to the patient, the medical assistant must calculate the correct dose. There are several methods for calculating the dose.

- dose on hand method
- ratio and proportion method
- fractional equation method

To understand these three methods, the following example will be applied.

Example

The physician orders medication to be given in the office, before the patient leaves, as follows:

Phenytoin 50 mg PO t.i.d.

The office only stocks the drug in the following dose and form:

Phenytoin 125 mg/5 mL (125 mg in every 5 mL unit).

For each method, the medical assistant must remember a formula containing these elements:

- D = dose ordered or desired dose
- H = dose on container label or dose on hand
- Q = amount, or quantity, in which the drug is available
- A = amount to give

Dose on hand method: To calculate the dose using the dose on hand method, the medical assistant must remember this formula:

$$\frac{D \times Q}{H} = A$$

$$\frac{50 \text{ mg} \times 5 \text{ mL}}{125 \text{ mg}} = A$$

$$\frac{250 \text{ mL}}{125} = 2 \text{ mL}$$

Ratio and proportion method: To calculate the dose using the ratio and proportion method, the medical assistant must remember this formula:

$$HA = DQ$$
$$125 \text{ mg} \times A = 50 \text{ mg} \times 5 \text{ mL}$$
$$125 \text{ mg} \times A = 250 \text{ mg/mL}$$
$$A = \frac{250 \text{ mg/mL}}{125 \text{ mg}}$$
$$A = 2 \text{ mL}$$

Fractional equation method: To calculate the dose using the fractional method, the medical assistant must remember this formula:

$$\frac{H}{Q} = \frac{D}{A}$$
$$\frac{125 \text{ mg}}{5 \text{ mL}} = \frac{50 \text{ mg}}{A}$$
$$125 \text{ mg} \times A = 50 \text{ mg} \times 5 \text{ mL}$$
$$A = \frac{50 \text{ mg} \times 5 \text{ mL}}{125 \text{ mg}}$$
$$A = 2 \text{ mL}$$

Using Conversions

If the dose on hand and the dose ordered are measured with different systems, the medical assistant must perform some conversions before he or she can calculate the correct dose. Virtually all medical offices have conversion tables readily available.

Example: If the order contains the dosage nitroglycerin gr 1/400 prn for angina pain and the dose on hand is nitroglycerin 0.3 mg tablets, the medical assistant must first convert grains to milligrams. Using conversion tables, the medical assistant will know that 1 grain equals 60 mg. Using this conversion, the medical assistant can calculate the dose using the dose on hand method:

$$1 \text{ grain} = 60 \text{ mg}$$
$$\frac{\text{gr } 1}{400} = \frac{60 \text{ mg}}{400} = \frac{3 \text{ mg}}{20} = 0.15 \text{ mg}$$
$$\frac{0.15 \text{ mg}}{0.3 \text{ mg}} = 0.5 \text{ tablet}$$

Also, some doses are measured with the same system but with different units within the system. The medical assistant must also perform conversions in this case.

Example: If the order says 0.5 g amoxicillin and the dose on hand is 250 mg tablets, the medical assistant must first convert grams to milligrams. Using conversion tables, the medical assistant will know that 0.5 g equals 500 mg. Using this conversion, the medical assistant can calculate the dose:

$$\frac{500 \text{ mg}}{250 \text{ mg}} = 2 \text{ tablets}$$

Calculating Infant and Child Dosages

The medical assistant must calculate dosages for pediatric patients according to the pediatric patient's body size. Administering an adult dose of a medication to an infant or child would increase the risk of overdose and would not be therapeutic. Two main methods of calculating pediatric dosages include the weight method and the body surface area method, although the weight method is the most common.

Weight Method

The medical assistant can calculate infant and child dosages according to the patient's weight. Because most dosages are expressed using kilograms (kg), the medical assistant must also convert pounds to kilograms in order to calculate correctly.

Example: The medical assistant is calculating a dosage for a 6-year-old patient who weighs 55 lb. The physician's order reads lidocaine 1 mg/kg. In order to provide the accurate dose, the medical assistant must convert 55 lb. into equivalent kilograms. Using the conversion table, she or he will know that 1 kg equals 2.2 lb. Using this conversion, the medical assistant can calculate the dose:

$$55 \div 2.2 \text{ kg} = 25 \text{ kg}$$
$$25 \times 1 \text{ mg} = 25 \text{ mg}$$

Routes of Administration

Drugs may be administered for either local or systemic effects. Generally, drugs that have local effects are applied directly to the skin, tissues, or mucous membranes. Drugs that produce systemic effects are administered by routes that allow the drug to be absorbed and distributed in the bloodstream throughout the body.

Oral Route

The oral, or enteral, route is defined as ingestion through the mouth and into the GI tract; it is the most common route of medication administration. It is safe and convenient and most patients are able to take medications in this manner. In addition, it requires no special equipment. However, a patient with **dysphagia** (difficulty swallowing) should not take oral medications because of the risk of aspirating an oral medication into the respiratory tract.

Oral drug forms include:

- Tablets—compressed, disk-like masses of medication manufactured from a powder form that require the patient to drink enough liquid so that the tablet does not stick in his or her throat.
- Capsules—medication surrounded by a gelatin container that will not dissolve until it reaches the acidic environment of the stomach, thus preventing the patient from tasting the medication.
- Syrups—concentrated solutions of sugar, water, and the medication that make it easier for the patient to tolerate swallowing drugs with a bitter flavor.
- Suspensions—solid particles mixed in a liquid but not dissolved that require shaking before use so that the medication will be equally dispersed in the liquid.

Physicians commonly prescribe syrups and suspensions to young children because young children may not be able to swallow tablets or capsules. When a liquid medication is poured into a container, the surface of the liquid, called the **meniscus**, will curve slightly due to surface tension with the sides of the container. When measuring a liquid dose, the medical assistant must be at eye level with the meniscus to ensure accurate dosing.

The stomach or small intestine digests and absorbs an oral drug. The rate of absorption for oral drugs is fairly slow (approximately 20 minutes). Other factors may cause acceleration or delay of oral drug action, including food in the stomach, the patient's emotions, or physical activity.

The medical assistant must pay careful attention to recommendations regarding food with oral medications. Some oral drugs can be irritating to the stomach, causing nausea or heartburn. Enteric-coated capsules or tablets are coated with a compound that does not dissolve until exposed to the fluids of the small intestine. The medication passes through the stomach into the intestines without causing irritation to the upper GI tract. The medical assistant must never cut an enteric-coated tablet or capsule or the medication could produce irritation and change the intended site for absorption.

Parenteral Routes

Any route other than oral is considered a **parenteral** route. Parenteral routes of administration include:

- sublingual
- buccal
- inhalation
- injection
- topical
- vaginal
- rectal

Sublingual (under the tongue) and **buccal** (between the cheek and gum): This type of administration of drugs involves placing the medication in the patient's mouth without the patient swallowing it. Unlike oral drugs, sublingual and buccal medications do not travel to the GI tract for absorption. Instead, the mucous membranes in the interior of the mouth absorb the drug and deliver it to the bloodstream. Thus, absorption through these routes is more immediate.

Examples: *Nitroglycerin, a strong vasodilator, is commonly administered sublingually for patients* experiencing acute angina pectoris. Opiate analgesics are commonly administered buccally for severe break-through pain in cancer patients.

Inhalation: Patients can inhale medications (inhalants) for delivery to the respiratory tract using a nebulizer, a machine that mixes room air with a medication. The nebulizer uses an atomizer to mix the medication with water to create a vapor that the patient can inhale. The patient can sleep or sit quietly in the room with the nebulizer and breathe in the medication with the humidified air. Patients with asthma or emphysema can also use portable metered-dose inhalers (MDIs) for immediate relief of respiratory distress.

Examples: *Nebulizers for asthma patients.*

Injection: For a parenteral administration given by injection, the medical assistant must first measure the correct amount of the drug by drawing it into a syringe from a vial, a small bottle with a thin metal or rubber top, or an ampule, small all-glass container. The medical assistant must also have an understanding of, and develop skill with, the different methods of injection, of which there are four:

- subcutaneous
- intradermal
- intramuscular (IM)
- intravenous (IV)

Information on these types of injections are covered in the section immediately following this one.

Topical: Topical medication can be administered by placing the medication on top of the skin, enabling absorption into the bloodstream through the skin. Examples of topical medications include creams and ointments. Cleaning the skin with soap and water enhances absorption of topical creams and ointments. Another method of topical medication administration is the transdermal method, which involves placing a patch made of a semipermeable membrane that releases the medication into the skin. Transdermal medication is absorbed more slowly, over a period of 12 to 24 hours.

Examples: *Nicotine smoking cessation patches, nitroglycerine patches for angina, and patches for contraception.*

Vaginal: The medical assistant may administer medications vaginally by inserting them into the vaginal cavity in the form of a cream, foam, or suppository. Patients may need specific instructions on inserting the medication. Administration of foams and creams involves insertion with an applicator. The medical assistant should be sure to give the patient the written instructions that accompany the medication. Insertion of suppositories, which are hard, is similar to the insertion of a tampon. The patient may need to lie in a recumbent position after inserting the medication to ensure absorption. Thus, physicians commonly order vaginal medication administration at bedtime.

Examples: *Antifungal creams and estrogen replacement therapy.*

Rectal: The medical assistant may administer medications by inserting them into the rectum for localized or systemic action. Rectal medications are in suppository form, which melt from the patient's body heat. Rectal administration is common for medications to treat nausea and vomiting when the patient cannot tolerate anything taken orally. Pain relievers and fever reducers are also available in suppository form.

Rectal drug action takes 15 to 30 minutes after insertion, so the patient should lie quietly for this time period. The medical assistant should always provide written instructions to the patient and instruct the patient to call the office if further questions arise. In addition, the patient should be advised to store the medication in a cool, dry place to avoid melting before administration.

Examples: *Anti-nausea medications; other drugs, such as pain relievers and fever, are also available in suppository form.*

Types of Injections and Injection Sites

Subcutaneous: When administering subcutaneous injections, the medical assistant injects the drug into the subcutaneous layer of the integument (skin), the fatty layer beneath the dermis and above the muscle tissue. Because the fatty layer is less vascular, meaning it has fewer blood vessels, than muscle, the drug absorption rate is moderate with this type of injection. However, the site of subcutaneous injection can affect the rate of absorption. For example, injection of a drug in the abdomen or arm offers quicker absorption than one in the thigh or upper buttocks. Subcutaneous injection sites are in areas where a substantial amount of connective tissue is present between the muscle and skin to absorb the medication without hitting nerves, muscle, bone, or blood vessels.

Examples: *Insulin is an example of a subcutaneously injected drug. Because patients or caregivers commonly administer subcutaneous insulin injections daily, they must rotate injection sites to prevent lipodystrophy (atrophy or hypertrophy of fat tissue), bruising, swelling, or infection.*

Intradermal: The medical assistant administers intradermal injections into the dermis, the layer of skin under the epidermis (surface of the skin). The quantity of medication given intradermally is small because the medication is not intended to be absorbed beyond the local site but should remain just under the surface for the patient's body to react to the allergen or TB test. The physician then reads the reaction on the surface of the skin.

Examples: *The intradermal route is most common in performing allergy testing or tuberculosis testing. Common intradermal injection sites are the upper arms for TB screening and the upper back for allergy testing.*

Intramuscular: When the medical assistant administers an intramuscular injection, he or she injects the drug directly into the muscle. Absorption happens quickly because of the rich blood supply of the muscle. The muscle can be injected with much more medication than in the intradermal or subcutaneous methods because the muscle is capable of retaining more liquid. Careful measurement of medications into syringes is necessary to ensure proper dosage. Common IM sites of administration include the **ventrogluteal, deltoid,** and **vastus lateralis** muscles.

The **z-track injection** method is a modification of IM injection technique. To use the z-track method, the medical assistant must pull the skin to one side and hold it while inserting the needle at a 90 degree angle. After administering the medication, he or she must wait 10 seconds and then withdraw the needle and release the skin. This technique leaves a zigzag needle track from the surface of the skin to the muscular layer, which stops the medication from leaking out into the subcutaneous tissue and onto the skin's surface. The preferred sites for the z-track method are the vastus lateralis and ventrogluteal muscles. This method is used for medications that may discolor or irritate subcutaneous tissues.

Examples: *Medications administered IM include antibiotics, vaccines, and drugs to treat a severe allergic reaction. When the medical assistant must administer multiple IM injections, he or she should use sites on hips, arms, and legs to avoid excessive soreness in one area.*

Patients with severe allergies to such foods as peanuts, tree nuts, or shellfish may need to carry an epinephrine injection (Epi-Pen), which is a device that delivers an IM injection of a premeasured amount of epinephrine to counteract the effects of a severe allergic reaction.

Prescriptions

Any drug that is not available over the counter (OTC) requires a prescription. According to the Controlled Substances Act, doctors may issue prescriptions for controlled drugs only in the schedules for which they are registered with the DEA.

Safekeeping

If a physician's office keeps a supply of controlled substances, the staff must conduct a controlled substances inventory at the date of DEA registration and every two years thereafter. In addition, the office must keep a separate inventory record for Schedule II drugs. With the inventories, the office must include the name of the physician or practice, the address of the medical office, the DEA number, and the date and time of inventories.

The office must keep these inventory records on file for two years. The office must keep controlled substances in a locked cabinet, separate from other drugs, such as samples and OTC drugs. Because the inventory must be complete and accurate, the medical assistant and other staff members should log the administration of a controlled substance in the inventory log at the time of administration to avoid forgetting to log the drugs. If an opioid analgesic is accidentally broken or spilled, two staff members must witness the disposal and sign the inventory log. The office must report any theft of a controlled substance to local police and the DEA and complete a police report and Form DEA-116.

Medication Record Keeping

In addition to obtaining a DEA registration number, physicians who prescribe controlled substances must keep records for two years of drugs dispensed, including the patient's full name and address, date prescribed, dosage (amount to be taken), route of administration, and the reason the drug was given. The physician must also maintain proper security for these records, which are subject to inspection by the DEA. In addition, the medical office must keep a progress note in the patient's medical record that includes the prescription.

Controlled Substance Guidelines

The Controlled Substances Act of 1990, which updated a 1970 law of the same name, identifies five schedules, or categories, of drugs that have potential for abuse and illegal use. Thus, when a physician prescribes opiates for severe pain, he or she must do so thoughtfully and cautiously. The legislation provides regulations for prescribing, refilling, dispensing, and medical use of these drugs. The drugs have mood-altering effects and the potential for physical dependence; therefore, they have the potential for abuse. For example, although physicians can prescribe opiates for severe pain, they should take care to avoid overprescribing opiates and causing addiction in the patient.

THE "SEVEN RIGHTS" OF DRUG ADMINISTRATION

Whenever administering drugs, the medical assistant must always confirm the "seven rights."

- Right patient—check the name of the patient with the physician's order to avoid medication errors.
- Right drug—check the drug label three times: when removing the drug container from storage, after preparing the medication, and before returning the drug container to storage.
- Right route—check the route the physician ordered against the route prepared.
- Right dose—check the dose on the physician's order against the dose prepared.
- Right time—check when the medication is to be given.
- Right technique—follow the procedure to administer the medication.
- Right documentation—record the procedure in the patient's medical record on completion. The medical assistant should be sure to include the date, time, drug, dose, route, site, lot number, expiration date, patient education, and how well the patient tolerated the procedure.

Immunizations

Immunization refers to the process by which the body is made immune, or unsusceptible, to a certain disease. The body uses its own immune system to protect against certain diseases, but immunization can also be introduced to the body in the form of vaccines. Vaccines work in one of two ways.

- **Active immunity:** the introduction of the small amounts of a weakened or dead version of organism that produces the disease, which results in the ability of immune system to produce antibodies that will fight disease if the individual is exposed; this method is slow-acting, in that it takes a while to become effective, but long-lasting, in some cases lasting a lifetime

Examples: *Vaccines against cholera, polio, and influenza.*

- **Passive immunity:** the direct introduction of antibodies to fight the disease, not relying on the immune system to create the antibodies, as with active immunity; in contrast to active immunity, the effects can be quick, but not long-lasting

Examples: *Vaccines for botulism, rabies, and tetanus.*

Natural immunity is a kind of active immunity that occurs frequently in the body; it refers to cases in which an individual is exposed to organisms of a disease, and develops the ability to fight it off in the future.

Childhood Vaccines

Routine childhood immunizations are state mandated and required for all children who attend public schools. When a patient comes to the office for immunizations during a well-child examination, the medical assistant should provide the parent with a recommended immunization schedule and a vaccine information sheet (VIS) for each vaccine administered during that visit.

The VIS explains the safety and efficacy of the vaccine as well as possible adverse reactions and when to contact a physician if the parent is concerned. The pediatrician is obligated by law to provide parents with a VIS statement that outlines the risks and benefits associated with vaccines. Some states also have informed consent laws that require a parent's signature before administration of a vaccine.

Adult Vaccines

The Centers for Disease Control and Prevention recommends the following immunizations for all adults:

- Tetanus booster every ten years, or sooner if the patient has an open wound.
- Measles, mumps, rubella (MMR) in one or two doses between the ages of 19 and 49 years for patients who do not have documentation of having the vaccine or for those who have never had the disease.
- The varicella vaccine (chickenpox) should be given in two doses between the ages of 19 and 49 years for patients who do not have documentation of having the vaccine or for those who have never had the disease.
- One injection of pneumococcal vaccine should be given at age 65.
- After age 50, an annual influenza vaccine should be given.
- Some doctors also recommend a series of three hepatitis B injections for any adult patient who has not received this immunization.

Storage and Record Keeping

Vaccine storage should follow specific manufacturer's guidelines. Some vaccines' preparations require refrigeration, freezing, reconstitution, or protection from light. The medical assistant must check the temperature settings to ensure proper storage of the vaccines.

Parents should be provided with an immunization record card at their infant's first well-child visit. They should be instructed to bring the card to every visit so that their child's immunization can be recorded.

An immunization flow sheet is used to account for vaccines given in the office, and according to federal law, information about a patient's vaccination history must be kept in his or her medical record. It must include:

- type of vaccine given
- date given
- route of administration
- vaccine lot number and manufacturer
- publication date of the VIS (found on a lower corner of each VIS)

Emergencies and First Aid

Emergencies

Most emergencies in the medical office are minor and include such events as a patient arriving unexpectedly with a nosebleed or fractured arm. However, emergencies of all types can and do occur in the medical office.

Therefore, the professional medical office team must always be ready for any emergency, small or large.

Policies and Procedures

Medical offices establish **protocols** that outline instructions on how to proceed in case of medical emergencies. Such a protocol might include supplies and equipment needed, the roles for each staff mem-

CONTROLLED SUBSTANCE SCHEDULE		
SCHEDULE	**DESCRIPTION**	**EXAMPLES**
I	■ no currently accepted medical use in the U.S. ■ high potential for abuse	heroin lysergic acid diethylamide (LSD) MDMA (ecstasy) marijuana mescaline peyote
II	■ currently accepted medical use in the U.S. with severe restrictions ■ high potential for abuse ■ written prescription must be provided to pharmacist within seven days ■ no refills allowed for prescription	cocaine hydromorphone (Dialaudid) meperidine (Demerol) methylphenidate (Ritalin) morphine (MS Contin) oxycodone (OxyContin)
III	■ currently accepted medical use in the U.S. ■ potential for abuse is less than for schedules I and II ■ telephone orders allowed ■ can be refilled five times within six months of prescription date	acetaminophen (Tylenol and codeine) acetaminophen and hydrocodone (Vicodin) anabolic steroids, such as oxandrolone (Oxandrin)
IV	■ potential for abuse is less than for schedule III ■ telephone orders allowed ■ can be refilled five times within six months of prescription date	diazepam (Valium) alprazolam (Xanax) zolpidem (Ambien) phentermine (Fastin)
V	■ potential for abuse is less than schedule IV ■ telephone orders allowed ■ number of refills determined by physician	cough suppressants with restricted amounts of codeine diphenoxylate and atropine (Lomotil)

The full schedule of controlled substances in the Controlled Substances Act of 1990 describes the medical uses, potential abuse level, prescription requirements, and safety of each group of drugs. The table shown here lists each schedule number along with a description of the drugs' uses and potential for abuse, and examples of the drugs included in that schedule.

ber, and the step-by-step procedure for responding to that particular emergency.

All members of the healthcare team should know where the emergency equipment is located and obtain proper training in its use. In some cases, a team captain is designated to guide members of the team throughout the emergency.

An important, but sometimes overlooked, part of emergency preparedness is the designation of a team member to document the emergency. This person should assume his or her role from the beginning of the emergency so he or she can accurately record the events in a chronological fashion. Otherwise, reconstructing events after the fact will be difficult, especially in a complex medical emergency.

During a medical emergency, the medical assistant is responsible for identifying the presence of serious conditions that threaten the patient's life. The medical assistant should take the appropriate actions that are within a medical assistant's scope of practice. The emergency must be documented in the patient's chart along with the patient's assessment.

Good Samaritan Principle and Laws

The Good Samaritan principle prevents a rescuer who has voluntarily helped a stranger in need of medical assistance from being sued for wrongdoing. In most of North America, one has no legal obligation to help a person in need. However, since governments want to encourage people to help others, they often pass Good Samaritan laws (or apply the principle to common laws). The person who offers medical assistance to a stranger in need is generally protected from liability as long as:

- he or she is reasonably careful
- he or she acts in "good faith" (not for a reward)
- he or she does not provide care beyond his or her skill level

If a medical assistant decides to help in an emergency, the medical assistant must not leave the injured person until someone who has the same or more skill and training in medical emergencies can take over.

Consent

A patient requiring first aid must give his or her consent, or permission, to receive treatment. This can come in two forms:

- Expressed consent: With patients who are responsive adults, caregivers should identify themselves, explain their level of training, and ask the patient for his or her permission to help.
- Implied consent: With unresponsive or unconscious patients, the permission to provide first aid treatment is implied, or assumed, since a reasonable person would be willing to be treated in emergency situations.

Common Emergency and First-Aid Supplies and Equipment

Not all medical offices keep emergency equipment on hand; however, many do. If an office does stock emergency equipment and medication, the medical assistant and other staff members must be familiar with its use.

Crash Cart

Many supplies are stored in a portable, wheeled supply cabinet, called a crash cart or code cart, which is specifically used for emergencies. The crash cart (or sometimes just a tray) contains basic drugs, supplies, and equipment for medical emergencies. Most crash carts also contain a first-aid kit with supplies for managing minor injuries and ailments. Specific equipment stored on the cart varies, depending on the type of patients seen by the doctor. The most common drugs included in a crash cart are as follows.

- Epinephrine has multiple uses in emergency situations. As a **vasoconstrictor**, it controls hemorrhage, relaxes the bronchioles to relieve acute asthma attacks, and is an emergency heart stimulant used to treat shock. Epinephrine should be in ready-to-use cartridge syringe and needle units. These are supplied in 1 mL cartridges.

- Atropine decreases secretions, increases respiration and heart rate, and is a smooth-muscle relaxant. It is administered in a cardiac emergency for asystole or can be used to treat bradycardia.

- Digoxin is a cardiac drug that treats arrhythmias and congestive heart failure (CHF) and is good for emergency use because it has a relatively rapid action.

- Nitroglycerin is a vasodilator that is given to relieve angina. It acts by dilating the coronary arteries so an increased volume of oxygenated blood can reach the myocardium.

- Lidocaine is used intravenously to treat a cardiac arrhythmia and is used locally as an anesthetic.

- Sodium bicarbonate corrects metabolic acidosis that typically occurs after a cardiac arrest.

- An emetic causes vomiting soon after swallowing.

- Activated charcoal is an antidote that is swallowed to absorb ingested poisons.

- Naloxone (Narcan) is a narcotic antidote that is administered intravenously for drug overdoses and acts to raise blood pressure and increase respiratory rate.

- Antihistamines for the treatment of allergic reactions and anaphylaxis should be available to treat potential allergic responses to medication administered in the facility. These can include diphenhydramine (Benadryl) for minor reactions and a corticosteroid (e.g., Solumedrol), for severe anaphylactic responses.

Other medications that may be found on a crash cart are:

- isoproterenol (for example, Isuprel, Medihaler-Iso, or Norisodrine), an antispasmodic that is used to treat bronchospasms (such as those experienced during an asthma attack) and is also effective as a cardiac stimulant

- metaraminol (Aramine) (50%, in a prefilled syringe) for severe shock

- phenobarbital, amobarbital sodium (Amytal), and diazepam (Valium) for convulsions and/or sedative effects

- furosemide (Lasix) for CHF

- glucagons, primarily used to counteract severe hypoglycemic reactions in diabetic patients taking insulin

Defibrillator

One item almost always present on a crash cart is defibrillator. This specialized device is used to deliver an electrical shock to a patient suffering from a life-threatening cardiac arrhythmia, such as ventricular

MOCK EMERGENCY DRILLS

Many facilities routinely run mock drills, which allow all members of the healthcare team to practice and develop their skills in responding to medical emergencies. Such drills rehearse the staff's response to bomb scares, fires, infant or child abduction, a threat of violence and, most commonly, a patient experiencing cardiac or respiratory failure.

After each mock drill, members of the team should debrief. This includes a discussion of the event among all team members to determine what worked during the event and what did not, so that appropriate changes can be made in the response plan.

fibrillation or ventricular tachycardia. During such arrhythmias, some or all heart muscle fibers contract in a disorganized fashion. Delivery of an electrical shock causes all cardiac muscle fibers to contract in unison, which sometimes stimulates the heart to convert back to normal sinus rhythm. Because some risk is associated with operating this device, all staff members who use it must be properly trained.

Automated external defibrillators: Automated external defibrillators (AEDs) make operation of this type of emergency equipment relatively easy. The AED's manufacturers have programmed the devices to give automatic, step-by-step instructions—through both voice and visual prompts—for their use. They are smaller and more portable than older defibrillators.

Healthcare providers, first responders, and other professional rescuers should practice cardiopulmonary resuscitation (CPR) and AED. (For more information on CPR, see the First Aid section of this chapter on page 217.)

There are many different brands of AEDs, but the same basic steps apply to all of them:

- Turn on the AED, and the voice prompts will be activated.
- Bare the patient's chest.
- Follow the voice and visual prompts.
- Remove the disposable electrode pads from the package. Look at the graphic images on each electrode as a guide for proper pad placement.
- Attach the electrodes to the patient's chest, after removing the adhesive backing.
- Most AEDs will automatically begin to analyze a patient's heart rhythm when the electrodes are fully attached. Some will prompt you to push a button to start the analysis; no one should be touching the patient while the AED is conducting its analysis of the heart rhythm.
- Once everyone is clear of the patient, the shock button can be pushed; and chest compressions can be resumed; see the section on Cardiac and Respiratory Arrest/CPR (page 218) for guidance on chest compressions.
- Perform five cycles of 30 compressions and two breaths and then very briefly reassess the rhythm. Continue as directed by the AED.

A ventricular fibrillation victim who gets his or her heart pattern restored immediately following a sudden cardiac arrest has about a two-thirds chance of recovery. Every minute that revival is delayed, the chances drop until there is little hope after ten minutes.

Triage

In the medical setting, **triage** involves making a quick determination about the nature of the patient's emergency, the type of immediate care needed, and the most appropriate response. If more than one patient is involved, triage involves determining which patient should be treated first. In many settings, a registered nurse performs triage; however, other staff members may perform this task, depending on their qualifications.

In some cases, medical assistants must perform triage. Most offices have written guidelines in place that guide the process. Even so, no guidelines are as valuable as experience and practice. Therefore, the person assigned triage duties should be an experienced healthcare provider.

Emergency Preparedness

All healthcare facilities must make an effort to create an environment that is safe for patients and staff alike. Workplace safety programs provide instruction in CPR, standard precautions, proper body mechanics, and other safety issues. New employees undergo safety training upon hire and are required to update their knowledge and regularly demonstrate competence (usually annually) on specific skills, such as CPR.

The appropriate response to an emergency depends on the nature of the emergency, the patient population being served, and the proximity of other medical facilities. Steps and principles to follow include:

- The physician or most highly trained clinician in the office should be summoned for immediate help.

- If the office has staff trained in advanced cardiac life support (ACLS) and the needed equipment is on hand, the staff can provide ACLS measures at the office.
- In the case of life-threatening emergencies, the staff should institute basic cardiac life support (BCLS) measures while summoning emergency medical service (EMS) personnel.
- EMS staff include experts experienced in evaluation, treatment, and transport of persons experiencing a medical emergency.

First Aid

First aid is treatment of individuals in emergency situations before professional medical care can be, or is, administered. In the medical office, the staff must be understand and be prepared to apply first-aid techniques for a range of conditions.

In all cases, the medical assistant should remember to identify him or herself as a medical assistant.

The first step in applying first aid is assessing the patient. The most basic assessment tool is the ABCs.

A—airway: Check for an open airway using the head-tilt/chin-lift method or the jaw thrust method (for suspected neck injuries).
B—breathing: Make sure the patient is breathing by looking for chest movement.
C—circulation: Check the patient's pulse.

In many emergency cases, the medical assistant, after assessing the patient, should follow the emergency preparedness guidelines discussed earlier in this section, including the activation of the office's emergency medical system.

Identification and the ABCs, along with activating the EMS when necessary, should be part of the medical assistant's response to all emergencies. The following sections describe the specific first-aid techniques for specific conditions.

In treating many of these conditions, the use of personal protective equipment is necessary. See the first section of this chapter, under Infection Control, for information on PPE and other precautions medical staff should take when in danger of exposure to potentially biohazardous material.

Severe Bleeding

Severe or excessive bleeding (hemorrhage) can result from a range of injuries and conditions. In all cases, it is important to locate the source of the bleeding.

- Clear away clothing from the area of the wound.
- Place an absorbent pad directly over the wound.
- Apply firm pressure on the wound, using a sterile gauze pad to absorb the blood.
- Wrap an elastic bandage over the gauze pad to keep it in place.
- If possible, position the part of the body containing the wound above the level of the heart.
- If needed—if blood soaks through the gauze pad—more should be applied.
- Pressure should be kept on the wound.

Applying pressure to pressure points, specific points on the body at which blood vessels are located close to the surface, can be helpful in reducing blood flow to a wound. Common pressure points are:

- brachial artery: located on the arm between shoulder and elbow
- femoral artery: located in the upper thigh, at the intersection with the groin area
- popliteal artery: located in the crease behind the knee

When using pressure points, the medical assistant should make sure he or she is pressing on a point closer to the heart than the wound. Pressing on a blood vessel further from the heart than the wound is will have no effect on the bleeding.

Shock

Shock can result from a range of conditions, such as severe bleeding, a severe allergic reaction (anaphylactic shock), hypoglycemia in diabetics (insulin shock), or massive internal infection (septic shock). Signs of shock include:

- skin that is cold and clammy to the touch
- drop in blood pressure
- weakened pulse, but elevated pulse rate
- elevated respiration rate
- sometimes behavioral changes, such as heightened anxiety or confusion

Guidelines to help manage shock include:

- Make sure an open airway exists for an adequate air supply.
- Keep the patient from becoming chilled or overheated.
- Administer oxygen, if you have the appropriate training.

In addition, the medical assistant staff should attempt to address the underlying cause of the shock. For instance, in the case of insulin shock, sugar should be administered, and in the case of anaphylactic shock, the allergen should be removed from touching, or any other interaction with, the patient.

Burns

Burns involve injury to the tissue caused not just by heat, but by chemicals, electricity, or radiation. Burns can cause massive injury to the body, and must be carefully handled.

The extent of a person's burns is estimated and reported by with the rule of nines: Each body part is considered 9% of the entire body, and individual percentages are added to arrive at a total percentage. For instance, in an adult, one arm is considered 9%, the chest is considered 9%, the abdomen is considered 9%, and so forth; if these parts were all burned, the total would be 27%.

Third-Degree Burn

The most severe burn, a third-degree burn, involves the layers of the skin—including the epidermis and dermis—and often underlying tissues. Signs include white, leathery, or blackened, charred skin.

Guidelines to handle third-degree burns:

- Clear away clothing covering the burned area; do not remove clothing that is stuck to the burned area.
- If clothing is stuck to the burn, do not remove it.
- Cover the burn area with clean moist sterile bandage, cloth, or towel.
- If possible, elevate the burned area above heart level.

Second-Degree Burn

A second-degree burn involves the epidermis and part of the dermis. Signs include pain, redness, blisters, and/or swelling.

Guidelines to handle second-degree burns include:

- Cool the burn with cool, running water or cold compresses.
- After cooling, use a sterile bandage or a clean dressing to cover the burned area and protect it.
- Wrap the bandage or dressing loosely but avoid putting pressure on the burned area.

First-Degree Burn

A first-degree burn involves the epidermis. Signs include redness, swelling, pain, and peeling of skin. First-degree burns should be treated by immersion in cool water or covering with cold compresses.

Cardiac and Respiratory Arrest/CPR

Cardiopulmonary resuscitation is an emergency treatment applied to individuals who are in cardiac arrest.

It combines breathing into the victim's lungs and compressing the victim's chest. Its object is to "buy some time," by getting some blood flowing to the heart and brain, after which restoration of full heart function can be achieved.

Steps for performing CPR on an adult are:

1. Try to rouse the victim.
2. Check for breathing: Open the victim's air passage by tilting the head back and lifting the chin; with your ear to the patient's mouth, listen for breathing, and with your cheek to the patient's mouth, feel for his or her breath.
3. Perform rescue breathing, if the victim is not breathing: Pinch the person's nose shut and cover his or her mouth completely with yours; breath fully into the mouth, watching for the chest to rise. Perform this rescue breathing twice.
4. Start chest compressions: Place the heel of your hand at the center of the patient's chest, with the other hand covering it; press down deeply—about two inches—and release, letting the chest fully relax before repeating the compression; the compressions should be done firmly and quickly, at a rate of about 100 times per minute, for a total of 30 compressions.
5. Perform rescue breathing again, followed by 30 chest compressions.
6. Continue this pattern until patient begins to breathe on his or her own, or until EMS providers arrive.

Choking

Choking—the blocking of the primary air passage from the mouth—happens in variety of situations. Small children often put small objects such as coins, toys, and candy in their mouth and then aspirate them. Adults sometimes aspirate food they are eating. In some cases, the obstruction of air flow is just partial, but in other cases, the blockage is complete, cutting off the supply of oxygen to the blood vessels, and therefore is life threatening.

Signs for choking include the inability to talk and labored, noisy, wheezing breathing. In severe cases, when oxygen supply is drastically reduced or cut off, the patient's lips and skin, including the skin under the nails, may take on a bluish cast.

Guidelines for handling choking in an adult include:

- First, encourage the patient to cough, since this may clear out the air passage.
- Perform back blows: Forcefully hit the patient's back with the heel of your hand, between the shoulder blades; this should be done five times.
- Perform abdominal thrusts, sometimes called the Heimlich maneuver, if choking has not cleared: Standing behind the patient with arms wrapped around him or her and hands clasped together in a fist, push in and up forcefully at the base of the diaphragm, just above the navel; perform five thrusts.
- Perform the five back blows and five abdominal thrusts continuously until the blockage clears or until EMS help arrives.
- With pregnant or obese patients, the Heimlich maneuver should be performed in the same way, except that the placement of the clenched fists is higher, just below the sternum, the point at which the lower ribs join.

Guidelines for handling choking in an infant include:

- Perform modified back blows: In a seated position, place the infant facedown on your forearm; push or thump the middle of the infant's back with the heel of your hand; perform five times.
- Perform chest compressions: Turn the infant over, so that he or she is facing up; position the infant with the head lower than the rest of the body; with two fingers at the infant's breast-

bone, push in quickly, delivering five chest compressions.

- Perform the five back blows and the five chest compressions continuously until the blockage clears or until EMS help arrives.

Emergencies for Diabetic Patients

Diabetes is a chronic disease characterized by the inability of the body to regulate the level of glucose in the blood. Two emergency situations can arise in patients with diabetes:

Insulin shock: Insulin shock is very severe hypoglycemia, in which a patient has too little glucose in the blood. Insulin shock occurs when insulin levels are so high that too much glucose is transported from the blood into the body's cells.

Symptoms include:

- rapid pulse
- shallow respiration
- hunger
- profuse sweating
- pale, cool, clammy skin
- double vision
- tremors
- restlessness
- confusion
- possible fainting

Insulin shock can usually be corrected with administration of some form of sugar (candy, juice, or regular soda for a conscious patient or a sprinkle of table sugar on the tongue for an unconscious patient).

Diabetic coma: Diabetic coma is the final stage of severe hyperglycemia, in which a patient has too much glucose in the blood. It occurs when insulin levels are insufficient to transport blood glucose into the cells of the body.

Symptoms include:

- rapid, deep gulping breaths
- flushed, warm, dry skin
- extreme thirst
- sweet or fruity-smelling breath
- disorientation or confusion

The medical assistant should notify the doctor at once and expect to arrange transport to the hospital if a diabetic coma is suspected.

If the cause of a diabetic emergency is not known, sugar in any form possible should be given to the patient. Once sugar is given, the patient will improve shortly if the cause is insulin shock. No harm will be done by the intake of sugar if the cause of the emergency is diabetic coma.

Fractures

A fracture is a break in a bone. Treatment of fractures depends on the nature of the injury and the patient's age and physical condition.

Types of fractures include:

- simple (closed) fracture: a fracture with no external wound caused by the bone
- compound (open) fracture: a fracture where the bone protrudes from the skin
- greenstick fracture: an incomplete break as when a fresh twig is bent; typical in children, whose bones are still relatively
- transverse fracture: a straight break straight across the bone
- spiral fracture: a break caused by a twisting force creating an "s" shaped fracture

Signs of fractures include tenderness, pain, swelling, and bruising. If the fracture is severe, deformity or external bleeding (in the case of a compound fracture) may occur.

The symptoms of other types of injuries to the musculoskeletal system, such as the following, might be confused with those of fractures.

- Dislocation: A bone is separated or displaced from its normal position at a joint.

- Sprain: Stretching or tearing of ligaments within a joint.
- Strain: Stretching or tearing of muscles or tendons.

Guidelines to handle open or closed fractures include:

- Apply ice to the area affected; this will reduce swelling, bleeding, and pain; use a cloth or thin towel between an ice pack and the skin to prevent frostbite.
- Elevate the affected limb, if possible.
- In the case of open, or compound, fracture, apply gentle pressure to control bleeding where the bone is protruding from the skin and use a sterile cloth or dressing to cover open wounds.
- Limit movement of the affected area; keep the patient from putting weight on the affected limb.

If a painful, deformed, or swollen limb is blue or extremely pale, EMS should be activated immediately.

Poisoning

Poisoning is the intake of toxic substances into the body. Poisons can be ingested, absorbed through the skin, or inhaled. Symptoms can be wide-ranging and can mimic many common illnesses.

One of the most important rules in dealing with cases of poisoning is to call the Poison Control Center to obtain instructions from an expert about the specific toxin the patient has encountered. Other guidelines to handle poisoning include:

- Put on PPE as soon as possible to protect from any toxin that is still present, and remove the toxin from the environment.
- Keep the containers holding the toxin with you and bring to the emergency room or give to EMS workers when they arrive; this is for the purpose of helping in the identification of the toxin if unknown.

- Do not administer water, milk, or antidote of any kind unless advised to do so by the poison control expert.
- Do not induce vomiting—with ipecac syrup, activated carbon, or another agent—unless advised to do so by the poison control expert.
- For toxins absorbed through the skin, thoroughly rinse the area of exposure with a large volume of water.

Seizures

A seizure is the sudden and abnormal incidence of involuntary muscle movements, which come in a series of contractions and relaxations. No matter what the underlying cause—which can include such factors as epilepsy, high fever, low sodium in the blood, head injury, and drug or alcohol abuse—the first aid used for individuals suffering from seizures is the same.

Guidelines for handling seizures in an adult include:

- Move objects—such as furniture—that the victim may hit.
- Do not insert anything in the victim's mouth.
- Do not restrain the victim; allow the seizure to take its course.
- Loosen tight clothing, if possible.
- When the seizure is over, the victim should be placed in, or helped into, the recovery position, which is on his or her side, to ensure an open air passage and prevent aspirating any liquid secreted orally during the seizure.

Stroke

A stroke, also referred to as a cerebrovascular accident (CVA), is a disturbance in, and potential loss of, brain function resulting from a lessening of the blood supply to the brain. A bursting of or blockage in a blood vessel is the usual cause of the reduced blood flow. Symptoms can include:

- weakness, numbness, or paralysis of a specific area, frequently on just one side of the body

- confusion and/or inability to communicate
- sudden and severe headache
- loss of balance and/or coordination
- dizziness

First aid guidelines call for simple supportive care, including keeping the patient calm, until EMS staff arrive. In a medical office, the medical assistant might prepare to administer oxygen upon direction from a physician, if the medical assistant has the appropriate training.

Syncope

Syncope, or fainting, results from a decrease in the blood flow to the brain. A fainting spell is usually brief and may have no medical significance.

When a patient faints and quickly comes to, the patient may become embarrassed by the attention that follows. It is important in these situations that the patient is evaluated by the doctor before he or she is allowed to leave. Fainting should be considered a medical emergency until proven otherwise. When a person feels faint, the medical assistant should help the individual sit or lie down and position his or head between the knees.

When a person faints, first aid guidelines include:

- Check for clear air passages.
- Loosen clothing and belts.
- The patient should be positioned on his or her back, with feet above the level of the head.

Wounds

Simply put, a wound is a break in the skin or other body tissue. The term, however, covers a wide range of conditions—from bruises and abrasions to punctures and complete amputations. In all cases, the basic role of first aid is to stop the bleeding and reduce the chance of infection.

Bruise

A contusion, or bruise, is a wound in which the surface skin has not been broken, but the blood vessels under the skin have been torn, causing a leakage of blood into the surrounding tissue. First aid treatment is to apply ice in order to reduce the swelling of the tissue and bleeding.

Open Wounds

There are several types of open wounds.

- An abrasion is an open wound in which the skin has been scraped open.
- A laceration is a jagged cut into the skin and surrounding tissue.
- An avulsion is a type of open wound characterized by a ripping away of the skin from bone; often a flap of loose skin remains connected to the skin.
- A puncture is an open wound in which an object has pierced the skin.
- An amputation is the complete removal of a body part.

First aid guidelines include:

- cleansing of the wound with soap and water to remove particles or residue
- application of an antiseptic to reduce the threat of infection
- covering the wound in sterile cloth or gauze
- If a laceration is deep, it may need to be closed up with adhesive strips (Steri-Strips) or sutures (by a qualified medical professional).
- The skin flap resulting from an avulsion can be replaced over the wound.
- In a puncture wound, if the object protruding from the skin remains, the object should be left in place.

Amputation

When resulting from trauma—amputation may also be surgically performed in rare cases if medically necessary—the procedure for open wounds should be followed, with one crucial added step. The amputated part should be wrapped in a sterile moistened dressing and brought to the hospital, since the severed part can often be surgically reattached and will successfully reconnect to the rest of the body during the healing process.

Nutrition

Nutrition is the study of how nutrients are taken into and used by the body. A nutrient is a chemical substance obtained from food and used in the body to provide energy, build structural materials, support growth and maintenance, or repair body tissues. Good nutrition is one of the most important factors in health maintenance.

Digestion

The digestive system plays a major role in proper nutrition. There are four processes that occur in the digestive system: ingestion, digestion, absorption, and elimination.

- **Ingestion** is simply taking food into the body. This occurs at the mouth.
- **Digestion** is the breaking down of food into smaller components that the body can absorb. This occurs both physically and chemically, and starts at the mouth with chewing and continues through the gastrointestinal tract to the small intestine.
- **Absorption** is the method the body uses to transfer nutrients from the gastrointestinal, or digestive, tract into the bloodstream.
- **Elimination** is the method through which the body removes, or excretes, waste.

Energy Nutrients

Energy is defined as the capacity to do work. The human body needs energy to do physical and chemical work, which is critical in metabolism, the set of physical and chemical processes that maintain life in an organism. The body uses energy, which is measured in calories, in foods for a variety of functions:

- to create body heat
- to move muscles
- to conduct nervous signals
- to produce hormones
- to regulate functions such as heart rate
- to repair damaged tissues

Three energy nutrients—carbohydrates, fats, and proteins—have one thing in common: All can be converted into energy.

Carbohydrates

Carbohydrates are the main source of energy. They are categorized as simple and complex, depending on the amount of energy needed to digest them.

Simple Carbohydrates

Simple carbohydrates, commonly referred to as simple sugars, are abundant in many foods we eat. Two categories of simple carbohydrates exist: monosaccharides and disaccharides.

Monosaccharides are single units of sugar. The most common monosaccharides in the human diet are glucose, fructose, and galactose.

- Glucose is the sugar that the body uses most efficiently; most ingested sugar is broken down in the intestines and converted to glucose in the liver.
- Fructose is found largely in fruits.
- Galactose is a product of the digestion of lactose (see next paragraph).

Three disaccharides constitute the main dietary sources of sugar for humans: sucrose, lactose, and maltose.

- Sucrose is one of the sweetest sugars. It occurs naturally in many fruits and vegetables as well as in sugar cane and the sugar beet. Table sugar, or refined sugar, is a form of sucrose.

- Maltose is a result of the breakdown of starch, a complex carbohydrate (see next section).
- Lactose is a disaccharide commonly found in milk products.

Complex Carbohydrates

Complex carbohydrates, also known as polysaccharides, are made up of many units of monosaccharides, the simple sugars. There are three types of complex carbohydrates:

- Starch is the most important dietary complex carbohydrate. Starch is found in plants. There are two kinds of starch molecules: amylase and amylopectin. Examples of foods that are sources of starch are wheat, rice, potatoes, and legumes.
- Glycogen is only ingested in small quantities, but is an important form of glucose as it is stored in the body. It releases glucose into the bloodstream to raise blood glucose levels.
- Fiber is a special polysaccharide because it cannot be digested. Fiber provides bulk to feces and promotes intestinal motility.

The American Cancer Society recommends a high-fiber diet to help prevent cancer. These recommendations include:

- eating high-fiber foods such as fruits, vegetables, and whole-grain cereals
- daily intake of five or more servings of vegetables and fruits
- consuming less processed and red meats
- maintaining a physically active lifestyle
- maintaining a healthy weight
- limiting the consumption of alcoholic beverages

Proteins

Proteins are a class of essential nutrients made up of amino acids linked together in chains and branching patterns by peptide bonds. Proteins and their component parts—amino acids—serve several important roles in the functioning of the body:

- as enzymes
- as hormones
- as the basic structural units in body tissues and cells

While proteins can be described as an energy nutrient, producing energy is not their main function. Ingesting foods that are high in protein is important for the healthy functioning of the body. Since the body cannot synthesize all amino acids on its own, it must get what are called **essential amino acids** from the food that is ingested.

Fats

Fats (which are also called lipids) perform important functions as part of a balanced diet.

Fatty acids are the building blocks of many fats and can be saturated or unsaturated.

- **Saturated:** when every carbon molecule in the fatty acid is saturated with, or holds, as many units of hydrogen as possible. Saturated fats can be found in meat, butter, and egg yolk and can increase blood cholesterol levels.
- **Unsaturated:** when the fatty acid's carbon molecules do not hold all the hydrogen atoms possible. The more unsaturated the fatty acid is, the more liquid the fat. Unsaturated fats are found in vegetable and olive oils and can decrease blood cholesterol levels.

There are three types of fats: triglycerides, phospholipids, and sterols, such as cholesterol.

Triglycerides and Phospholipids

Calories taken in through ingestion that are not immediately used are stored in the form of triglycerides. Most fat in the body—and in food—is stored in the form of triglycerides, which contain three fatty acids and a glycerol molecule. The more saturated the molecule, the larger it is and the more likely it will contribute to stagnation in the bloodstream and the formation of fatty streaks.

Phospholipids are similar to triglycerides. However, they contain two fatty acids and a phosphate group.

- The phosphate group on the phospholipids makes the molecule soluble in water.
- The fatty acid component makes it soluble in fat.

This property of dual solubility—unique in the body—allows phospholipid molecules to form cell membranes.

Sterols

Sterols are lipids that contain a sterol group, which is made up of four carbon structures. The most common type of sterol is cholesterol, which is derived only from animal sources, such as eggs, meat, fish, and poultry. Cholesterol becomes harmful when it forms deposits of fatty streaks and fibrous plaque along artery walls.

There are two types of cholesterol:

- High-density lipoproteins (HDLs) help carry cholesterol to the liver for breakdown and secretion.
- Low-density lipoproteins (LDLs) circulate in the bloodstream and transport cholesterol and triglycerides from the liver to the peripheral tissues.

For more information on lipids, see the Lipid Profile section on page 195.

Vitamins

Vitamins are organic compounds vital to human nutrition. Needed in small amounts, they support a range of metabolic functions that are critical to the proper functioning of the human body.

There are two general classifications: fat-soluble and water-soluble.

Fat-Soluble Vitamins

Fat-soluble vitamins are absorbed into the body through lipids, or fat, in the intestines. They are more easily stored in the body than water-soluble vitamins and have the potential for a unsafe higher buildup.

- **Vitamin A:** promotes vision and supports growth; obtained primarily from fortified milk and dairy products, such as cheese, and some vegetables, such as carrots
- **Vitamin D:** supports bone development; obtained primarily from sunlight and fortified milk and dairy products such as cheese, some seafood such as salmon and sardines, and some meat such as veal and beef
- **Vitamin E:** antioxidant that protects cellular structure; obtained primarily from nuts, seeds, vegetable oils, and leafy green vegetables
- **Vitamin K:** essential for blood clotting; obtained primarily from leafy green vegetables, such as spinach and kale

Water-Soluble Vitamins

Water-soluble vitamins, as the name indicates, can be readily dissolved in water, and are generally easily excreted in urine. Because of this, specified daily intake levels must be maintained.

- **Vitamin B1 (thiamine):** necessary for energy metabolism; obtained primarily from sunlight and milk
- **Vitamin B2 (riboflavin):** necessary for energy metabolism; obtained primarily from milk and dairy products, eggs, spinach, and broccoli
- **Vitamin B3 (niacin):** necessary for energy metabolism; obtained primarily in foods high in proteins, such as meats, poultry, and some seafood, such as shrimp, halibut, and tuna; peanuts are also a good source

- **Vitamin B6:** necessary for a range of health-related functions, including protein metabolism; obtained primarily from beans, meat, poultry, some seafood, and some fruits, such as bananas
- **Vitamin B12:** necessary for red blood cell production and supports nerve function and DNA synthesis; obtained primarily from fish, meat, poultry, milk, and other dairy products
- **Vitamin C:** plays an important role in the immune system; necessary for synthesis of collagen, a vital part of connective tissue; supports protein metabolism and has antioxidant properties; obtained primarily from citrus fruits, tomatoes, and red and green peppers

Some standard foods, such as cereals and milk, are routinely fortified to include essential vitamins and minerals.

Minerals

Minerals are inorganic elements that are generally needed in larger quantities relative to vitamins. They help in the formation of hard bones, as is the case with calcium, and also are an important part of metabolic function.

Two general classifications include the major minerals and trace minerals. Major minerals, such as calcium and sodium, are needed in larger quantities than the trace minerals, such as iron and copper.

Major Minerals

- **Calcium (Ca):** supports bone and teeth structure; necessary for muscle and blood vessel function; obtained primarily from milk and other dairy products; deficiencies can cause osteoporosis in adults, especially women, and rickets in children
- **Chlorine (Cl):** important part of stomach acid and critical to electrolyte balance; obtained primarily from table salt and meat; no known disorders result from deficiency

- **Magnesium (Mg):** helps support nerve and muscle function, important in maintaining heart rhythm; supports bone development and the immune system; obtained primarily from beans and peas (legumes), green vegetables such as spinach, nuts and seeds, and unrefined grains; deficiencies can cause muscle weakness and twitching, confusion and hallucinations, dysphagia, and lack of growth in children
- **Phosphorus (P):** important for energy metabolism, bone and teeth development, and obtained primarily from meats and fish; deficiencies can cause weakness, bone pain, and bone loss
- **Potassium (K):** supports nerve and muscle function and important to electrolyte balance; obtained primarily from citrus fruits, tomatoes, potatoes, soybeans, and some dried fruits, such as dates and raisins; deficiencies can cause muscle weakness, paralysis, confusion; disorders include hypokalemia, low levels of potassium, and hyperkalemia, high levels of potassium
- **Sodium (Na):** helps maintain fluid balance; obtained primarily from table salt and meat; disorders include hypertension, due to high levels of sodium
- **Sulfur (S):** important part of protein structure; obtained primarily from milk, other dairy products, meats, eggs, and other foods containing protein; no known disorders result from deficiency

Trace Minerals

- **Copper (Cu):** important in many enzymes, necessary for the absorption of iron; obtained primarily from whole grains, nuts, beans and peas, and seafood; deficiencies can cause bone loss and anemia
- **Iodine (I):** critical component of thyroid hormone, which regulates growth and development; obtained primarily from iodized table salt and saltwater seafood; deficiencies can cause goiter

- **Iron (Fe):** critical part of the hemoglobin protein that carries oxygen to tissues, important for cellular development; obtained primarily from red meat, poultry, seafood, beans, and dark green leafy vegetables, such as spinach; deficiencies can cause anemia and fatigue
- **Zinc (Zn):** supports the immune system, important in protein and DNA development, helps wound healing, and supports the senses of taste and scent; obtained primarily from oysters, red meats, and some whole grains, nuts, and beans; deficiencies can cause stunted growth in children, hair loss, night blindness, slow wound healing, and skin problems

Other trace elements include chromium, molybdenum, selenium, cobalt, and fluorine.

Water

Water is an essential non-energy yielding nutrient. Water is the most abundant molecule in the body and makes up 65% of body weight in males and 55% in females. Without adequate water intake, the body cannot survive. Water is critical in a range of functions.

- part of intracellular fluids that allow chemical reactions to occur within cells
- part of extracellular fluids that allow transport of nutrients to cells
- removal of toxic waste from the body
- major component of blood
- control of bodily temperature by eliminating excess heat through the evaporation in the form of perspiration

The recommended amount of water that should be consumed in one day is eight eight-ounce glasses.

Dietary Guidelines

A variety of dietary guidelines exist to help people obtain proper nutrition, reduce the occurrence of disease, and control weight. These recommendations suggest the types and quantities of food that people should eat each day. They may also contain recommendations about which types of foods to limit and which types of foods to increase, given the specific health status of an individual.

USDA Dietary Guidelines for Americans

The U.S. Department of Agriculture (USDA) and the U.S. Department of Health and Human Services (HHS) have established dietary guidelines. These guidelines encourage people to eat a balanced diet, limit consumption of less nutritious foods, increase physical activity, and make good nutritional decisions consistently. Much of the information on these guidelines—and in this section—can be found in *Dietary Guidelines for Americans,* published jointly by the USDA and HHS, and can be found at http://www.health.gov/dietaryguidelines.

Key Recommendations

The USDA dietary guidelines recommend that individuals balance the food they eat with physical activity. The USDA guidelines also recommend that individuals maintain or reduce their weight to help reduce the possibility of high blood pressure, heart disease, stroke, some types of cancer, and diabetes.

Specific recommendations in the USDA guidelines include:

- Maintain an adequate nutrient intake while monitoring caloric needs.
- Consume a variety of nutritious foods from the basic food groups.
- Avoid foods that contain saturated fat, trans fat, sugar, and salt.
- Restrict alcoholic beverages.
- Maintain body weight in a healthy range.
- Exercise regularly and reduce sedentary activities.
- Balance calorie consumption with physical activity.
- Prevent gradual weight gain over time.

Food group recommendations by the USDA include:

- Eat a lot of fruits and vegetables, and a wide variety of them, each day while staying within energy requirements.
- Consume three or more servings of whole grains per day.
- Consume three cups of fat-free or low-fat milk or equivalent each day.
- Limit amounts of fats and oils that are high in saturated and/or trans fatty acids.

Carbohydrate recommendations from the USDA:

- Stick with fiber-rich fruits, vegetables, and whole grains.
- Stay away from foods that are high in simple sugars.

In addition, the USDA advises individuals who drink alcoholic beverages to do so in moderation. Alcoholic beverages should not be consumed by pregnant or lactating women, individuals who take medication that can interact with alcohol, and children and adolescents. Avoid alcoholic beverages if engaging in activities that require skill and coordination.

USDA Food Guide Pyramid

Continued research on obesity by the U.S. Department of Agriculture and the U.S. Department of Health and Human Services led to the 2005 redesign of the food pyramid, which was initially introduced in 1988, to include emphasis on eating more fruits, vegetables, whole grain foods, beans, and nuts, and to include less emphasis on carbohydrates.

The new food pyramid can be found at http://www.mypyramid.org. It is designed to help balance nutritional and physical activity needs, and the medical assistant can use the pyramid and its guidelines, scheduled to be updated in 2010, as a source of information on maintaining a healthy diet.

The new pyramid presents color-coded vertical wedges, with each color representing a food group and the size of the wedge suggesting the relative amount of food to be eaten from each group.

- The orange, green, and red wedges—representing grains, vegetables, and fruits respectively—are the largest.
- The blue wedge is also relatively large; this represents milk and other calcium-rich foods, which the guidelines caution should be limited to low-fat or fat-free.
- The purple wedge is somewhat smaller than the blue wedge and represents beans and meats.
- The yellow wedge is the smallest and it represents oils.

To help patients plan a balanced diet, the medical assistant will need to know how much of a food equals a serving. For example, one serving of fruit equals one medium apple or orange, $\frac{1}{2}$ cup canned fruit, or $\frac{3}{4}$ cup (6 ounces) of fruit juice.

The food guide pyramid is a general guideline, and lists ranges of serving amounts. It does not provide exact information about what to eat. Nutritional needs vary from person to person, depending on age, gender, and activity level.

Some patients may have special dietary preferences or choices. For example, vegetarians do not eat meat, poultry, and fish. In order to provide vegetarians with guidelines for healthful eating, the American Dietetic Association has developed a food guide pyramid specifically for these individuals.

Special Diets

Nutritional needs vary for people in different stages of life depending on their health status.

Pregnancy

During the second and third trimesters of pregnancy, calorie needs are increased. Pregnant teenagers and underweight women may require even more of an increase. Extra calories should be nutrient-dense foods with an emphasis on increasing levels of nutrients needed for fetal development and growth.

The medical assistant should advise pregnant women to limit processed foods, because nutrients are less available in those foods than in whole foods. Problems associated with pregnancy can include nausea and constipation. The pregnant woman can lessen nausea by eating small, frequent meals; eating dry toast or crackers; and avoiding foods with strong odors.

Children

From infancy through adolescence, children's nutritional needs change. The medical assistant must have an understanding of a child's nutritional status in relation to overall nutritional health in the developing child. A child's nutritional needs can be summarized in three basic phases: infancy, age two to 12, and adolescence.

Infancy to age two: This age group is further broken down into three age groups.

- From birth to age six months, an infant should be fed breast milk or formula exclusively. Studies have shown that introducing solid foods before six months leads to an increased risk of food allergies.
- From age six months to one year, breast milk or formula should still make up most of an infant's diet. However, at six months, the parent or caregiver can begin introducing solid foods, such as cereals, vegetables, and fruit.
- By age one, the child can transition from breast milk or formula to whole milk and eat an expanded diet that includes whole wheat crackers, cheese, applesauce, bananas, scrambled or hard boiled eggs, vegetables, fruits, and meats.

Ages two to twelve: Starting at age two, the child's diet should include a variety of dairy products, meats, beans, vegetables, fruits, bread, pasta, and cereals. As the child ages and tastes vary, the diet can grow to include more seasonings and varied flavors. Portion sizes will increase as the child grows, requiring more calories.

Adolescence: Adolescents undergo periods of rapid growth, such as the onset of puberty, that require more energy. The appetite of teenagers varies, but their diet should always include healthy foods, not empty calories that offer limited nutritional value. The medical assistant can advise his or her young patients to drink milk to build strong bones and to avoid soda, which adds unnecessary sugar to the diet. The medical assistant can also advise adolescent female patients that additional iron in the diet is necessary to replace iron lost in menstrual blood; this additional dietary iron may help symptoms of fatigue during menses.

Older Adults

As a person ages, he or she may become less active. A decrease in activity slows metabolism and, thus, decreases the need for calories. If eating habits of early adulthood do not change, weight gain will ensue. A decrease in activity is commonly due to painful arthritis or other medical complications. The medical assistant should encourage patients to exercise within their ability in order to avoid weight gain and promote good health. Special nutritional concerns of the aging adult include:

- **Dentition**—Patients with ill-fitting dentures may have trouble chewing and swallowing. High-nutrition soft foods (such as yogurt or soft cheese) provide the needed calcium.
- **Income**—Patients on a fixed income are sometimes forced to reduce food expenditures. Because carbohydrates are inexpensive, these patients may not get the protein and fresh fruits and vegetables needed for good health. The medical assistant can investigate government assistance (such as food stamps) for patients in need.
- **Sense of taste**—As people age, their sense of taste decreases. Because the sweet taste is strongest for elderly patients, they may crave sweets. Thus the medical assistant should emphasize the

importance of controlling the amount of sweets in the diet.

■ **Digestive disorders**—Digestive enzymes and stomach acids decrease as a person ages. These changes may create symptoms of heartburn, gas, and acid reflux that can discourage eating. Treatment for digestive disorders will allow more balanced food choices.

Dietary Restrictions
Sodium-Restricted Diet

Patients with kidney disease, high blood pressure, edema, or cardiovascular disease may benefit from a sodium-restricted diet. Because many processed foods contain a lot of sodium, the diet consists of natural foods and no addition of table salt. Although there are low-sodium processed foods available, such as tomato sauces, soups, and pretzels, patients must read labels and understand the amount of sodium included in each serving of the food.

Patients must pay close attention to the salt content of any condiments they may use. High-sodium condiments include ketchup, pickles, mustard, mayonnaise, and salad dressing. Spices can be added to foods to enhance flavor as long as no sodium is added.

Weight-Loss Diets

Weight-loss diets are numerous and can vary in approach. Low-fat or low-carbohydrate diets can yield weight loss; however, patients may tolerate them differently.

A healthy weight-loss diet does not promise dramatic weight loss in a short period of time and must not compromise nutrient supply. Patients should focus on losing weight safely by focusing on balanced nutrition and exercise; this approach will more likely allow a patient to keep weight off in the future.

Lactose Sensitivity

Lactose, the sugar contained in human and animal milk, must be broken down in the body by the enzyme lactase to enable the body to digest dairy products. In people from some parts of the world, lactase is present in the body until age three or four, after which it all but disappears. As a result, after early childhood, many people have trouble digesting foods that contain lactose and eliminate these foods from their diets. People who are especially sensitive to dietary lactose are often referred to as being lactose intolerant.

Chemical preparations can help a person digest lactose. Those preparations may be added to certain foods, such as ice cream, for lactose-sensitive people. If people with a lactose sensitivity choose to avoid dairy products, they need to be sure to obtain protein and calcium from other sources.

Heart Disease

Coronary heart disease that is caused by atherosclerosis usually results from hyperlipidemia, or an excess of lipids in the bloodstream. Left untreated, this condition can lead to angina (chest pain), heart attack, or stroke.

Patients can significantly lower their risk by reducing their blood cholesterol levels and losing weight if they are overweight. Patients who have coronary heart disease usually must reduce their consumption of fats to a level that provides less than 30% of their total caloric intake. Saturated fats should provide less than 10% of caloric intake. Patients who have had a heart attack or are at increased risk for a heart attack are also encouraged to increase their consumption of soluble fiber.

The medical assistant should encourage patients to follow the nutritional regimen prescribed by the doctor. The medical assistant must not recommend other dietary changes. Instead, the medical assistant should educate patients about ways to reduce the amount of fat in their diets, such as by substituting skim milk for whole milk.

Soft Diets

Soft diets include foods that are easy to digest and are commonly prescribed for gastrointestinal problems to reduce strain on the GI tract. The diet consists of milk, yogurt, and soft cheese; cooked and pureed vegetables and fruits; pastas; and ground beef or chicken.

Diabetes

The physician will prescribe a diabetic diet to focus on frequent, small meals—a regimen that will decrease fluctuations in blood glucose levels. The diet also emphasizes foods with a lower glycemic index, meaning foods that take less time to raise blood glucose levels. Foods to avoid include candy, donuts, cakes, syrups, and alcohol.

Practice Questions

Infection Control

1. Which of the following situations causes incomplete sterilization in an autoclave?
   a. allowing air to enter the chamber
   b. keeping the temperature too high
   c. using distilled water in the reservoir
   d. venting after the pressure is equalized
   e. letting the sterilized packs cool on a cold surface

2. Which of the following bacteria is normally found in the intestinal tract, but can cause infection if it gains entry into the urinary tract?
   a. *Staphylococcus*
   b. *Chlamydia*
   c. *Giardia lamblia*
   d. *Escherichia coli*
   e. prions

3. Which of the following is the most common vehicle for spreading infectious agents in the medical office?
   a. air circulation ducts
   b. contaminated supplies
   c. hands of employees
   d. improper autoclaving
   e. soiled examination tables

4. Which of the following is an example of personal protective equipment?
   a. bandage
   b. gloves
   c. hand soap
   d. puncture-proof sharps container
   e. suture

5. When the medical assistant is using an autoclave, which of the following is the minimum temperature necessary to sterilize medical instruments?
   a. 48.9°C (120°F)
   b. 82.2°C (180°F)
   c. 107.2°C (225°F)
   d. 121.1°C (250°F)
   e. 137.7°C (280°F)

6. Which of the following is NOT a form of barrier protection?
   a. condoms
   b. face masks
   c. gloves
   d. gowns
   e. hand washing

7. An acute infection
   a. persists for a long period of time.
   b. is asymptomatic.
   c. has periods of relapse and remission.
   d. has a rapid onset of symptoms, but lasts a short time.
   e. is caused by the herpes simplex virus.

8. A nosocomial infection is
   a. acquired in a healthcare setting.
   b. often caused by lack of standard precautions at the facility.
   c. caused by not washing one's hands.
   d. caused by not disinfecting instruments.
   e. caused by not wearing gloves.

9. Medical asepsis means
   a. free from all microbiobial life.
   b. hand washing.
   c. sanitization.
   d. sterilization.
   e. both hand washing and sanitization.

10. To break the chain of infection, the medical assistant should teach patients
   a. to cover their mouths when coughing.
   b. that immunizations are not necessary anymore.
   c. to wash hands only when they are visibly soiled.
   d. that an infection cannot be spread by sneezing.
   e. that an infection cannot be spread by coughing.

Preparing and Maintaining the Treatment Area

1. The top of the crutch pad should be how many inches from the axillary (underarm) areas?
   a. one
   b. two
   c. three
   d. four
   e. five

2. Electrocardiograms are most commonly recorded at which of the following speeds?
   a. 15 millimeters per second
   b. 25 millimeters per second
   c. 35 millimeters per second
   d. 60 millimeters per second
   e. 80 millimeters per second

3. Spirometry tests the function of which of the following organ systems?
   a. cardiovascular
   b. integumentary
   c. musculoskeletal
   d. neurologic
   e. respiratory

4. Which of the following instruments is used by the physician to determine the presence or absence of bowel sounds?
   a. audiometer
   b. colposcope
   c. dosimeter
   d. onychograph
   e. stethoscope

5. When measuring blood pressure, the medical assistant should place the stethoscope over which artery?
   a. apical
   b. brachial
   c. carotid
   d. pedal
   e. radial

6. The best method for delivering deep heat to tissues is to use
   a. a paraffin bath.
   b. a heat lamp.
   c. a whirlpool.
   d. TENS.
   e. an ultrasound.

Patient Preparation and Assisting the Physician

1. What instrument is used to measure blood pressure?
   a. audiometer
   b. pulse oximeter
   c. sphygmomanometer
   d. spirometer
   e. ophthalmoscope

2. A patient's use of tobacco and alcohol should be recorded in which of the following parts of his or her medical record?
   a. family history
   b. history of present illness
   c. past medical history
   d. review of systems
   e. social history

3. In a patient's medical record, which of the following complaints is subjective?
   a. abdominal distention
   b. high blood pressure
   c. irregular heart rate
   d. nausea
   e. swollen ankles

4. In healthy adults, which of the following is the normal range for rates of respiration per minute?
   a. 6 to 9
   b. 10 to 11
   c. 12 to 20
   d. 22 to 28
   e. 30 to 32

5. Assessing range of motion is part of which type of exam?
   a. auscultation
   b. mensuration
   c. percussion
   d. manipulation
   e. palpation

6. When measuring blood pressure, the medical assistant should place the stethoscope over which artery?
   a. radial
   b. brachial
   c. carotid
   d. apical
   e. femoral

7. The common pulse pressure points are
   a. abdominal, aorta, popliteal, and iliac.
   b. carotid, axillary, and hypogastric.
   c. apical (apex), brachial, and radial.
   d. anterior tibialis, sciatic, and brachial.
   e. brachial, pedal, and apex.

8. Which of the following positions is most appropriate for a patient with severe hypotension?
   a. knee-chest
   b. lithotomy
   c. Trendelenburg
   d. semi-Fowler
   e. dorsal recumbent

Collecting and Processing Specimens and Laboratory Testing

1. When obtaining a capillary blood sample by finger puncture, a medical assistant should NOT perform which of the following steps?
   a. Cleanse the puncture site with 70% alcohol.
   b. Massage the finger to promote circulation to the tip.
   c. Squeeze the puncture site with alcohol wipe.
   d. Wipe away the first drop of blood with sterile gauze.
   e. Position the device to cut perpendicular to the lines of the fingerprints.

2. A urine sample that cannot be processed immediately should be placed in which of the following?
   a. centrifuge
   b. freezer
   c. incubator
   d. refrigerator
   e. 24-hour collection container

3. When determining an erythrocyte sedimentation rate (ESR), the tubes must stand in a sedimentation rack for exactly how many minutes?
   a. 60
   b. 75
   c. 90
   d. 105
   e. 120

4. Which of the following steps is most likely to reduce bruising after venipuncture?
   a. applying pressure to the puncture site
   b. applying heat to the puncture site
   c. leaving the tourniquet in place for 30 seconds after the venipuncture
   d. placing a bandage over the puncture site
   e. wiping the puncture site with alcohol

5. Heterophile antibodies are
   a. produced by persons who have rubella.
   b. produced in response to an infection with Epstein-Barr virus.
   c. used in a pregnancy test kit to detect pregnancy.
   d. the antibodies produced in the response to syphilis.
   e. the antibodies produced in the response to HIV.

6. Which of the following evacuated tubes is routinely used for hematology testing?
   a. lavender-topped
   b. red-topped
   c. green-topped
   d. light blue-topped
   e. gray-topped

7. In performance of a microhematocrit, which of the following is true?
   a. Clotted blood must be used.
   b. The capillary tube must be completely filled and sealed on both ends.
   c. The open end of the capillary tube should be placed against the rubber gasket of the centrifuge.
   d. The capillary tube should be centrifuged in a labeled, sealed evacuated tube.
   e. The serum blood is placed in the capillary tube for testing.

8. WBCs include all of the following EXCEPT
   a. neutrophils.
   b. monocytes.
   c. basophils.
   d. platelets.
   e. lymphocytes.

Preparing and Administrating Medications

1. Calculate the following dosage:
   The physician orders 250 mg of ceftriaxone. The vial on hand contains ceftriaxone at a concentration of 500 mg/mL. How much medication will be administered?
   a. 0.2 mL
   b. 0.3 mL
   c. 0.4 mL
   d. 0.5 mL
   e. 0.6 mL

2. Calculate the following dosage:
   The physician orders promethazine 12.5 mg by mouth. The medical assistant has on hand promethazine syrup that has a concentration of 25 mg/5 mL. How many milliliters should the medical assistant give the patient?
   a. 0.5 mL
   b. 1.0 mL
   c. 1.5 mL
   d. 2.0 mL
   e. 2.5 mL

3. Calculate the following dosage:
   The physician has ordered 500 units of vitamin B12. The medical assistant has on hand vitamin B12 at a concentration unit of 1,000 units/mL. How many units should the medical assistant give the patient?
   a. 0.1 mL
   b. 1.5 mL
   c. 0.2 mL
   d. 0.5 mL
   e. 1.5 mL

4. Calculate the following dosage:
   The physician orders erythromycin q6h for an infant weighing 12 lbs. 6 oz. The label states that there are 200 mg of the drug in 5 cc of suspension. The recommended medication for infants is 30 mg/kg/day. How much medication should the infant receive?
   a. 0.1 cc
   b. 1.1 cc
   c. 1.2 cc
   d. 2.0 cc
   e. 2.1 cc

5. Essential medication guidelines include all of the following EXCEPT
   a. following the "seven rights."
   b. asking the patient if he or she is allergic to any medication.
   c. storing medication at the appropriate temperature.
   d. preparing the medication in front of the patient.
   e. checking the medication label three times.

6. Which of the following steps is appropriate for inventory control of a controlled substance in a physician's office?
   a. Count the supply twice a day.
   b. Place the supply order on duplicate order forms.
   c. Maintain inventory records for three years.
   d. Report theft or loss to the regional health department.
   e. Store all controlled substances in a locked cabinet.

7. Which of the following is the process through which the body inactivates a drug after the drug has been used in order to eliminate the drug from the body?
   a. bioavailablilty
   b. potentiation
   c. metabolism
   d. anatagonism
   e. synergism

8. All of the following statements about immunization are true EXCEPT
   a. immunization provides immunity with active and passive vaccines.
   b. immunization protects individuals against specific infectious diseases.
   c. all immunization is given by injection.
   d. immunization is state mandated for children.
   e. adults should have a tetanus booster every 10 years.

9. Which of the following statements accurately describes an epinephrine autoinjector?
   a. It counteracts the effects of a severe allergic reaction.
   b. It counteracts the effects of a heart attack.
   c. It protects against infection.
   d. It is administered to patients in insulin shock.
   e. It is administered to patients who are having a CVA.

10. Insulin injection sites must be rotated
    a. because the dermis will atrophy.
    b. to avoid an adverse reaction to the insulin.
    c. because the muscle tissue will atrophy.
    d. to avoid lipodystrophy.
    e. to avoid staining of the medication.

Emergencies and First Aid

1. Triage means
   a. using proper body mechanics.
   b. the process of screening patients based on medical condition.
   c. expected behavior during a situation.
   d. an emergency situation.
   e. consent to perform CPR.

2. The Good Samaritan law means that the medical assistant is protected from liability in all of the following situations EXCEPT
   a. when helping a stranger.
   b. when the medical assistant sustains a physical injury.
   c. when the medical assistant is reasonably careful.
   d. when the medical assistant acts in good faith.
   e. when the medical assistant does not provide care beyond his or her skill level.

3. A crash cart contains all of the following EXCEPT
   a. first aid supplies.
   b. AED.
   c. epinephrine autoinjectors.
   d. immunizations.
   e. emergency medication.

4. Expressed consent means
   a. that permission to treat the patient is assumed.
   b. consent to release medical information.
   c. that consent has been given by the patient.
   d. that consent has been given in an emergency situation.
   e. that consent has been denied.

5. Minor office emergencies include the following EXCEPT
   a. nosebleed.
   b. syncope.
   c. asthma.
   d. vomiting.
   e. hematemesis.

6. A first degree burn can cause all of the following symptoms EXCEPT
   a. redness.
   b. swelling.
   c. pain.
   d. broken skin.
   e. peeling of the skin.

7. A person with a severe airway blockage will show which of the following signs and symptoms?
   a. blue lips, nails, and skin
   b. strong coughing
   c. high-pitched squeaking noise
   d. wheezing
   e. can breathe in and out but cannot speak

8. Syncope is
   a. septic shock.
   b. a shock caused by an allergic reaction.
   c. insulin shock.
   d. a stroke.
   e. fainting.

9. The assessment and treatment of an unconscious person includes the ABC. What does ABC stand for?
   a. assessment, basic first aid, and care
   b. airway, breathing, and circulation
   c. airway, basic first aid, and circulation
   d. assessment, basic life support, and care
   e. assessment, basic life support, and CPR

10. Seizures can be caused by all of the following EXCEPT
   a. head injury.
   b. drug or alcohol use.
   c. very high fever.
   d. very high blood pressure.
   e. very low blood sugar.

Nutrition

1. Which mineral is part of the hemoglobin protein that carries oxygen to tissues?
   a. potassium
   b. iron
   c. phosphorus
   d. selenium
   e. calcium

2. Metabolism means
   a. unit of energy that produces heat.
   b. taking in of nutrients; eating and drinking.
   c. the set of physical and chemical processes that maintain life in an organism.
   d. transfer of digested nutrients from the gastrointestinal system to the blood circulation.
   e. digestion.

3. A lack of which mineral will cause weakness and bone pain or loss?
   a. niacin
   b. vitamin K
   c. phosphorus
   d. vitamin E
   e. zinc

4. Which of the following is an example of saturated fat?
   a. butter
   b. egg whites
   c. nuts
   d. tuna
   e. bread

5. Which of the following is not a water-soluble vitamin?
   a. riboflavin
   b. vitamin B6
   c. thiamin
   d. vitamin D
   e. vitamin C

6. All of the following are minerals EXCEPT
   a. iron.
   b. zinc.
   c. niacin.
   d. chromium.
   e. phosphorus.

7. All of the following minerals have Dietary Reference Intakes (DRIs) EXCEPT
   a. calcium.
   b. zinc.
   c. iodine.
   d. magnesium.
   e. thiamine.

8. The American Cancer Society recommends a high-fiber diet to prevent cancer. A high fiber diet would include all of the following EXCEPT
   a. fish.
   b. oranges.
   c. broccoli.
   d. peas.
   e. whole-grain cereals.

9. A patient who is diagnosed with hypertension will usually benefit from a diet low in which of the following?
   a. protein
   b. sugar
   c. iron
   d. sodium
   e. calcium

10. A patient who is sensitive to lactose needs to
   a. avoid salt.
   b. avoid high fat foods.
   c. eat only soft foods.
   d. avoid foods that contain sugar.
   e. avoid dairy products.

Answers and Explanations

Infection Control

1. a. Allowing air to enter the chamber causes incomplete sterilization in an autoclave. The air in the chamber will prevent the autoclave from reaching the pressure it needs in order to sterilize.

2. d. *Escherichia coli* is the bacteria found in the intestinal tract that can cause urinary tract infection. *Staphylococcus* is sphere-shaped bacteria that live on the skin and mucous membranes. *Chlamydia* is a genus of bacteria known as a parasite, which are organisms that must live inside another living organism in order to survive. *Giardia lamblia* is a single-celled parasite called a protozoa. Prions are infectious protein particles that destroy brain tissue and cause fatal conditions, such as Creutzfeld-Jakob disease.

3. c. The hands of employees are the most common vehicle for spreading infectious agents in the medical office. Medical employees are in direct contact with pathogenic organisms, and in order to break the chain of infection and protect everyone, the employee must wash his or her hands frequently. The medical employee's hands have more direct contact with pathogens and with patients than an air circulation duct would. Because not everyone in the medical office needs supplies, even if the supplies were contaminated, they would pose less of a risk to patients than medical employees' hands do. Also, because not all patients or medical office employees are in direct contact with autoclave supplies or with soiled examination tables, improper autoclaving and soiled examination tables pose less of a risk to patients than medical employees' hands do.

4. b. Gloves are an example of personal protective equipment. Gloves are used to prevent the risk of contact with blood or body fluids. A bandage holds a dressing in place and helps maintain pressure on a wound. A suture is a surgical stitch used to close a wound. The other choices, hand soap and sharps containers, while important in implementing standard precautions to reduce the transmission of infectious diseases, are not items that an individual wears on his or her person.

5. d. When the medical assistant uses an autoclave, the minimum temperature necessary to sterilize medical instruments is 121.1°C (250°F). In order to ensure sterilization, the items must be exposed to steam pressure of 121.1°C (250°F) with 15 pounds of pressure for a specific amount of time.

6. e. While an important standard precaution, hand washing is not a form of barrier protection. Hand washing is a way to sanitize one's hands. It does not prevent exposure of the skin to a pathogen. Condoms, face masks, gloves, and gowns are all forms of barrier protection since they prevent the exposure of the skin to pathogens.

7. d. An acute infection is characterized by rapid onset and lasts for only a short period of time. "Asymptomatic" indicates that a condition does not manifest symptoms, and an acute infection does manifest symptoms, even though they are generally nonspecific. An acute infection does not have periods of relapse and remission, whereas a latent infection does. Herpes simplex virus is a latent infection because it has periods of relapse and remission.

8. a. A nosocomial infection is acquired in a healthcare setting and is often caused by a lack of standard precautions within the facility. It can be caused by not washing one's hands or by not disinfecting instruments.

9. e. Medical asepsis means both hand washing and sanitization. Sanitization of an object is the removal of microorganisms. The single most effective standard precaution is proper hand hygiene and sanitization.

10. a. To break the chain of infection, the medical assistant should teach patients to cover their mouths when coughing, to exercise daily and stay up-to-date on their immunizations, to cover their wounds, to wash their hands, and to use a tissue when they sneeze. Maintaining these healthy habits prevents the means of exit and mode of transmission in the chain of infection.

Preparing and Maintaining the Treatment Area

1. b. The top of the crutch pad should be two inches away from the axillary (underarm) areas to prevent the patient from developing back pain, nerve damage, and injuries to the axillae (underarms) and to the palms of the hands. If the distance between the crutch pad and the axillary areas is too short, the patient will need to bend over to use the crutches, which would be uncomfortable and awkward. If the distance between the crutch pad and the axillary areas is too long, the patient may injure the radial nerve in the brachial plexus, which can lead to muscular weakness in the forearm, wrist, and hand.

2. b. Electrocardiograms are most commonly recorded at 25 millimeters per second. Each small square measures 1 millimeter on each side of the ECG graph paper. Every fifth line, both vertically and horizontally, is darker than the other lines and creates a larger square measuring 5 millimeters on each side. When the ECG runs at normal speed, one small 1 millimeter square passes the stylus every 0.04 seconds, which means that one large 5 millimeter square passes the stylus every 0.2 seconds. In one second, five large squares pass the stylus, which equals to 25 millimeters per second.

3. e. Spirometry, used to test the function of the respiratory system, measures air taken into and expelled from the lungs.

4. e. The stethoscope, an instrument used to amplify and hear sounds produced by the body, is used by the physician to determine the presence or absence of bowel sounds. An audiometer is a machine used to evaluate hearing loss. A colonoscope is an instrument used in a colonoscopy (an examination of the colon). A dosimeter measures exposure to ionizing radiation noise or other environmental factor. An onychograph is an instrument for recording the capillary blood pressure.

5. b. When measuring blood pressure, the medical assistant should place the stethoscope over the brachial artery. The brachial pulse is felt at the antecubital space (inner forearm) in both arms. The apical pulse, or heartbeat at the apex of the heart, can be heard with the stethoscope. The carotid pulse is the pulse located between the larynx and the sternocleidomastoid muscle in the front and to the side of the neck. The pedal pulse is in the foot. The radial pulse is the most frequently used site for counting the pulse rate; it is found on the thumb side of the wrist.

6. e. The most effective way for delivering deep heat to tissues is to perform an ultrasound. An ultrasound is a treatment modality that uses high- or low-frequency sound waves transmitted to surrounding tissue. The sound waves penetrate the muscles, causing deep tissue or muscle warming. Therefore, ultrasounds are often used to treat muscle tightness and muscle spasms. A paraffin bath is useful in treating chronic joint inflammation. A heat lamp is used to relieve muscle pain. A whirlpool is used to improve circulation and to perform range of movement exercises. Transcutaneous electrical nerve stimulation (TENS) is a machine that uses electricity, with electrodes applied to the affected area. The electrical signal disrupts the pain signal being sent from the affected area so that the patient experiences less pain.

Patient Preparation and Assisting the Physician

1. c. A sphygmomanometer is an instrument for measuring arterial blood pressure. An audiometer is an instrument for testing hearing. A pulse oximeter is an instrument used for measuring the oxygen saturation of arterial blood. A spirometer is an instrument for measuring air taken into and expelled from the lungs. An ophthalmoscope is an instrument for examining the interior components of the eye.

2. e. The social history section of the health history includes information on the patient's lifestyle, such as health habits and living environment. Family history is the review of the health status of the patient's blood relatives. History of present illness is a full description of the patient's current illness from time of onset. Past medical history is a review of the patient's past medical status. Review of systems is a systemic examination of each body system.

3. d. Nausea is a subjective symptom, which means it is felt by the patient, but is not observable by an examiner. Abdominal distention, high blood pressure, irregular heart rate, and swollen ankles are all objective symptoms because the can be observed by the examinser.

4. c. Respirations rates will vary with age, but the average adult respiration rate is 12 to 20 respirations per minute.

5. d. Range of motion refers to the extent to which a joint has mobility, measured in terms of the distance and direction a joint can move. The physician will manipulate a joint to see the distance and direction the joint can move. Auscultation is the process of listening to the sounds produced within the body to detect signs of disease. Mensuration refers to the measuring of a body part. Percussion involves tapping the patient with fingers and listening to the sounds produced to determine the size, density, and location of an organ. Palpation is the process of feeling with the hands to detect signs of disease.

6. b. The brachial pulse is taken at the inside of the elbow (a location called the antecubital space). The radial artery is on the inside of the wrist, on the thumb side, about one inch from the thumb's base. The carotid artery is at the throat, in the groove between the larynx (Adam's apple) and the long muscle on the front side of the neck (called the sternocleidomastoid muscle). The apical artery is at the apex of the heart. The femoral pulse is in the middle of the groin.

7. c. The apical, brachial, and radial pulse sites are the most commonly used sites: the apical on infants, the brachial for blood pressures, and the radial for pulse assessment. The other choices include one or more terms that do not relate to pulse sites.

8. c. For this position, the patient lies with his or her head approximately 30 degrees lower than the outstretched legs and feet. In the knee-chest position, the patient sits on his or her knees with the chest and face resting forward on a pillow. Lithotomy requires the patient to lie on his or her back with the feet in stirrups. The semi-Fowler position is used to examine the upper body of patients with cardiovascular and respiratory problems. The dorsal recumbent position requires the patient to lie on his or her back and bend the knees.

Collecting and Processing Specimens and Laboratory Testing

1. b. When obtaining a capillary blood sample by finger puncture, a medical assistant should not massage the finger to promote circulation to the tip. Massaging the finger would cause tissue fluid to get into the sample, thereby altering the test results.

2. d. A urine sample that cannot be processed immediately should be placed in the refrigerator. Refrigerating the specimen will slow down the multiplication of bacteria in the urine sample. Centrifuging the specimen is spinning the specimen down; this will not slow the multiplication of bacteria. Freezing the specimen would make the test invalid for a urinalysis. Placing the sample in an incubator, an apparatus that controls temperature and humidity, will not slow the multiplication of bacteria. Placing the sample in a 24-hour urine collection would make the sample too diluted for testing.

3. a. When determining an erythrocyte sedimentation rate, the tubes must stand in a sedimentation rack for 60 minutes.

4. a. Applying pressure to the puncture site is most likely to reduce bruising after venipuncture. Applying direct pressure to the site is the best method for stopping the bleeding and to avoid bruising. Applying heat to the site will increase circulation, causing more bleeding. Leaving the tourniquet in place for 30 seconds after the venipuncture will not prevent bruising. Placing a bandage over the puncture site will not prevent bruising. Wiping the puncture site with alcohol will cause a burning sensation and will not prevent bruising.

5. b. Heterophile antibodies are antibodies produced in response to an infection of mononucleosis, which is caused by the Epstein-Barr virus. Antibodies produced by a person who has rubella are rubella antibodies. Human chorionic gonadotropin (HCG) is the hormone used in pregnancy test kits to detect pregnancy. The antibodies produced in the response to syphilis are called anti-deoxyriboneucleoprotein antibodies. The antibodies produced in the response to the HIV virus are enzyme-linked anti-human gamma globulin antibodies.

6. a. Lavender-topped evacuated tubes are routinely used for hematology testing. A lavender topped tube contains EDTA, which removes calcium to prevent blood from clotting and is used for hematology testing. A red-topped tube contains no preservative and is used for chemistry and serology testing. A green-topped tube contains heparin and is used for chemistry testing. A light blue-topped tube contains sodium citrate and is used for coagulation testing. A gray-topped tube contains potassium oxalate and sodium fluoride and is used for chemistry and alcohol testing.

7. c. In performance of a microhematocrit, the sealed end is placed in the centrifuge against the gasket. If the sealed end were not placed in the centrifuge first, the blood would spin out of the capillary tubes. Clotted blood should not be used since whole blood is required for the microhematocrit. Only one end of the capillary tube needs to be sealed for the microhematocrit. The microhematocrit requires a capillary tube; a labeled, sealed evacuated tube is not required. Serum does not contain the RBCs that are needed for the hematocrit testing.

8. d. White blood cells do not contain platelets. Platelets are cell fragments that circulate in the blood and assist in clot formation. White blood cells contain neutrophils, monocytes, basophils, and lymphocytes.

Preparing and Administrating Medications

1. d. The dosage will be 0.5 mL.
$$\frac{250 \text{ mg}}{500 \text{ mg}} \times 1 \text{ mL} = 0.5 \text{ mL}$$

2. e. The medical assistant should give the patient 2.5 ml of promethazine syrup.
$$\frac{12.5 \text{ mg}}{25 \text{ mg}} \times 5 \text{ mL} = 2.5 \text{ mL}$$

3. d. The medical assistant should give the patient 0.5 mL of vitamin B12.
$$\frac{500 \text{ units}}{1,000 \text{ units}} \times 1 \text{ mL} = 0.5 \text{ ml}$$

4. b. The infant should receive 1.1 cc of medication. First calculate the infant's weight in kilograms (kg):
$$\frac{6 \text{ oz.}}{16 \text{ oz.}} = 0.375 \text{ converted to } 0.4 \text{ lbs} + 12$$
$$= 12.4 \text{ lbs.}$$
$$\frac{12.4 \text{ lbs.}}{2.2 \text{ lbs.}} = 5.6 \text{ kg}$$
The total daily dose of the medication = 30 mg times the weight in kilograms.
$$30 \times 5.6 = 168 \text{ mg/day}$$
A single dose of the drug is the total daily dose divided by 4, since there are four 6-hour time periods in a 24 hour day, and the request was q6h, every 6 hours.
$$\frac{168 \text{ mg}}{4} = 42 \text{ mg/dose}$$
The amount of medication that should be administered in a single dose is determined by the drug label, which states that there are 200 mg in every 5 cc of the suspension.
$$\frac{42 \text{ mg}}{200 \text{ mg}} \times 5 \text{cc} = 1.05, \text{ rounded up to } 1.1 \text{ cc}$$

5. d. It is not necessary to prepare the medication in front of the patient. Following the "seven rights" is necessary since these are essential medication guidelines. Asking the patient if he or she has any allergies to medication will prevent adverse reactions. Storing medication at the appropriate temperature will ensure the medication is viable when it is needed. Checking the medication label three times will verify that it is the correct medication.

6. e. Storing all controlled substances in a locked cabinet is appropriate for inventory control of a controlled substance in a physician's office. Counting the supply twice a day will not help the inventory control. Placing the supply order on a duplicate order form will verify what was ordered, but it will not help maintain the inventory control. It is required by the DEA that the medical office maintain inventory records of controlled substances for two years. It is not appropriate to report theft or loss of a controlled substance to the regional health department; theft or loss of a controlled substance must be reported to the DEA.

7. c. Metabolism is the process through which the body inactivates a drug after the drug has been used in order to eliminate the drug from the body. Metabolism is a chemical reaction that breaks down the drug into different substances that the body can easily use and excrete. Bioavailability is the percentage that expresses the amount of the drug that reaches the bloodstream and the length of time needed for the drug to reach the bloodstream. Potentiation is an interaction between two drugs that enhances the effect of either drug. Antagonism is a drug effect that occurs when drugs work in opposition to one another. Synergism is a drug effect that occurs when two drugs taken together have a greater therapeutic effect together than the expected effects of each drug used alone.

8. c. It is not true that all immunization is given by injection. Some immunizations are oral or nasal. Immunization is indeed state mandated for children, and adults should have a tetanus booster every ten years.

9. a. An epinephrine autoinjector is a small device that holds epinephrine, a medicine that counteracts the effects of a severe allergic reaction by relaxing the smooth muscles (bronchodilation).

10. d. Insulin injection sites must be rotated to avoid lipodystrophy, which is atrophy or hypertrophy of the fat tissue. Insulin injections are given subcutaneously and not intradermally. Rotation of the injection sites will not prevent a reaction to the drug. Insulin injections are given subcutaneously, not in the muscle. Insulin does not stain the skin.

Emergencies and First Aid

1. b. Triage is a process of screening patients to determine which need immediate medical treatment and in what order each patient must be seen, and which patients must go to the emergency room or if they can be worked into the schedule.

2. b. The Good Samaritan law does not address the medical assistant's physical injury. The Good Samaritan law protects the medical assistant from being sued when he or she helps a stranger as long as he or she is reasonably careful, acts in good faith, and does not provide care beyond his or her skill level.

3. d. A crash cart does not contain immunizations. Immunizations are given to protect an individual from disease.

4. c. Expressed consent means that the patient has given consent.

5. e. Hematemesis is vomiting blood. It is not considered minor. The patient may go into shock and an IV may need to be started to replace lost fluids. Minor office emergencies include nosebleed, syncope, asthma, and vomiting.

6. d. A first-degree burn does not cause broken skin. Broken skin can be found with third-degree burns. Redness, swelling, pain, and peeling of skin can all be caused by first-degree burns.

7. a. Blue lips, nails, and skin are signs and symptoms of a severe airway blockage.

8. e. Syncope is fainting. Septic shock is caused by an overwhelming infection affecting major body systems. Anaphylactic shock is caused by a severe allergic reaction that results in respiratory distress. Insulin shock is caused by severe hypoglycemia in diabetics. A stroke is caused a cerebrovascular accident in which there is occlusion, or blocking, of a blood vessel in the brain.

9. b. ABC stands for airway, breathing, and circulation. The airway is checked to see if it is clear, then breathing is checked (if the patient is not breathing, the medical assistant should administer two "rescue" breaths), and then circulation is checked by taking the patient's pulse.

10. d. A seizure cannot be caused by very high blood pressure. Very high blood pressure can lead to a stroke. A seizure can be caused by head injury, drug or alcohol use, very high fever, or very low blood sugar.

Nutrition

1. b. Iron is the part of the hemoglobin protein that carries oxygen to tissues. Potassium supports nerve and muscle function and is important to electrolyte balance. Phosphorus helps the support the development of bones and teeth and is important in energy metabolism. Selenium is an antioxidant and regulates thyroid hormones. Calcium supports bone and teeth structure and is necessary for the functioning of muscles and blood vessels.

2. c. Metabolism means the set of physical and chemical processes that maintain life in an organism. A calorie is the unit of energy that produces heat. Ingestion is taking in of nutrients. Absorption is the transfer of digested nutrients from the gastrointestinal system to the blood circulation. Digestion is the breaking down of food (both physically and chemically) into smaller particles that the body can absorb.

3. c. A lack of phosphorus will cause weakness and bone pain or loss. Niacin is a B vitamin that is important in energy metabolism. Vitamin K is a vitamin that aids blood clotting. Vitamin E is an antioxidant that protects cellular structure. Zinc is a mineral important for a several functions, including supporting protein and DNA development.

4. a. Butter is an example of a saturated fat; saturated fats are solid at room temperature.

5. d. Vitamin D is a fat-soluble vitamin, not a water-soluble vitamin. The other choices are all vitamins that are all water-soluble. Riboflavin and thiamin are different names for two of the B vitamins, all of which are water-soluble, as is vitamin C.

6. c. Niacin is vitamin B3. Iron, zinc, chromium, and phosphorus are minerals.

7. e. Thiamine is vitamin B1. Calcium, zinc, iodine, and magnesium are minerals that have a DRI.

8. a. A high-fiber diet would include oranges, broccoli, peas, and whole grain cereals. Fish is not high in fiber as fruits and vegetables are, so it would not be included in a high-fiber diet.

9. d. A patient who is diagnosed with hypertension (high blood pressure) will usually benefit from a diet low in sodium. Sodium is responsible for maintaining fluid balance, so a diet low in sodium may help lower blood pressure by decreasing fluid retention.

10. e. A patient who is sensitive to lactose needs to avoid dairy products. Lactose is the sugar contained in human and animal milk. Those who are lactose intolerant have a problem digesting foods that contain lactose.

6 ▶ CMA PRACTICE EXAM

This practice exam is designed to help you practice for the Certified Medical Assistant exam by including questions not only in academic and clinical areas in which you have command of important information, but also in areas in which you need more review. Because the format mimics that of the CMA exam, it will also help you familiarize yourself with the format of the actual exam.

One of the main reasons for taking this practice exam, in addition to getting more practice in answering the kinds of questions on the CMA exam, is to identify your strengths and weaknesses. Make a note of the types of questions you missed and the topics on which you need to concentrate your study time further. Do not neglect any subject area unless you have an almost-perfect score in that area. Remember to refer back to Chapter 2 to design a study plan that fits in with your schedule and lifestyle. Good luck!

CMA Practice Exam

1. (a) (b) (c) (d) (e)
2. (a) (b) (c) (d) (e)
3. (a) (b) (c) (d) (e)
4. (a) (b) (c) (d) (e)
5. (a) (b) (c) (d) (e)
6. (a) (b) (c) (d) (e)
7. (a) (b) (c) (d) (e)
8. (a) (b) (c) (d) (e)
9. (a) (b) (c) (d) (e)
10. (a) (b) (c) (d) (e)
11. (a) (b) (c) (d) (e)
12. (a) (b) (c) (d) (e)
13. (a) (b) (c) (d) (e)
14. (a) (b) (c) (d) (e)
15. (a) (b) (c) (d) (e)
16. (a) (b) (c) (d) (e)
17. (a) (b) (c) (d) (e)
18. (a) (b) (c) (d) (e)
19. (a) (b) (c) (d) (e)
20. (a) (b) (c) (d) (e)
21. (a) (b) (c) (d) (e)
22. (a) (b) (c) (d) (e)
23. (a) (b) (c) (d) (e)
24. (a) (b) (c) (d) (e)
25. (a) (b) (c) (d) (e)
26. (a) (b) (c) (d) (e)
27. (a) (b) (c) (d) (e)
28. (a) (b) (c) (d) (e)
29. (a) (b) (c) (d) (e)
30. (a) (b) (c) (d) (e)
31. (a) (b) (c) (d) (e)
32. (a) (b) (c) (d) (e)
33. (a) (b) (c) (d) (e)
34. (a) (b) (c) (d) (e)
35. (a) (b) (c) (d) (e)

36. (a) (b) (c) (d) (e)
37. (a) (b) (c) (d) (e)
38. (a) (b) (c) (d) (e)
39. (a) (b) (c) (d) (e)
40. (a) (b) (c) (d) (e)
41. (a) (b) (c) (d) (e)
42. (a) (b) (c) (d) (e)
43. (a) (b) (c) (d) (e)
44. (a) (b) (c) (d) (e)
45. (a) (b) (c) (d) (e)
46. (a) (b) (c) (d) (e)
47. (a) (b) (c) (d) (e)
48. (a) (b) (c) (d) (e)
49. (a) (b) (c) (d) (e)
50. (a) (b) (c) (d) (e)
51. (a) (b) (c) (d) (e)
52. (a) (b) (c) (d) (e)
53. (a) (b) (c) (d) (e)
54. (a) (b) (c) (d) (e)
55. (a) (b) (c) (d) (e)
56. (a) (b) (c) (d) (e)
57. (a) (b) (c) (d) (e)
58. (a) (b) (c) (d) (e)
59. (a) (b) (c) (d) (e)
60. (a) (b) (c) (d) (e)
61. (a) (b) (c) (d) (e)
62. (a) (b) (c) (d) (e)
63. (a) (b) (c) (d) (e)
64. (a) (b) (c) (d) (e)
65. (a) (b) (c) (d) (e)
66. (a) (b) (c) (d) (e)
67. (a) (b) (c) (d) (e)
68. (a) (b) (c) (d) (e)
69. (a) (b) (c) (d) (e)
70. (a) (b) (c) (d) (e)

71. (a) (b) (c) (d) (e)
72. (a) (b) (c) (d) (e)
73. (a) (b) (c) (d) (e)
74. (a) (b) (c) (d) (e)
75. (a) (b) (c) (d) (e)
76. (a) (b) (c) (d) (e)
77. (a) (b) (c) (d) (e)
78. (a) (b) (c) (d) (e)
79. (a) (b) (c) (d) (e)
80. (a) (b) (c) (d) (e)
81. (a) (b) (c) (d) (e)
82. (a) (b) (c) (d) (e)
83. (a) (b) (c) (d) (e)
84. (a) (b) (c) (d) (e)
85. (a) (b) (c) (d) (e)
86. (a) (b) (c) (d) (e)
87. (a) (b) (c) (d) (e)
88. (a) (b) (c) (d) (e)
89. (a) (b) (c) (d) (e)
90. (a) (b) (c) (d) (e)
91. (a) (b) (c) (d) (e)
92. (a) (b) (c) (d) (e)
93. (a) (b) (c) (d) (e)
94. (a) (b) (c) (d) (e)
95. (a) (b) (c) (d) (e)
96. (a) (b) (c) (d) (e)
97. (a) (b) (c) (d) (e)
98. (a) (b) (c) (d) (e)
99. (a) (b) (c) (d) (e)
100. (a) (b) (c) (d) (e)

CMA Practice Exam

101.	ⓐ	ⓑ	ⓒ	ⓓ	ⓔ	136.	ⓐ	ⓑ	ⓒ	ⓓ	ⓔ	171.	ⓐ	ⓑ	ⓒ	ⓓ	ⓔ
102.	ⓐ	ⓑ	ⓒ	ⓓ	ⓔ	137.	ⓐ	ⓑ	ⓒ	ⓓ	ⓔ	172.	ⓐ	ⓑ	ⓒ	ⓓ	ⓔ
103.	ⓐ	ⓑ	ⓒ	ⓓ	ⓔ	138.	ⓐ	ⓑ	ⓒ	ⓓ	ⓔ	173.	ⓐ	ⓑ	ⓒ	ⓓ	ⓔ
104.	ⓐ	ⓑ	ⓒ	ⓓ	ⓔ	139.	ⓐ	ⓑ	ⓒ	ⓓ	ⓔ	174.	ⓐ	ⓑ	ⓒ	ⓓ	ⓔ
105.	ⓐ	ⓑ	ⓒ	ⓓ	ⓔ	140.	ⓐ	ⓑ	ⓒ	ⓓ	ⓔ	175.	ⓐ	ⓑ	ⓒ	ⓓ	ⓔ
106.	ⓐ	ⓑ	ⓒ	ⓓ	ⓔ	141.	ⓐ	ⓑ	ⓒ	ⓓ	ⓔ	176.	ⓐ	ⓑ	ⓒ	ⓓ	ⓔ
107.	ⓐ	ⓑ	ⓒ	ⓓ	ⓔ	142.	ⓐ	ⓑ	ⓒ	ⓓ	ⓔ	177.	ⓐ	ⓑ	ⓒ	ⓓ	ⓔ
108.	ⓐ	ⓑ	ⓒ	ⓓ	ⓔ	143.	ⓐ	ⓑ	ⓒ	ⓓ	ⓔ	178.	ⓐ	ⓑ	ⓒ	ⓓ	ⓔ
109.	ⓐ	ⓑ	ⓒ	ⓓ	ⓔ	144.	ⓐ	ⓑ	ⓒ	ⓓ	ⓔ	179.	ⓐ	ⓑ	ⓒ	ⓓ	ⓔ
110.	ⓐ	ⓑ	ⓒ	ⓓ	ⓔ	145.	ⓐ	ⓑ	ⓒ	ⓓ	ⓔ	180.	ⓐ	ⓑ	ⓒ	ⓓ	ⓔ
111.	ⓐ	ⓑ	ⓒ	ⓓ	ⓔ	146.	ⓐ	ⓑ	ⓒ	ⓓ	ⓔ	181.	ⓐ	ⓑ	ⓒ	ⓓ	ⓔ
112.	ⓐ	ⓑ	ⓒ	ⓓ	ⓔ	147.	ⓐ	ⓑ	ⓒ	ⓓ	ⓔ	182.	ⓐ	ⓑ	ⓒ	ⓓ	ⓔ
113.	ⓐ	ⓑ	ⓒ	ⓓ	ⓔ	148.	ⓐ	ⓑ	ⓒ	ⓓ	ⓔ	183.	ⓐ	ⓑ	ⓒ	ⓓ	ⓔ
114.	ⓐ	ⓑ	ⓒ	ⓓ	ⓔ	149.	ⓐ	ⓑ	ⓒ	ⓓ	ⓔ	184.	ⓐ	ⓑ	ⓒ	ⓓ	ⓔ
115.	ⓐ	ⓑ	ⓒ	ⓓ	ⓔ	150.	ⓐ	ⓑ	ⓒ	ⓓ	ⓔ	185.	ⓐ	ⓑ	ⓒ	ⓓ	ⓔ
116.	ⓐ	ⓑ	ⓒ	ⓓ	ⓔ	151.	ⓐ	ⓑ	ⓒ	ⓓ	ⓔ	186.	ⓐ	ⓑ	ⓒ	ⓓ	ⓔ
117.	ⓐ	ⓑ	ⓒ	ⓓ	ⓔ	152.	ⓐ	ⓑ	ⓒ	ⓓ	ⓔ	187.	ⓐ	ⓑ	ⓒ	ⓓ	ⓔ
118.	ⓐ	ⓑ	ⓒ	ⓓ	ⓔ	153.	ⓐ	ⓑ	ⓒ	ⓓ	ⓔ	188.	ⓐ	ⓑ	ⓒ	ⓓ	ⓔ
119.	ⓐ	ⓑ	ⓒ	ⓓ	ⓔ	154.	ⓐ	ⓑ	ⓒ	ⓓ	ⓔ	189.	ⓐ	ⓑ	ⓒ	ⓓ	ⓔ
120.	ⓐ	ⓑ	ⓒ	ⓓ	ⓔ	155.	ⓐ	ⓑ	ⓒ	ⓓ	ⓔ	190.	ⓐ	ⓑ	ⓒ	ⓓ	ⓔ
121.	ⓐ	ⓑ	ⓒ	ⓓ	ⓔ	156.	ⓐ	ⓑ	ⓒ	ⓓ	ⓔ	191.	ⓐ	ⓑ	ⓒ	ⓓ	ⓔ
122.	ⓐ	ⓑ	ⓒ	ⓓ	ⓔ	157.	ⓐ	ⓑ	ⓒ	ⓓ	ⓔ	192.	ⓐ	ⓑ	ⓒ	ⓓ	ⓔ
123.	ⓐ	ⓑ	ⓒ	ⓓ	ⓔ	158.	ⓐ	ⓑ	ⓒ	ⓓ	ⓔ	193.	ⓐ	ⓑ	ⓒ	ⓓ	ⓔ
124.	ⓐ	ⓑ	ⓒ	ⓓ	ⓔ	159.	ⓐ	ⓑ	ⓒ	ⓓ	ⓔ	194.	ⓐ	ⓑ	ⓒ	ⓓ	ⓔ
125.	ⓐ	ⓑ	ⓒ	ⓓ	ⓔ	160.	ⓐ	ⓑ	ⓒ	ⓓ	ⓔ	195.	ⓐ	ⓑ	ⓒ	ⓓ	ⓔ
126.	ⓐ	ⓑ	ⓒ	ⓓ	ⓔ	161.	ⓐ	ⓑ	ⓒ	ⓓ	ⓔ	196.	ⓐ	ⓑ	ⓒ	ⓓ	ⓔ
127.	ⓐ	ⓑ	ⓒ	ⓓ	ⓔ	162.	ⓐ	ⓑ	ⓒ	ⓓ	ⓔ	197.	ⓐ	ⓑ	ⓒ	ⓓ	ⓔ
128.	ⓐ	ⓑ	ⓒ	ⓓ	ⓔ	163.	ⓐ	ⓑ	ⓒ	ⓓ	ⓔ	198.	ⓐ	ⓑ	ⓒ	ⓓ	ⓔ
129.	ⓐ	ⓑ	ⓒ	ⓓ	ⓔ	164.	ⓐ	ⓑ	ⓒ	ⓓ	ⓔ	199.	ⓐ	ⓑ	ⓒ	ⓓ	ⓔ
130.	ⓐ	ⓑ	ⓒ	ⓓ	ⓔ	165.	ⓐ	ⓑ	ⓒ	ⓓ	ⓔ	200.	ⓐ	ⓑ	ⓒ	ⓓ	ⓔ
131.	ⓐ	ⓑ	ⓒ	ⓓ	ⓔ	166.	ⓐ	ⓑ	ⓒ	ⓓ	ⓔ						
132.	ⓐ	ⓑ	ⓒ	ⓓ	ⓔ	167.	ⓐ	ⓑ	ⓒ	ⓓ	ⓔ						
133.	ⓐ	ⓑ	ⓒ	ⓓ	ⓔ	168.	ⓐ	ⓑ	ⓒ	ⓓ	ⓔ						
134.	ⓐ	ⓑ	ⓒ	ⓓ	ⓔ	169.	ⓐ	ⓑ	ⓒ	ⓓ	ⓔ						
135.	ⓐ	ⓑ	ⓒ	ⓓ	ⓔ	170.	ⓐ	ⓑ	ⓒ	ⓓ	ⓔ						

General Medical Assisting Knowledge

1. Which of the following planes divides the body into anterior and posterior portions?
   a. sagittal
   b. median
   c. midsagittal
   d. frontal plane
   e. transverse

2. Which of the following systems pumps and distributes blood throughout the body?
   a. nervous
   b. respiratory
   c. sensory
   d. cardiovascular
   e. integumentary

3. The four major types of tissue in the body are
   a. muscle, nervous, epithelial, and connective.
   b. nervous, connective, vascular, and epithelial.
   c. epithelial, nervous, vascular, and epidermis.
   d. muscle, epithelial, blood, and connective.
   e. muscle, epithelial, nervous, and vessels.

4. The upper respiratory tract includes all of the following EXCEPT the
   a. nose.
   b. pharynx.
   c. bronchi.
   d. upper trachea.
   e. larynx.

5. The accessory organs include the
   a. gallbladder, liver, and pancreas.
   b. pancreas, anus, and liver.
   c. liver, mouth, and esophagus.
   d. large intestine, anus, and stomach.
   e. esophagus, gallbladder, and pancreas.

6. Hydrocele means
   a. inflammation of the prostate.
   b. inflammation of the cervix.
   c. swelling of the testes.
   d. inflammation of the testes.
   e. impotence.

7. All of the following are true about leukocytes EXCEPT
   a. leukocytes are white blood cells.
   b. leukocytes fight infection.
   c. leukocytes produce antibodies.
   d. leukocytes are part of the circulatory system.
   e. leukocytes are responsible for blood clotting.

8. Tendonitis is a(n)
   a. broken bone.
   b. inflammation of a tendon.
   c. injury to a muscle.
   d. progressive wasting of muscle tissue.
   e. muscle pain.

9. The function of the skin includes all of the following EXCEPT
   a. protection from sunlight.
   b. lubrication.
   c. protection from microorganisms.
   d. regulation of temperature.
   e. transportation of immune cells.

10. The nucleus is
    a. the control center that directs the activity of the cell.
    b. a gel-like fluid in the cell.
    c. a lysosome.
    d. a tissue.
    e. a cell membrane.

11. Cholelithiasis is
   a. inflammation of a joint.
   b. inflammation of the stomach.
   c. gallstones.
   d. inflammation of the gallbladder.
   e. chronic degenerative disease of the liver.

12. The sensory organs include all the following EXCEPT
   a. the pharynx.
   b. the eyes.
   c. the nose.
   d. the tongue.
   e. the ears.

13. Which of the following terms means "the surgical removal of the kidney"?
   a. appendectomy
   b. cholecystectomy
   c. hysterectomy
   d. nephrectomy
   e. splenectomy

14. The combining form *cost/o* refers to which of the following anatomic structures?
   a. bone marrow
   b. clavicle
   c. joint
   d. ligament
   e. rib

15. All of the following components are a part of Sigmund Freud's theories of psychology EXCEPT
   a. id.
   b. subconscious.
   c. ego.
   d. behaviorism.
   e. superego.

16. Which of the following terms means "difficulty swallowing"?
   a. dyscrasia
   b. dyspepsia
   c. dysphagia
   d. dyspnea
   e. dysuria

17. Cognitive theory offers an approach to psychology that encourages individuals to examine
   a. their dreams.
   b. errors in their thinking.
   c. rational beliefs.
   d. grief and loss.
   e. needs and desires.

18. Which suffix means "surgical repair"?
   a. *opsy*
   b. *rrhea*
   c. *plasty*
   d. *tome*
   e. *lysis*

19. Which of the following conditions is commonly known as a bruise?
   a. ecchymosis
   b. epistaxis
   c. hematoma
   d. lesion
   e. thrombosis

20. Each of the following identifies one of Elizabeth Kübler-Ross's five stages of grief EXCEPT
   a. denial.
   b. anger.
   c. shock.
   d. bargaining.
   e. depression.

21. The most accurate definition of "defense mechanisms" in psychology is
   a. a means to bring upsetting emotions to the surface of an individual's consciousness.
   b. ways to strike out in anger in difficult situations.
   c. strategies individuals use to avoid difficult or painful feelings.
   d. one type of mood swing experienced by individuals suffering from bipolar disorder.
   e. a way for humans to avoid talking to each other.

22. All of the following statements about renewing the CMA credential are true EXCEPT
   a. the CMA credential must be renewed every five years.
   b. the CMA credential may be renewed by retaking the certifying examination.
   c. the CMA credential is required in order to practice in the medical assisting profession.
   d. the CMA credential may be renewed by earning continuing education units (CEUs).
   e. a current CMA credential may help in career advancement and financial compensation.

23. Which certifying agency allows a medical assistant to use the CMA credential?
   a. Registered Medical Assistants (RMA)
   b. Commission on Accreditation of Allied Health Education Programs (CAAHEP)
   c. American Medical Association (AMA)
   d. American Association of Medical Assistants (AAMA)
   e. American Medical Technologists (AMT)

24. Which type of resume is written specifically for an advertised job?
   a. letter of recommendation
   b. targeted
   c. chronological
   d. functional
   e. cover letter

25. Which of the following incoming calls should the medical assistant transfer immediately to the physician?
   a. a new patient demanding to speak with the physician before making an appointment
   b. the emergency room calling about admitting an established patient with chest pain
   c. the intensive care unit requesting a diet order for tomorrow on one of the physician's patients
   d. a pharmaceutical representative excited about a new discovery in medicine
   e. a patient requesting a prescription refill

26. A physician who specializes in disorders of the eye is known as which of the following?
   a. ophthalmologist
   b. oncologist
   c. orthodontist
   d. osteologist
   e. otolaryngologist

27. When the medical assistant is preparing to answer incoming calls, what supplies or items should he or she have readily available?
   a. patient medical records, coding books, and office policy manual
   b. appointment book, calendar, message pad or notepad, and pen and pencil
   c. reminder cards, appointment book, and pen and pencil
   d. new patient registration forms and change of address forms
   e. notepad, medical dictionary, and pen and pencil

28. The information needed to make a return appointment for an established patient includes all of the following EXCEPT
   a. reason for the visit.
   b. daytime phone number.
   c. type of insurance.
   d. name of the patient.
   e. patient's employer.

29. A patient's neighbor calls, stating that she is concerned about her friend and would like to know what is wrong with the patient. The medical assistant should
   a. give just basic information because the neighbor is such a good friend to the patient.
   b. tell the neighbor that she should know better than to be prying into someone else's business.
   c. tell the neighbor she needs to come into the office to discuss any information about the patient because the phone lines are not secure.
   d. tactfully refuse to release any patient information without the patient's written permission.
   e. ask the neighbor to accompany the patient on her next office visit.

30. When responding to a hearing-impaired caller, the medical assistant should
   a. speak a little more slowly and a little more loudly.
   b. shout so that he or she will not have to repeat the information too many times.
   c. ask to speak to a family member to be sure that the information is received correctly.
   d. tell the patient that he or she will mail a response to the patient's questions as soon as possible.
   e. spell out each word so that the patient can write down the information.

31. The best way to handle an unidentified caller who insists on speaking with the physician but refuses to give her phone number or the reason for her call would be to
   a. transfer the call to the physician because the patient is becoming upset.
   b. transfer the call to the office manager, who may be able to get the patient's name and phone number.
   c. ask the caller not to call back until she is prepared to give the requested information.
   d. tell the caller that unidentified calls are never transferred to the physician and then hang up.
   e. ask the caller to send a letter to the physician.

32. Which of the following conditions is most characteristic of an asthma attack?
   a. dyspareunia
   b. dysphagia
   c. dysphasia
   d. dyspnea
   e. dystonia

33. To obtain confidential patient information, which caller does NOT need a patient's written consent?
   a. insurance carrier
   b. lawyer
   c. patient's neighbor
   d. referring physician
   e. member of the patient's family

34. Which of the following situations is NOT considered to be a reportable incident?
   a. a gunshot wound
   b. a sexually transmitted disease
   c. a negative result for HIV
   d. a case of pertussis
   e. child abuse

35. Which of the following terms means "the thing speaks for itself" when applied to the law of negligence?
a. malfeasance
b. res ipsa loquitur
c. nonfeasance
d. jurisprudence
e. respondant superior

36. Which type of insurance would cover the medical expenses of an employee injured on the job?
a. major medical
b. TRICARE
c. Medicare
d. workers' compensation
e. health maintenance organization

37. All of the following are reasons for proper documentation of procedures performed in a medical office EXCEPT
a. information documented in the medical record may be used to reassure an employer about the health of an employee.
b. information documented in the medical record may be used in a court of law in the defense of a physician being sued.
c. information documented in the medical record may be used to provide information to referring physicians.
d. information documented in the medical record may be used to gather statistical information for research.
e. information documented in the medical record allows physicians to keep track of the medical treatments and care provided to a patient.

38. Which of the following terms refers to the narrowing of the urethra?
a. urethralgia
b. urethritis
c. urethrorrhagia
d. urethroscope
e. urethrostenosis

39. Which of the following is the correct spelling of the term for an enlarged spleen?
a. spleenamegly
b. spleenomegaly
c. splenamegaly
d. splenomegaly
e. splenomeglly

40. The Personnel Record Act prohibits an employer from keeping information about
a. an employee's job performance.
b. an employee's political affiliation.
c. recent disciplinary actions against the employee.
d. recent work incidences.
e. an employee in a locked file.

41. Which of the following is an example of an open-ended question?
a. "How are you today, Mrs. Jones?"
b. "Do you have any questions about your diet?"
c. "Would you please describe the exercises you do each day that tend to cause the chest pain you are experiencing?"
d. "Do you enjoy the foods on the low-sodium list the nutritionist gave you?"
e. "Are you happy with the progress you are making?"

42. When should the W-2 form, the wage and tax statement, be given to an employee?
  a. annually in April
  b. annually in January
  c. biannually in January and June
  d. quarterly in March, June, September, and December
  e. every time there is a change in the employee's work status

43. All of the following may interfere with a therapeutic relationship between the patient and the healthcare provider EXCEPT
  a. stress.
  b. physical disabilities.
  c. anger.
  d. empathy.
  e. mistrust.

44. Which of the following statements would be an example of stereotyping?
  a. All elderly patients have difficulty walking.
  b. Some elderly patients have difficulty hearing.
  c. Many patients have some type of vision impairment.
  d. A lot of patients have memory lapses.
  e. A few elderly patients have high blood pressure.

45. Which of the following terms refers to the surgical removal of a lymph node?
  a. lymphadenectomy
  b. lymhadenitis
  c. lymphadenopathy
  d. lymphadenotomy
  e. lymphectasia

46. Which of the following is NOT considered a special accessibility alteration designed just for disabled patients coming to the physician's office?
  a. mats on the floors near entryways to prevent patient falls because of wet floors
  b. widened corridors enabling easy movement of wheelchairs
  c. bathroom stalls with handrails
  d. Braille signs to mark the elevator levels
  e. examining rooms designed to allow easy movement of wheelchairs

47. Which organization registers physicians to prescribe controlled substances?
  a. Joint Commission on the Accreditation of Healthcare Organizations (JCAHO)
  b. Drug Enforcement Administration (DEA)
  c. Occupational Safety and Health Administration (OSHA)
  d. Health Insurance Portability and Accountability Act (HIPAA)
  e. Food and Drug Administration (FDA)

48. Which of the following describes a wrong and unlawful act performed by a physician?
  a. malfeasance
  b. misfeasance
  c. nonfeasance
  d. feasance
  e. disfeasance

49. A legal, valid contract may include all of the following EXCEPT
  a. offer and acceptance.
  b. a legal subject matter.
  c. signatures made by mentally competent emancipated minors.
  d. a valid consideration or something of value.
  e. any two individuals.

50. Which of the following terms describes written statements made to damage an individual's reputation?
    a. libel
    b. negligence
    c. battery
    d. slander
    e. bias

51. All of the following actions may result in revocation of a physician's license EXCEPT
    a. impersonating another physician.
    b. providing substandard care.
    c. practicing without a license.
    d. prescribing legal drugs.
    e. substance abuse.

52. A healthcare agent with durable power of attorney is
    a. an individual who will be responsible for all decisions should the patient become physically and mentally incapable of making decisions.
    b. considered to be the patient's primary care physician.
    c. an attorney who will be able to make the best legal decisions for the patient.
    d. the person chosen to make the final decisions about the patient's end-of-life healthcare.
    e. the medical assistant in the physician's office who is charge of billing and insurance reimbursement.

53. Which of the following situations is NOT considered to be a reportable incidence?
    a. accidental stabbing
    b. spousal abuse
    c. a positive result for HIV
    d. a case of rubeola
    e. a case of bronchitis

54. The Occupational Safety and Health Act was legislation passed to ensure all of the following EXCEPT
    a. more control for employers over employee non-working hours.
    b. safer and healthier working environments for employees.
    c. enforcements of its safety regulations.
    d. training and education on safety issues for employers and employees.
    e. compliance assistance to worksites.

55. Which of the following federal agencies was formed as the first attempt to establish consumer protection in the manufacture of drugs and foods?
    a. OSHA
    b. HIPAA
    c. FDA
    d. DEA
    e. CLIA

56. The Clinical Laboratory Improvement Act of 1988 was developed for all of the following reasons EXCEPT
    a. to increase the waiting time for specimen results.
    b. to develop comprehensive standards for better accuracy.
    c. to improve reliability of testing in smaller facilities.
    d. to categorize lab tests by complexity for better regulation.
    e. to decrease waiting time for specimen results.

57. All of the following accommodations may be made to comply with the regulations recommended in the Americans with Disabilities Act EXCEPT
   a. providing ramps for easier access to buildings
   b. providing elevators in buildings having more than one level
   c. widening doorways to accommodate wheelchairs
   d. replacing stairs with elevators in all buildings
   e. placing handrails and grip bars in bathrooms

58. Which of the following terms states that a physician is liable for the negligent actions of any employee working under his or her supervision?
   a. malfeasance
   b. *res ipsa loquitur*
   c. nonfeasance
   d. jurisprudence
   e. *respondeat superior*

Administrative Medical Assistant Knowledge

59. The process of preparing documents by converting dictated physician notes into written documents is called
   a. typing.
   b. transcription.
   c. modified block.
   d. outsourcing.
   e. memoranda.

60. Which of the following would be the best salutation to use in a business letter?
   a. *Best regards*
   b. *Dear Dr. Smith*
   c. *Yours truly*
   d. *Sincerely*
   e. *To whom it may concern*

61. Which device protects a computer from electrical damage?
   a. central processing unit
   b. modem
   c. surge protector
   d. motherboard
   e. cursor

62. All of the following are examples of computer hardware EXCEPT
   a. a keyboard.
   b. a printer.
   c. a monitor.
   d. system software.
   e. a central processing unit.

63. Which of the following is a pointing device that notifies the user where the next letter, number, or symbol will be placed?
   a. flash drive
   b. cursor
   c. motherboard
   d. disk
   e. prompter

64. Which of the following is NOT a subjective symptom?
   a. backache
   b. headache
   c. stomach cramps
   d. fever
   e. chest pain

65. Who owns a patient's medical record?
 a. The patient owns the actual paper medical record and the information it contains.
 b. The information in the record is owned by the patient, and the physician or medical facility that created the record owns the paper medical record.
 c. The patient's insurance company has ownership of the record because they are the third-party payer.
 d. The medical office has the sole ownership of the paper medical record and its content.
 e. The archives of the hospital become the owner of the patient's medical record after three years.

66. Medical records are used for all of the following reasons EXCEPT
 a. for research.
 b. for legal documentation.
 c. to determine health patterns that signal a patient's needs.
 d. to keep track of the patient's financial transactions.
 e. to manage patient care.

67. Medical records are classified as
 a. closed, open, or miscellaneous.
 b. incomplete, active, or closed.
 c. closed, active, or inactive.
 d. inactive, open, or active.
 e. incomplete, inactive, or active.

68. Which type of medical record filing system offers the most privacy?
 a. subject
 b. numeric
 c. chronological
 d. alphabetic
 e. color-coded

69. All of the following are advantages of the numeric filing system EXCEPT
 a. easy expansion.
 b. an alphabetic card system.
 c. no patient names listed on record.
 d. no need to shift or move files.
 e. more confidentiality.

70. All of the following statements describe strict chronological filing EXCEPT
 a. all incoming patient information is filed with the most recent information on top.
 b. there are no separate sections for subject matter.
 c. the problem list is arranged according to the patient's past history.
 d. it may be difficult to locate specific patient information.
 e. information is filed according to date.

71. Which of the following would be considered an example of objective clinical evidence?
 a. elevated temperature, headache, and back pain
 b. high blood pressure, elevated temperature, and swollen ankle
 c. stomach cramps, swollen ankle, and back pain
 d. headache, stomach pain, and painful ankle
 e. back pain, joint pain, and headache

72. All of the following should be considered when selecting new file cabinets for a medical office EXCEPT
 a. size of the area available for record storage.
 b. cost of the equipment.
 c. requirements for confidentiality.
 d. estimated record volume.
 e. whether or not the office uses color-coded files.

73. Which type of mail should be used when proof is needed that a patient received a letter sent by a physician's office?
a. certificate of mailing
b. registered mail
c. certified mail
d. media mail
e. standard mail A

74. How many digits are contained in the ZIP + 4?
a. five
b. six
c. seven
d. eight
e. nine

75. Where on an envelope should notations such as "Confidential" and "Personal" be included?
a. typed directly below the return address
b. aligned with right edge of letter
c. written in the lower right-hand corner
d. written in red ink
e. written directly under the postage stamp

76. The correct USPS abbreviation for the state of Maine is
a. MA.
b. MI.
c. M.N.
d. N.M.
e. ME.

77. The procedure to follow when opening mail is to
a. arrange mail by size.
b. place all payments from patients and insurance companies on top.
c. place the most important mail on top.
d. place mail in alphabetical order.
e. place all drug samples on top to be stored in a locked cabinet as soon as possible.

78. Annotating is
a. jotting down notes about an action needed to be taken in the letter's margins.
b. sorting the mail by importance.
c. another word for "release mark."
d. the first step in filing.
e. keeping a record of all mail received.

79. Which of the following should be placed on the top when sorting incoming mail?
a. the latest edition of a medical journal
b. a letter marked "Personal"
c. a letter with no return address
d. reports from the laboratory
e. pharmaceutical updates about drug recalls

80. Which of the following patients should be seen first if all of them arrived at the walk-in center at approximately at the same time?
a. a 35-year-old female with a sore throat for two days
b. a 55-year-old male with a poison ivy rash on his arms
c. a 56-year-old male with dyspnea
d. a 14-year-old teenager with a swollen ankle
e. an 82-year-old female with anorexia and confusion

81. Which type of scheduling system schedules three patients at the beginning of each hour?
a. double-booking
b. stream
c. modified wave
d. clustering
e. wave

82. CPT codes are used to code
a. diagnoses.
b. procedures.
c. symptoms.
d. illnesses.
e. allergies.

83. Medicare Part B covers all of the following EXCEPT
   a. inpatient hospital visits.
   b. durable medical equipment.
   c. ambulance service.
   d. preventive care.
   e. X-rays.

84. Which part of Medicare provides prescription coverage?
   a. Part A
   b. Part B
   c. Part C
   d. Part D
   e. Part E

85. TRICARE was formerly known as
   a. Medicare.
   b. Medicaid.
   c. CHAMPUS.
   d. CHAMPVA.
   e. PPO.

86. Which of the following coding systems is used to identify and code diseases on insurance claims?
   a. CPT
   b. CMS
   c. HCFA
   d. ICD-9-CM
   e. NUUC

87. Which type of ICD-9-CM code is used to classify external causes of poisoning and injuries?
   a. E codes
   b. M codes
   c. V codes
   d. modifying codes
   e. N codes

88. Which term is used when describing the amount of money owed by the medical office for products and services purchased on credit?
   a. accounts receivable
   b. billing accounts
   c. accounts payable
   d. monthly accounts
   e. credit card accounts

89. The role of the medical assistant when checking in a patient is to
   a. explain the advantages of different types of medical insurance.
   b. explain the insurance claim form.
   c. confirm office coverage for patient's insurance plan.
   d. explain the patient's insurance policy.
   e. explain diagnoses.

90. When an insurance policy pays a percentage of the balance after application of the deductible, it is referred to as
   a. coordination of benefits.
   b. coinsurance.
   c. a co-pay.
   d. the deductible.
   e. the birthday rule.

91. When more than one policy pays on a claim, it is called
   a. coordination of benefits.
   b. coinsurance.
   c. a co-pay.
   d. the deductible.
   e. the birthday rule.

92. When both parents (married) are covered by health insurance, claims for the family are paid according to the
   a. coordination of benefits.
   b. coinsurance.
   c. co-pay.
   d. deductible.
   e. birthday rule.

93. A method of containing hospital costs has been adopted with a system called
   a. OPPS.
   b. DRGs.
   c. fee for service.
   d. allowable amounts.
   e. ICDs.

94. Which of the following is NOT a federal health insurance program or a state health insurance program?
   a. Medicaid
   b. Medicare Part A
   c. CHAMPUS
   d. MCOs
   e. workers' compensation

95. What percentage will Medicare pay on an allowed claim?
   a. 50%
   b. 60%
   c. 70%
   d. 80%
   e. 90%

96. Mrs. Lee, a patient of Dr. Chad, is charged $80 for a visit. Medicare allows $60 for this visit and paid $48. Because Mrs. Lee has already met her yearly deductible, how much will she have to pay the physician?
   a. $48
   b. $32
   c. $12
   d. $80
   e. $0

97. Which volumes of the ICD-9-CM books are needed for coding diagnoses in the medical office?
   a. Volumes I and III
   b. Volumes II and III
   c. Volumes I and II
   d. Volumes I, II, and III
   e. Volume III only

98. Place the following medical records in alphabetic order.
   1. Scoville   Francis   J   Sr.
   2. Scoville   Frances   J
   3. Scoville   Francis   J   III
   4. Scoville   Francis   J   Jr.
   a. 1, 2, 3, 4
   b. 3, 1, 4, 2
   c. 4, 1, 3, 2
   d. 2, 3, 4, 1
   e. 2, 1, 3, 4

99. Codes that cannot stand alone are
   a. modifier codes.
   b. V codes.
   c. E codes.
   d. preventive care codes.
   e. ICD-9-CM.

100. Insurance policies that include coverage on a fee-for-service basis are called
a. traditional insurance policies.
b. managed care policies.
c. Medicare.
d. Medicaid.
e. TRICARE.

101. Which of the following will happen to an insurance claim when the coding is incorrectly entered on the insurance form?
a. The claim will be denied, and the physician will not receive payment.
b. The incorrect information on the claim will not affect payment to the physician.
c. The claim will be destroyed without payment.
d. The patient will be billed instead of the physician.
e. The insurance carrier will notify the patient that a claim in his or her name was incorrect.

102. Which of the following is the final step to the aging and collection process for a patient with private insurance?
a. Send an itemized statement.
b. Send an overdue notice with the intent of turning the bill over to a collection agency if not paid promptly.
c. Turn the account over to a collection agency.
d. Call the patient to request payment.
e. Call the patient's employer to notify patient about the overdue bill.

103. Non-duplication of benefits means that
a. benefits will not cover preexisting conditions.
b. benefits will cover conditions covered by a previous insurance policy.
c. the physician may not bill more than one insurance company.
d. benefits will be coordinated between two separate insurance companies.
e. the insurance benefits will not cover the same condition twice.

104. Medical expenses for a patient injured at his or her place of employment should be sent to
a. the patient's private insurance carrier.
b. the patient's employer.
c. the patient.
d. the state insurance commissioner.
e. workers' compensation insurance.

105. Which of the following information would be listed on the front portion of a patient's Medicare card?
a. the name of the beneficiary and the patient's ID number
b. the patient's ID number and the address of the patient's insurance company
c. the name of the patient and the patient's current address
d. the name of the participating physician and his or her ID number
e. the name and age of the patient and the expiration date of the patient's insurance

106. Which of the following individuals would require the consent of an adult before treatment may be given by a physician?
a. a mentally sound 75-year-old woman
b. an emancipated 17-year-old male
c. an unconscious 45-year-old patient brought into the emergency room
d. a 22-year-old single woman
e. a 15-year-old girl living with her parents

107. Which of the following criteria is an example of the clustering style of scheduling?
a. scheduling three patients for follow-up visits each hour throughout the workday
b. scheduling a well-baby clinic for Tuesday mornings from 10:00 a.m. to 11:00 a.m. and performing school physicals one morning per week
c. leaving one morning free of appointment times for patients to walk in at their convenience
d. scheduling two patients every 20 minutes
e. scheduling two patients at the top of the hour and one patient at half past the hour

108. Which scheduling style utilizes any method or combination of methods that works best for the individual office?
a. open hours
b. stream
c. clustering
d. practice-based
e. double-booking

109. Which of the following best describes the prior permission or approval needed from an insurance carrier before a patient may be treated or have a specific procedure performed by the physician?
a. referral
b. protocol
c. prepayment
d. precertification
e. capitation

110. Which of the following would be an example of an accounts receivable?
a. charges for a patient's office visit
b. charges from the electric company
c. payment made for the maintenance of the computer
d. charges for a new ink cartridge for the printer
e. payment made to the maintenance person

111. A one-write, or write-it-once, bookkeeping system is also referred to as a
a. POMR system.
b. SOMR system.
c. balance statement system.
d. pegboard system.
e. encounter form.

112. All of the following are ways to help in the collection process of accounts receivable EXCEPT
a. asking the patient if he or she will be paying by cash, check, or credit card.
b. enclosing an addressed return envelope with the patient bill.
c. making the patient aware of the payment policy prior to an appointment.
d. allowing three months to pass before billing the patient for the office visit.
e. making a call to the patient about an overdue bill.

113. Which of the following is the safest type of check endorsement?
  a. blank endorsement
  b. total endorsement
  c. restrictive endorsement
  d. insurance endorsement
  e. private endorsement

114. Payroll documents of employees need to be kept for a minimum of
  a. one year.
  b. two years.
  c. four years.
  d. five years.
  e. seven years.

115. The money collected through contributions to the Federal Insurance Contribution Act (FICA) is used for all of the following EXCEPT
  a. retirement income.
  b. Medicare coverage.
  c. disability insurance.
  d. unemployment insurance.
  e. benefits for survivors.

116. Which type of insurance is usually purchased to cover catastrophic illness and injuries?
  a. Medicare
  b. Medicaid
  c. major medical
  d. HMOs
  e. CHAMPVA

117. The usual fee charged by a physician is
  a. the amount charged for an exceptionally difficult or complex procedure requiring more time and effort on the part of a provider.
  b. the amount allowed by an insurance carrier.
  c. the amount charged by a provider in a specific geographical area for a specific service or procedure.
  d. the amount allowed by the government.
  e. the amount a physician charges for a service or procedure.

118. Which law protects consumers by requiring full disclosure of any additional charges that may apply to a bill, such as interest?
  a. Equal Opportunity Law
  b. Truth-in-Lending Act
  c. Good Samaritan Law
  d. Americans with Disabilities Act
  e. Fair Debt Collection Practices Act

119. Which of the following statements is NOT true about patient referrals?
  a. They may be classified as an urgent referral.
  b. They may be classified as a regular referral.
  c. They may be requested by a patient.
  d. They may be classified as a stat referral.
  e. They may be made without pre-authorization from the insurance carrier.

120. Which of the following statements describes a patient advocate?
  a. a liaison between patient and healthcare provider
  b. a person selected to make healthcare decisions for the patient
  c. a type of living will
  d. an advance directive
  e. an attorney for the patient during a lawsuit

121. Which of the following terms may be defined as the science of designing equipment in a workplace to help workers reach maximum productivity and reduce fatigue and discomfort?
   a. ergonomics
   b. kinesiology
   c. physiology
   d. body mechanics
   e. etiology

122. Which of these laws or organizations developed rules regarding the proper handling of blood products and other infectious material such as wearing gloves, gowns, and goggles?
   a. Controlled Substances Act of 1970
   b. Centers for Disease Control and Prevention
   c. Occupational Safety and Health Administration
   d. universal precautions
   e. Food and Drug Administration

123. All of the following are requirements for safety in the medical office EXCEPT
   a. a working fire extinguisher.
   b. a working smoke alarm.
   c. exits marked only in Braille.
   d. a written plan for exposure to bloodborne pathogens.
   e. safety training for all employees.

124. Which of the following is NOT an example of a biohazardous substance?
   a. synovial fluid
   b. cerebrospinal fluid
   c. pleural fluid
   d. blood and blood products
   e. perspiration

125. All of the following are bookkeeping guidelines EXCEPT
   a. writing numbers legibly.
   b. lining up columns of numbers when adding or subtracting.
   c. checking math carefully, especially the placement of decimal points.
   d. completing bookkeeping once every two weeks.
   e. using dark blue or black ink for easier viewing.

126. All of the following statements are true about the encounter form EXCEPT
   a. an encounter form is also called a super bill or a charge slip.
   b. an encounter form provides an itemized list of charges.
   c. an encounter form comes in triplicate.
   d. an encounter form provides documentation that may be easily placed in the patient's medical record.
   e. an encounter form is considered the universal insurance claim form.

Clinical Medical Assistant Knowledge

127. Which of the following medications should be included on a crash cart?
   a. fluocinonide (Lidex)
   b. furosemide (Lasix)
   c. pantoprazole (Protonix)
   d. pravastatin (Pravachol)
   e. promazine (Prozine)

128. After delivering a shock with the AED, the medical assistant should
  a. check the patient's pulse.
  b. immediately resume chest compressions cycled with rescue breathing.
  c. give 30 chest compressions and deliver another shock.
  d. turn off the AED.
  e. deliver a series of abdominal thrusts.

129. An AED is used to treat which of the following?
  a. CVA
  b. diabetic coma
  c. seizures
  d. heart arrhythmias
  e. stroke

130. The medical assistant is protected from liability during an emergency situation for all of the following reasons EXCEPT
  a. reasonable care is given to the patient.
  b. the patient agrees to treatment.
  c. the medical assistant does not go beyond his or her skill level.
  d. he or she stays with the injured person until someone who has the same or more skill takes over.
  e. acts in good faith.

131. The medical assistant is caring for a child with a painful, blistered burn on the arm from a hot liquid. The medical assistant should
  a. cool it with cold water as quickly as possible and continue cooling until the pain is relieved.
  b. quickly pop each blister, then apply cold water until the pain is relieved.
  c. apply triple antibiotic ointment to the burn and cover it with an adhesive bandage.
  d. apply ice directly to the burn and keep it there until the pain is relieved.
  e. apply direct pressure with an absorbent pad.

132. According to basic cardiac life support procedures, which of the following describes appropriate rescue breathing for an adult patient?
  a. one breath every three seconds
  b. one breath every five seconds
  c. two breaths every three seconds
  d. two breaths every five seconds
  e. one breath every two seconds

133. To control bleeding or hemorrhaging, the medical assistant should initially
  a. apply heat over the wound.
  b. apply ice over the wound.
  c. apply direct pressure.
  d. apply a tourniquet above the injury.
  e. immobilize the body part.

134. Which burn destroys the epidermis and dermis, including the nerve endings?
  a. third-degree
  b. first-degree
  c. second-degree
  d. minor
  e. acid burn

135. A strain is a
  a. fracture.
  b. ligament injury.
  c. broken blood vessel.
  d. muscle injury.
  e. cartilage injury.

136. Which of the following should be assessed first when rendering first aid?
  a. pulse
  b. capillary action
  c. pain or injury to limbs
  d. emotional state
  e. airway

137. All of the following are common causes of breathing emergencies EXCEPT
    a. choking.
    b. obstruction.
    c. strains.
    d. asthma.
    e. allergic reaction.

138. According to the rule of nines, the amount of body surface represented by the head and neck is
    a. 1%
    b. 4.5%.
    c. 9%.
    d. 18%.
    e. 36%.

139. Shock is caused by
    a. a tear in a ligament.
    b. a lack of blood flow and oxygen to body tissues.
    c. a heart attack.
    d. a stroke.
    e. epistaxis.

140. What is a seizure?
    a. a type of myocardial infarction
    b. a syncope
    c. an involuntary muscle contraction/relaxation
    d. a hemorrhage
    e. an abrasion

141. Insulin shock causes
    a. hyperkalemia.
    b. severe hypoglycemia.
    c. severe hyperglycemia.
    d. hypokalemia.
    e. syncope.

142. When using an autoclave, which of the following is the minimum temperature necessary to sterilize medical instruments?
    a. 120°F (48.9°C)
    b. 180°F (82.2°C)
    c. 225°F (107.2°C)
    d. 250°F (121.1°C)
    e. 280°F (137.7°C)

143. Which of the following is one of the agencies that regulates the disposal of infectious waste outside the workplace?
    a. Association for Professionals in Infection Control
    b. Centers for Disease Control and Prevention
    c. Environmental Protection Agency
    d. Exposure Control Plan
    e. Department of Health and Human Services

144. Which of the following terms describes complete destruction of all microorganisms?
    a. antiseptic
    b. aseptic
    c. disinfection
    d. sanitization
    e. sterilization

145. When a patient has taken a drug for an extended period of time, the desired effect may lessen or will not occur at all. This is called
    a. toxic effect.
    b. idiosyncratic effect.
    c. tolerance.
    d. vasoconstrictor.
    e. potentiation.

146. Which of the following agencies is responsible for enforcing the Controlled Substance Act?
   a. American Medical Association
   b. Drug Enforcement Administration
   c. Food and Drug Administration
   d. Federal Trade Commission
   e. Physician's Desk Reference

147. Which of the following is a drug used to lessen or prevent the effects of a disease?
   a. curative
   b. prophylactic
   c. replacement
   d. therapeutic
   e. supplemental

148. Which of the following food types is the best protein source?
   a. meats
   b. raw vegetables
   c. citrus
   d. oils
   e. butter

149. Which of the following is the best source of calcium and vitamin D?
   a. meats and nuts
   b. raw vegetables
   c. citrus fruits
   d. dairy products
   e. oils

150. Which type of pathogen survives in the absence of oxygen?
   a. spores
   b. aerobes
   c. anaerobes
   d. vectors
   e. fomites

151. Which of the following is an effective disinfectant used in the medical office to destroy blood-borne pathogens?
   a. alcohol
   b. bleach
   c. chlorhexidine gluconate
   d. formaldehyde
   e. phenol

152. Which of the following is an example of a standard precaution for infection control?
   a. disinfecting the examination table after each patient
   b. emptying the garbage can weekly
   c. recapping used needles with the two-hand method
   d. wearing heavy gloves to remove instruments from the autoclave
   e. wearing two sets of gloves when cleaning surgical instruments

153. Which of the following describes a drug that is not protected by a trademark but is registered by the Food and Drug Administration?
   a. controlled
   b. generic
   c. research
   d. over-the-counter
   e. trademark

154. A physician prescribes amoxicillin 500 mg capsules po qid for 10 days. How many capsules should be dispensed?
   a. 10
   b. 20
   c. 30
   d. 40
   e. 50

155. A drug from which of the following classes is used for a heart condition?
   a. antacids
   b. antiarrhythmic
   c. anesthetics
   d. antibiotics
   e. analgesics

156. The food guide pyramid suggests that patients plan a balanced diet by doing all of the following EXCEPT
   a. eating more fruits.
   b. eating nuts.
   c. eating more carbohydrates.
   d. eating whole grain foods.
   e. eating more vegetables.

157. Which of the following is an example of a fat-soluble vitamin?
   a. vitamin B
   b. vitamin C
   c. vitamin B6
   d. vitamin E
   e. vitamin B12

158. Which of the following terms means "all of the factors required for infectious disease to spread"?
   a. chain of infection
   b. droplet transmission
   c. infection control
   d. inflammatory response
   e. nosocomal infection

159. Which of the following is the first line of defense in the practice of medical asepsis?
   a. cleaning the examination table
   b. sanitizing the patient's skin
   c. sterilizing instruments
   d. washing hands
   e. wearing gloves

160. The medical assistant is to obtain the history of a patient who is suspected to have active tuberculosis. For protection, which of the following articles is essential for the medical assistant to wear before entering the room?
   a. gloves
   b. goggles
   c. gown
   d. mask
   e. laboratory coat

161. Substances that prevent or inhibit the growth of a fungus are known as
   a. antiseptics.
   b. disinfectants.
   c. germicides.
   d. fungicides.
   e. analgesics.

162. A drug that is given sublingually is
   a. injected into the deltoid muscle.
   b. placed under the tongue.
   c. administered buccally.
   d. injected into the muscle.
   e. injected under the intradermal layer of the skin.

163. Calculate the following drug dosage: *Ampicillin 0.5 g.* The unit dose packet reads *250 mg/cap.*
   a. one-half capsule
   b. one capsule
   c. two capsules
   d. two and one-half capsules
   e. three capsules

164. High-protein diets are often used
   a. before surgery.
   b. when an infection is present.
   c. with hypothermia.
   d. with hyperthermia.
   e. to treat hypertension, or high blood pressure.

165. The recommended amount of water to ingest daily is
   a. two eight-ounce glasses.
   b. eight eight-ounce glasses.
   c. six eight-ounce glasses.
   d. four eight-ounce glasses.
   e. ten eight-ounce glasses.

166. Biohazardous waste must be collected in impermeable polyethylene bags that are which color?
   a. black
   b. blue
   c. green
   d. red
   e. yellow

167. Which of the following body parts is considered the lower limit of a sterile surgical field?
   a. ankles
   b. knees
   c. shoulders
   d. waist
   e. neck

168. Gloves, gowns, and face shields or masks, are examples of
   a. asepsis.
   b. personal protective equipment.
   c. engineering controls.
   d. sterilization.
   e. decontamination.

169. Which of the following types of infection has a quick onset and a short duration, similar to the common cold?
   a. chronic infection
   b. acute infection
   c. latent infection
   d. purulent infection
   e. congenital infection

170. Which of the following are liquid at room temperature and may help reduce blood cholesterol?
   a. saturated fats
   b. lipids
   c. unsaturated fats
   d. fatty acids
   e. amino acids

171. Where is the most common intramuscular injection site for infants less than seven months old?
   a. deltoid
   b. gluteus maximus
   c. vastus lateralis
   d. epidermis
   e. dorsogluteal

172. What is the subscription part of a prescription?
   a. directions for the patient
   b. refill information
   c. directions for the pharmacist
   d. information that is included on the medication label
   e. the DEA number

173. Calculate the following drug dosage: An infant who weighs 12 pounds 5 ounces is ordered fluconazole qid for treatment of thrush. The label reads 150 mg in 3 cc of suspension. The recommended range of the medication is 3 mg/kg/day. How much should the infant receive per dose?
   a. 0.2 cc
   b. 0.4 cc
   c. 0.6 cc
   d. 0.8 cc
   e. 1.0 cc

174. A VIS is
  a. a form to request a DEA number.
  b. a form used to document vaccinations.
  c. a form that explains the safety and efficacy of the vaccine and adverse reactions caused by the vaccine.
  d. a form that tells the patient the immunization schedule.
  e. a form used to request controlled substances from the pharmacy.

175. In which of the following parts of the patient interview should the medical assistant ask the patient about drug allergies?
  a. chief complaint
  b. family history
  c. past medical history
  d. present illness
  e. social history

176. Which of the following positions is more comfortable for a patient who has dyspnea?
  a. dorsal recumbent
  b. lithotomy
  c. Trendelenburg
  d. semi-Fowler
  e. supine

177. A newborn's pulse is most accurately measured at which of the following sites?
  a. behind the knee
  b. inside the forearm
  c. over the apex of the heart
  d. side of the neck
  e. side of the wrist

178. The dorsalis pedis pulse is detected in which of the following areas of the body?
  a. back of the knee
  b. inner aspect of the elbow
  c. neck
  d. thumb side of the wrist
  e. top of the foot

179. If a mass is felt in a patient's neck, the finding is classified as which of the following?
  a. constitutional
  b. diagnostic
  c. functional
  d. objective
  e. subjective

180. A patient who has orthostatic hypotension should be helped from the supine position to the sitting position to prevent which of the following?
  a. defecation
  b. incontinence
  c. syncope
  d. pyrexia
  e. colic

181. The usual sequence of the general physical examination involves moving
  a. from the head toward the feet.
  b. from the center of the body.
  c. from the area where there is a complaint.
  d. from the trunk outward to the limb.
  e. from the feet toward the head.

182. Which of the following is an instrument used to inspect the inner structures of the eye?
  a. audiometer
  b. ophthalmoscope
  c. otoscope
  d. stethoscope
  e. tympanometer

183. A patient with chronic obstructive pulmonary disease has difficulty breathing. What term indicates this condition?
   a. bradypnea
   b. tachypnea
   c. eupnea
   d. apnea
   e. dyspnea

184. Which of the following would allow the medical assistant to document a firm, moveable abdominal mass?
   a. auscultation
   b. mensuration
   c. palpation
   d. manipulation
   e. observation

185. Which of the following is the documentation that is gathered regarding a patient's address and insurance information?
   a. chief complaint
   b. demographics
   c. family history
   d. medical history
   e. medications

186. The physician orders the medical assistant to draw a blood sample for a hematology test and a chemistry test. What is the correct order of draw?
   a. lavender, then gold-topped tubes
   b. green, then lavender-topped tubes
   c. gold, then lavender-topped tubes
   d. light blue, then gold-topped tube
   e. yellow, then gold-topped tubes

187. A positive result on a human chorionic gonadotropin (HCG) test in a 23-year-old woman most likely indicates which of the following conditions?
   a. anemia
   b. appendicitis
   c. diabetes mellitus
   d. hepatitis
   e. pregnancy

188. Which of the following refers to a combination of activities designed to ensure reliable and valid test results?
   a. infection control
   b. safety education
   c. quality control
   d. standard precautions
   e. sensitivity training

189. Measurement of which of the following is the most effective method to monitor a patient who takes warfarin (Coumadin)?
   a. bleeding time
   b. clotting time
   c. partial thromboplastin time (PTT)
   d. prothrombin time (PT)
   e. lipid profile

190. Which of the following serum levels can be measured to assess a patient's kidney function?
   a. amylase
   b. blood urea nitrogen
   c. cholesterol
   d. glucose
   e. hemoglobin

191. Which of the following organisms causes yeast infection?
a. *Aspergillus*
b. *Candida*
c. *Escherichia*
d. *Staphylococcus*
e. *Streptococcus*

192. The Mantoux test is used to determine the presence of which of the following?
a. mononucleosis
b. pregnancy
c. strep throat
d. blood in stool
e. tuberculosis

193. A stethoscope is required for a patient reporting which chief complaint?
a. constipation and abdominal pain
b. numbness and tingling in his or her right hand and fingers
c. rheumatoid arthritis
d. a skin lesion that has increased in size in the last two months
e. a sore throat

194. Which of the following procedures measures the amount of air moving into and out of the lungs?
a. bronchoscopy
b. intubation
c. spirometry
d. thoracentesis
e. nebulizer

195. To ensure proper ambulation, a walker should be level with the patient's
a. elbows.
b. hips.
c. waist.
d. wrists.
e. axillary.

196. Spore test monitoring in an autoclave is used to determine
a. whether an autoclave has an air leak.
b. whether the instruments were cleaned properly before sterilization.
c. whether the instruments were wrapped properly.
d. whether the autoclave is sterilizing instruments properly.
e. the sterility of the autoclave itself.

197. Which of the following is the name for the blood pressure value when the heart is contracting?
a. mean arterial pressure
b. systolic pressure
c. diastolic pressure
d. pulse pressure
e. high heart tension

198. How often should medical assistants check the expiration dates on supplies stored in examination rooms?
   a. daily
   b. weekly
   c. monthly
   d. annually
   e. bimonthly

199. Which of the following parts of a microscope holds the slide?
   a. condenser
   b. diaphragm
   c. eyepiece
   d. objective
   e. stage

200. An infant with a rectal temperature of 103.6°F would have an oral temperature of
   a. 100.6°F.
   b. 105.6°F.
   c. 101.6°F.
   d. 102.6°F.
   e. 98.6°F.

Answers and Explanations

General Medical Assistant Knowledge

1. e. The transverse plane divides the body into anterior and posterior portions. The sagittal plane divides the body into left and right parts. The midsagittal (or median) plane divides the body into left and right halves or into left and right halves. The frontal (or coronal) plane divides the body into front and back parts.

2. d. The cardiovascular system pumps and distributes blood throughout the body and delivers oxygen and other nutrients to every organ, tissue, and cell of the body. The nervous system serves to identify and evaluate internal and external environmental changes for the appropriate response. The respiratory system distributes oxygen and eliminates carbon dioxide. The sensory system works with the nervous system by acting as a medium through which external stimuli are transmitted to and interpreted by the brain. The integumentary system (the skin) provides protection, secretion, sensation, thermoregulation, and excretion functions.

3. a. The four major types of tissue of the body are muscle, nervous, epithelial, and connective. Vascular tissue is part of the cardiovascular system. The epidermis is the surface layer of the skin. Blood is part of the cardiovascular system. Vessels are part of the cardiovascular system.

4. c. The upper respiratory tract does not include the bronchi. The bronchi are part of the lower respiratory system. The nose, the pharynx, the upper trachea, and the larynx are all part of the upper respiratory system.

5. a. The accessory organs include the gallbladder, liver, and pancreas. The pancreas makes digestive juices called enzymes, which help to digest food further. The gallbladder stores bile (which is made in the liver), and the bile helps to digest fatty acids. The liver is where the blood that is carrying the nutrients, vitamins, and minerals from the small intestine enters. The liver is a "food processor," because it stores, changes, and releases the nutrients to the blood. The mouth, the esophagus, the large intestines, and the anus are part of the digestive system.

6. c. Hydrocele means swelling of the testes. Inflammation of the prostate is prostatitis. Inflammation of the cervix is cervicitis. Inflammation of the testes is orchitis. Impotence is the inability to maintain an erection.

7. e. Platelets, not leukocytes, are responsible for blood clotting.

8. b. Tendonitis is an inflammation of a tendon. A broken bone is a fracture. An injury to a muscles is a strain. Progressive wasting of muscle tissue is muscular dystrophy. Muscle pain is myalgia.

9. e. The function of the skin does not include transportation of immune cells. Leukocytes transport immune cells.

10. a. The nucleus is the control center that directs the activity of the cell. The cytoplasm is gel-like fluid in the cell. Lysosomes are organelles that contain digestive enzymes. There are four primary tissues: epithelial, connective, nervous, and muscle tissue. A cell membrane serves as a barrier by enclosing the cell contents.

11. c. Cholelithiasis are gallstones. Inflammation of a joint is called arthritis. Inflammation of the stomach is called gastritis. Inflammation of the gallbladder is cholecystitis. Cirrhosis is chronic degenerative disease of the liver.

12. a. The sensory organs do not include the pharynx. The pharynx is part of the digestive system.

13. d. Nephrectomy. *Nephr/a* = "kidney" + *ectomy* = "removal of."

14. e. *Cost/o* refers to the rib.

15. d. Behaviorism is a theory of behavior distinct from Freud's; it originated after Freud's theories, in response to them. All other choices—the id, subconscious, ego, and superego—are parts of human personality and psychology, according to Freud.

16. c. Dysphagia. *Dys* = "bad" + *phagia* = "swallowing."

17. b. Through cognitive theory, psychologists have developed approaches to help their patients analyze and understand errors in their thinking. Uncovering these cognitive errors helps an individual adapt to more realistic expectations and adjust his or her behavior and emotional responses to events accordingly. Examining dreams is part of the approach developed by Freud to explore the unconscious. Grief and loss is a concern of many psychologists, and needs and desires are general terms that may also be of concern to many psychologists and their patients.

18. c. *Plasty* means "surgical repair."

19. c. Hematoma. *Hema* = "blood" + *oma* = "mass" or "collection."

20. c. While a person who is undergoing trauma and loss may experience shock, it is not one of the stages described by Kübler-Ross in her theory of the five stages of grief. The five stages, in order, are denial, anger, bargaining, depression, and acceptance.

21. c. Defense mechanisms are strategies individuals use to avoid difficult or painful feelings; they are means to submerge upsetting emotions into an individual's subconscious. This is the opposite of choice **a**: a means to bring upsetting emotions to the surface of an individual's consciousness. Defense mechanisms is not a term used to describe a mood swing in an individual with bipolar disorder, despite the fact that bipolar patients may use defense mechanisms for other reasons. The other two choices—**b** and **e**—may sound like plausible definitions, but they are not technically exact definitions.

22. c. The CMA credential is not required in order to practice in the medical assisting profession because credentialing is a voluntary process. Most graduating medical assistants choose to get credentialed, earning either the CMA or the RMA credential, because most employers prefer to hire credentialed medical assistants. Credentialing is a way of indicating to others that the graduate has met the high standards set forth by the accrediting agencies.

23. b. The Commission on Accreditation of Allied Health Education Programs (CAAHEP) is the accrediting agency for the CMA credential. The American Medical Technologists (AMT) is the accrediting agency for the RMA. The American Medical Association (AMA) is the professional organization for physicians, and the American Association of Medical Assistants (AAMA) is the professional organizations for the CMA, although an RMA may join the organization.

24. a. A targeted resume is written specifically for an advertised job. A functional resume emphasizes the most valuable parts of the candidate's experience. A cover letter is usually sent with a resume to provide additional information explaining why the applicant feels he or she is the right person for the position being offered. A letter of recommendation is a note from a reference stating why the person writing the letter feels the applicant is suitable for the offered position.

25. b. The medical assistant should transfer the emergency room call about admitting an established patient with chest pain to the physician. Chest pain can be a life-threatening condition, so this call should be put through to the physician. Requesting a diet change for the next day—even for a patient in the intensive care unit—is not an emergency. A new patient may request a call back from the physician before scheduling an appointment, but it is up to the physician if he or she will make the call. Although the pharmaceutical representative is enthusiastic about a new drug, his or her business is to encourage the physician to use his or her company's drugs. The pharmaceutical representative's call is not an emergency, so the physician should not be interrupted.

26. a. Ophthalmologist. *Ophthal* = "eyes" + *ologist* = "one who studies."

27. b. Most of the incoming calls in a medical office are requests to make or cancel appointments or involve taking messages that need further action. It is necessary for a medical assistant to have the following supplies in order to handle incoming calls successfully: an appointment book (with which to make or cancel appointments), a calendar to check dates, a message pad or notepad to record messages, a pencil to use with a manual appointment book and with which to record messages. A telephone is obviously essential to handle incoming calls and should be placed in a location that ensures privacy. Many offices have a glass partition between the reception area and the office where the medical assistant answers the phone. Although the other items listed can be helpful when answering incoming calls, they are not essential.

28. e. Information about the patient's employer is not necessary when making an appointment for an established returning patient. The patient's daytime phone number and insurance information may have changed because his or her previous visit, so it is always necessary to make sure this information is updated with each visit. Without a correct, up-to-date phone number, the patient would not be able to be reached, if needed, prior to the appointment. It is always a good idea to request information about an insurance change to be sure the physician is a participating physician in the patient's insurance if the patient expects financial reimbursement from his or her insurance carrier for the office appointment. Patients get married or divorced, often changing their names when they do so.

29. d. It is against the law to release information about a patient to a friend, neighbor, lawyer, insurance company, unauthorized family member, employer of the patient, or any third party without the patient's written permission or consent to do so. The medical assistant should politely and tactfully inform the caller that patient information is restricted and can be released only with written permission.

30. a. Speaking clearly, a little more loudly, and a bit more slowly will make it easier for the hearing-impaired caller to understand the information being spoken by the medical assistant. Shouting is disrespectful to the patient. Slowing down the speed of one's speech and very carefully articulating the words will help clarify the spoken word and will be easier to hear and understand by the hearing-impaired caller.

31. e. The medical assistant should ask the caller to send a letter to the physician. Unidentified callers are not put through to the physician. The call may be from a salesperson trying a new tactic in order to get to speak directly to the physician. If the issue is important enough, the caller may send a letter to the physician about the matter he or she wished to discuss. The call should not be put through to the office manager because he or she probably won't be able to get the name and number of the caller either; it is not necessary to interrupt the office manager for this type of call. The medical assistant must always be courteous and polite regardless of the attitude and responses of the caller.

32. d. Dyspnea is the sensation of inadequate breathing, which is characteristic of an asthma attack.

33. d. Patient information can be shared with the referring physician. The referring physician, as a member of the healthcare team, may call a medical facility and request an appointment for one of his or her patients or call to get information on his or her patient. Patient information can be shared with healthcare team members. More than one physician can be actively involved in the care of the patient, and an attending physician is also considered a "needing to know" team member; therefore, he or she does not need the patient's written permission in order to obtain confidential patient information. Insurance carriers, lawyers, neighbors, and family members of the patient are not entitled to patient information without written permission of the patient.

34. c. A negative result for HIV indicates that the patient is not contagious, and therefore, it does not needed to be reported, although a positive HIV test *would* need to be reported. A gunshot wound, child abuse, spousal abuse, and elder abuse are violent crimes against members of society and are reportable incidences. A sexually transmitted disease needs to be reported. Pertussis, or whooping cough, is a contagious disease and needs to be reported.

35. b. *Res ipsa loquitur* is the Latin term meaning "the thing speaks for itself" when explaining negligent actions. *Respondeat superior* is the Latin term for the law that states that physicians are liable for the negligent acts of people under their supervision. Malfeasance is performing a wrong or unlawful act, such as selling signed prescription forms to a patient. Nonfeasance is failure to perform a required duty or obligation, such as a physician not ordering a test for a patient that a reasonable physician would order. Jurisprudence is a department of law that deals with legal issues and decisions.

36. d. Workers' compensation is a state insurance plan purchased by the employer to cover medical expenses for an employee injured on the job. Major medical and health maintenance organizations are private insurances. TRICARE and Medicare are government insurances.

37. a. Information documented in the medical record may not be used to reassure an employer about the health of an employee, because the employer is not entitled to private information about a patient unless the patient has provided written consent giving the employer access to his or her medical records. General information may be used for statistical and research purposes. Information in a patient's medical record should be kept current to record treatment provided to the patient by the primary physician and any other physicians involved in patient care. The law states that if a procedure or treatment is not documented, it was not done. A current, fully documented medical record is often the best defense for a physician being sued.

38. e. Urethrostenosis. *Urethra/o* = "ureter" + *stenosis* = "narrowing."

39. d. Splenomegaly. *Splen/o* = "spleen" + *megaly* = "enlargement."

40. b. Keeping information about an employee's political affiliation (or about any activity or organizational membership occurring off the premises of the place of employment) is not allowed under the Personnel Record Act. Records should be kept in a locked file for privacy. Information older than four years may not be divulged to inquiring future employers.

41. c. "Would you please describe the exercises you do each day that tend to cause the chest pain you are experiencing?" is an open-ended question because it requires more than a one-word answer. Open-ended questions encourage the patient to elaborate, thus giving the medical assistant information that may be useful in the patient's treatment plan. All of the other questions listed can be answered with only a yes-or-no or one-word response.

42. b. The W-2 form is issued once a year, by the end of January.

43. d. Empathy is understanding another's situation and being sensitive to the needs of another person by putting oneself in someone else's position. When a medical assistant has empathy and a caring attitude toward the patient, he or she will be in a position to establish a therapeutic relationship with the patient. Physical disabilities such as hearing and vision impairments may make communication more difficult. Stress may prevent a therapeutic relationship because the patient is so engrossed with worry that he or she does not hear the conversation. Mistrust prevents the patient from believing what is being said and, therefore, may interfere with the therapeutic relationship.

44. a. Stereotyping is making a generalized assumption of a group of individuals, which can be either positive or negative. Saying all elderly patients have difficulty walking is making an assumption about all elderly patients that is not true. Not all elderly patients have difficulty walking. Using the terms *some, many, a few,* or *a lot* do not group all elderly patients or all patients into a limited category, so those statements would not be considered stereotyping.

45. a. Lymphadenectomy. *Lympha/o* = "lymph node" + *ectomy* = "removal of."

46. a. Mats on the floors near entryways to prevent patient falls because of wet floors may be used for all patients and are not considered a special accessibility alteration for disabled patients. Widened corridors, bathroom handrails, Braille signs, and examination rooms made larger to accommodate wheelchairs are considered special alterations needed by individuals with physical impairments.

47. b. The Drug Enforcement Administration is responsible for registering physicians who write prescriptions for controlled substances such as narcotics. JCAHO is in charge of accreditation for healthcare organizations, OSHA is involved with safety issues in the workplace, HIPAA ensures the confidentiality of private information, and FDA regulates the manufacture of drugs and cosmetics.

48. a. Malfeasance is when a physician performs a wrong and unlawful act, such as selling signed prescription slips. Misfeasance is improperly performing a legal act such as amputating the wrong leg of a patient. Non-feasance is failure to perform a required duty or obligation, such as neglecting to order an EKG on a patient experiencing severe left-sided chest pain indicating a heart attack. Feasance is defined as performing an act and does not specify right or wrong. Disfeasance is not a medical term.

49. e. A contract cannot be made between any two individuals because individuals participating in a contract need to be mentally sound and of legal age. The contract must be of a legal nature for something of value (medical care) and made with a competent adult or emancipated minor (an individual no longer under the care, supervision, or custody of parents).

50. a. Libel is writing false statements that may harm or damage an individual's reputation, and slander is speaking falsely about someone in a way that may harm or damage the person's reputation. Battery is unlawful or unwanted touching. Bias is a predetermined attitude about a person or situation, usually one that can interfere with impartial judgment. Negligence is failing to use a reasonable amount of care, resulting in harm or damage to an individual.

51. d. Prescribing legal drugs will not result in the revocation of a physician's license. Impersonating another physician, providing substandard care, practicing without a license, and being addicted to chemical substances—either legal or illegal—are all reasons why a physician's license to practice medicine may be revoked.

52. d. A healthcare agent with durable power of attorney is the person chosen to make the final decisions about an individual's end-of-life healthcare. A durable power of attorney for healthcare does not have any legal rights to make decisions about any area of an individual's life other than heathcare. The person chosen to be the durable power of attorney does not have to be an attorney, a physician, or a medical assistant, but should be a trusted friend or family member of the patient's choosing.

53. e. Bronchitis is not a reportable incidence. Reportable incidences include contagious diseases such as rubeola (measles) or a positive HIV test result. Crimes against others such as spousal abuse and a stabbing (even if accidental or self imposed) are reportable incidences.

54. a. More control of employers over employee non-working hours was not part of the legislation passed in OSHA. The main goal of OSHA is to provide a safer and healthier environment in the workplace for both the employer and the employees. OSHA trains, educates, and offers consulting services to achieve the goal of a safer and healthier workplace.

55. c. The Food and Drug Administration (FDA) was the first attempt to establish consumer protection in the manufacture of drugs and foods. It was created by the Pure Food and Drug Act of 1906, which was the first in a series of acts designed to regulate foods and patent medicines. The Drug Enforcement Administration regulates controlled substances. The Clinical Laboratory Improvement Act regulates the standards for laboratory testing to ensure accurate test results. The Health Insurance Portability and Accountability Act involves patient privacy regulations. The Occupational Safety and Health Act was developed to ensure a safe and healthy environment in the workplace.

56. a. CLIA was not developed to increase the waiting time for specimen results. One of the goals of CLIA was to decrease the waiting time for specimen results so that the physician would be able to use the results of the test sooner when providing care to the patient. CLIA regulates lab tests done in smaller facilities to ensure their accuracy and to be sure that the facility is following the standards set by CLIA. CLIA categorizes lab tests according to complexity to ensure that only qualified employees perform the complex tests.

57. d. Replacing stairs with elevators in all buildings is not a regulation of the ADA. Handrails, widened doors, ramps, and elevators are some of the recommendations made by the ADA for accommodating disabled individuals and complying with the ADA.

58. e. *Respondeat superior* is the Latin term for the law that states that physicians are liable for the negligent actions of any employee working under the physician's supervision. Malfeasance is performing a wrong or unlawful act, misfeasance is improperly performing a legal act, and *res ipsa loquitur* means "the thing speaks for itself" when applied to the law of negligence.

Administrative Medical Assistant Knowledge

59. b. Transcription is the preparing of accurate reports by converting dictated physician notes into written documents. Typing is using a piece of equipment such as a typewriter or computer keyboard to produce documents. Modified block is a formatting style of letter writing. Outsourcing is a newer trend whereby larger medical facilities send out paperwork to companies that specialize in transcription.

60. a. *Dear Dr. Smith* is an example of a salutation. *To whom it may concern* is used only in situations when a communication is addressed to a company or organization for whom a specific contact is not known. *Best regards,* *Yours truly,* and *Sincerely* are examples of complimentary closings.

61. c. A surge protector is a device, such as an electrical power strip, used to help prevent damage caused by a sudden rise of current or increased voltage flowing into electrical equipment. The central processing unit (CPU) of a computer allows the computer to perform all operations. The motherboard is a circuit board that allows all computer parts to communicate with one another. A modem is a device that converts electronic signals allowing them to travel across telephone or cable lines, or even by satellite. A cursor is a device used to point to or to highlight a specific area on the computer screen.

62. d. System software operates the computer hardware; it is not considered computer hardware. Computer hardware is made up of the computer itself (the central processing unit) and devices that are connected to the computer, such as a printer, monitor, keyboard, or speaker. Computer software consists of programs that perform various tasks on the hardware.

63. b. A cursor is a blinking symbol used to point to a specific area on the computer screen. As the cursor is moved, it shows where the next letter, number, or symbol will be placed. A flash drive is a type of memory storage unit. The motherboard is a circuit board in the computer that allows all other parts in the computer to communicate with one another. A prompter is a symbol on a computer indicating that the computer is ready for input.

64. d. A fever is measurable by taking the patient's temperature, so it is not considered a subjective symptom. A subjective symptom is a symptom only the patient experiences, such as a headache or a backache. A subjective symptom cannot be seen or measured by others. Backache, stomach cramps, and chest pain cannot be seen or measured by anyone other than the patient. A patient may be asked to rate the degree of pain he or she is experiencing by using a number from one to ten, with ten being the most painful, but no one else can validate the extent of the pain he or she is feeling. An objective symptom is one that is measurable or can be seen by others, such as bleeding, bruises, fever, or blood pressure.

65. b. The law states that whoever created the medical record, which is considered a piece of property, owns the physical medical record. The patient owns the information contained in the medical record and is entitled to receive a copy of any or all information in the medical record.

66. d. Financial transactions are not part of the patient's medical record. The medical record can contain a listing of the patient's employer, insurance carrier, and insurance identification number, but it does not list any charges or payments made to the office for treatment. The medical record can be used as legal documentation to provide protection to the patient and the medical staff in cases of lawsuits. It is important to have accurate and complete documentation of all missed appointments, no-shows, and all other pertinent information. By keeping a continual record of the patient's medical care, patterns of illness, for example, can be detected and signal a need for intervention by the physician to manage the problem.

67. c. Active, inactive, and closed are the classification of files used in a medical office. Active files include patients currently being treated in the office; these records should be readily accessible. Inactive files include patients who have not been treated in the office recently, usually for the last two or three years. It is up to the individual office to decide when patient records become inactive. Inactive records can be removed from the currently used active records, but must be kept in a safe, secure location. Closed files are records that will not become active again. For example, records of deceased patients become closed files once the account has been paid. Closed records are also kept in a safe, secure area for an indefinite period of time.

68. b. A numeric filing system offers the most privacy for patients because there are no names on the file folders, only numbers. To find the patient's medical record, the name must be looked up in an alphabetic card file to obtain the number of the medical record, creating an addition step in the filing process. Patient medical records are not filed under subject. An alphabetic file system interferes with privacy by placing the patient's name on the outside of the medical record. New patient medical records are added to the numeric filing system in chronological order, meaning every new patient is added on to the last record in the system. Chronological filing is used to place the newest material on top when placed in the medical record.

69. b. The disadvantage of the numeric filing system is that it uses an alphabetic card system to locate the chart number of the patient, adding an extra step and taking more time. Advantages of the numeric filing system include easy expansion—adding on new records after the last record is easier than shifting the records to another area to adjust for overcrowding. Because there are no names on the record and only a number, the patient's privacy is maintained. Numeric files are not always arranged using color-coding, and if they are, color-coded file folders are not commonly used.

70. c. In chronological filing, there is not a problem list. Strict chronological filing means that regardless of the type of patient information coming into the office, the most recent item is added on the top. Items are not separated according to surgical reports, lab reports, or X-ray reports. Strict chronological filing makes it difficult to locate patient data unless a specific date is given.

71. b. High blood pressure, an elevated temperature, and a swollen ankle are all clinical complaints or symptoms that can be seen by others and measured, and are therefore referred to as objective clinical evidence. Temperature can be measured with a thermometer; blood pressure can be measured with a BP cuff and stethoscope; and a swollen ankle can be seen by observing the condition of the ankle. Symptoms such as headache, back pain, stomach cramps or stomach pain, and ankle pain are considered subjective symptoms because they can be felt only by the patient and cannot be seen or measured by others.

72. e. Whether or not the offices uses color-coded files should not be a consideration in choosing new cabinets for the medical office. There should be enough room for the cabinet's drawers to open or to turn a rotary file easily. The cabinets should be able to hold the estimated number of records expected and to provide patient confidentiality if the cabinet will be in view of patients. Locking devices or retractable doors for lateral shelving are more expensive, but if the cabinets are to be located in a separate locking room, the cost can be contained by purchasing cabinets without the locking mechanisms.

73. c. Certified mail should be used when proof is needed that a patient received a letter sent by a physician's office. Certified mail will prove that the letter was received, and the receipt will be kept at the post office for two years. For an additional fee, a return receipt request may be added to the letter. A return receipt means that the signature of the person accepting the letter will be obtained, and the receipt with the signature will be returned to the medical office, where it can be placed in the patient's medical record for documentation. Standard mail A and media mail are slower methods of mailing that do not provide proof of receipt.

74. e. Nine digits make up the ZIP + 4. The first three digits identify a major city or specific location in the city and the first five digits identify an individual post office. The last four digits identify street addresses.

75. a. Notations such as "Confidential" or "Personal" should be typed directly below the return address, aligned with the left, not the right, edge of the envelope, and should be underlined. Notations such as "Special Delivery" or "Certified" are typed directly below the stamp on the envelope.

76. e. ME is the correct USPS abbreviation for the state of Maine. State abbreviations need to be two capital letters, with no periods, to be read by the OCR scanner.

77. c. The medical assistant should place the most important mail on top, such as telegrams, registered mail, or certified letters. If mail were arranged by size or in alphabetical order, important mail may not be opened as soon as possible. Samples from drug companies should not be placed on top because the samples are not the most important pieces of mail.

78. a. To annotate means to jot down notes in the margin of a letter as a reminder of an action needing to be done. Annotating saves time because the letter does not have to be reread to perform the action, making the office run more efficiently. For example, if the letter needed information from the physician about material recorded in the patient's medical record, the record would be pulled and the annotated letter would be attached to the patient's record when the medical assistant gives it to the physician, so that he or she may provide the needed information.

79. b. A letter marked "Personal" would be placed on top of the sorted incoming mail. Other types of incoming mail that would be considered important enough to be placed at the top of the incoming mail would be telegrams or mail marked "Registered" or "Certified." Reports from the laboratory and pharmaceutical updates about drugs come to the office almost every day, and unless they are marked urgent, they would not be considered top priority. A letter with no return address is not necessarily an urgent or private letter and would not be considered a priority.

80. c. The 56-year-old male with dyspnea would be seen first. Patients with breathing problems are considered to be in life-threatening situations, so these patients would be treated ahead of the other patients listed in this question. Although a severe poison ivy rash, if located on the face, could interfere with breathing, the poison ivy rash is located on the patient's arms, and if no problem with breathing is indicated, the rash is uncomfortable but not life-threatening. A severe sore throat could also cause swelling in the throat and perhaps interfere with breathing, but if the patient doesn't indicate difficulty breathing, his or her condition is not life-threatening. A swollen ankle, although uncomfortable, does not present as a compound fracture, so it isn't considered life-threatening. The elderly female's symptoms of anorexia and confusion, although important, are not considered an emergency.

81. e. The wave system schedules three patients for the beginning of each hour, for example, three patients at 10:00 A.M. and three patients at 11:00 A.M. The goal of this scheduling style is to treat three patients per hour. Because each patient may not take the same amount of time for his or her visit with the physician, a more flexible schedule can be done. Double-booking is scheduling two patients for every time slot. The only time double-booking should be used is if two patients scheduled for the same time slot were to see different staff members; for example, one patient could be having an EKG procedure by the medical assistant, while the other patient is being examined by the physician. The modified wave style schedules two appointments on the hour and one appointment half past the hour. Clustering styles set aside blocks of time for patients with similar procedures or reasons for the visit, such as immunizations or well-baby clinic.

82. b. CPT (Current Procedural Terminology) codes are used for reporting medical services and procedures. Diagnoses, symptoms, illnesses, and allergies would be coded using the ICD (International Classification of Disease, 9th revision, Clinical Modifications) coding system.

83. a. Medicare Part B does not cover inpatient hospital visits. Medicare Part A covers inpatient hospital services. Medicare Part B covers most necessary physician services, preventive care, hospital outpatient services, durable medical equipment, laboratory testing, X-rays, mental healthcare, and some types of home care and ambulance services.

84. d. Medicare Part D provides for prescription coverage. Medicare Part A is hospital insurance. Medicare Part B covers outpatient services. Medicare Part C, also known as Medicare Advantage Plan, allows private insurance carriers to offer the same benefits that are offered by regular Medicare, using different rules. There is no Medicare Part E.

85. c. TRICARE was formerly known as CHAMPUS (Civilian Health and Medical Program of the Uniformed Services) and was designed to provide healthcare to dependants of military personnel.

86. d. International Classification of Diseases, 9th revision, Clinical Modification (ICD-9-CM) is used to identify and code diseases on insurance claims. Current Procedural Terminology is used to code services and procedures provided to the patient. The CMS-1500 form is the universal claim form for submitting insurance claims and was formally known as the HCFA 1500 form. The National Uniform Claims Committee (NUCC) is a voluntary organization that was developed to institute changes in the claim forms used in the reimbursement process.

87. a. External cause codes (E codes) classify poisoning and injuries and identify medications. E codes provide additional information for a diagnosis and cannot be used alone. V codes, or supplementary health factor codes, are used to classify factors that influence the health status of a patient. Morphology codes (M codes) are used mainly for cancer registries.

88. c. Accounts payable describes the amount of money owed by the medical office for products and services purchased on credit. Accounts receivable describes the amount of money owed to the office by patients.

89. c. The role of the medical assistant when checking in a patient is to confirm office coverage for patient's insurance plan. Confirming insurance coverage is important if the office expects to be reimbursed by the insurance carrier. The patient has the responsibility to learn about his or her own insurance plan because it is difficult for a medical assistant to know all the details about every insurance plan or to explain details to patients about individual insurance plans. If the patient has a question regarding his or her diagnosis, the medical assistant should encourage the patient to discuss this matter with the physician.

90. b. When an insurance policy pays a percentage of the balance after application of the deductible, it is referred to as the coinsurance. Many coinsurances split the cost of service 80/20, meaning that the insurance will pay 80% of the bill while the patient is responsible for 20% of the bill. The deductible is the predetermined amount that the patient must pay yearly before the insurance carrier provides reimbursement for medical services. The co-pay is the set amount that the patient must pay at each visit to the medical office. Coordination of benefits occurs when two insurance carriers will pay only a maximum of 100% of the charges for medical care.

91. a. When more than one policy pays on a claim, it is referred to as coordination of benefits. When an insurance policy pays a percentage of the balance after application of the deductible, it is referred to as coinsurance. Many coinsurances split the cost of service 80/20, meaning that the insurance will pay 80% of the bill while the patient is responsible for 20% of the bill. The deductible is the predetermined amount that the patient must pay yearly before the insurance carrier provides reimbursement for medical services. The co-pay is the set amount the patient must pay at each visit to the medical office. The birthday rule states that, with a married couple, the parent whose birthday comes first in the year is the guarantor for the medical expense of the child and his or her insurance is the primary insurance carrier.

92. e. When both parents (married) are covered by health insurance, claims for the family are paid according to birthday rule. The birthday rule states that, with a married couple, the parent whose birthday comes first in the year is the guarantor for the medical expense of the child and his or her insurance is the primary insurance carrier. When more than one policy pays on a claim, it is called a coordination of benefits. When an insurance policy pays a percentage of the balance after application of the deductible, it is referred to as coinsurance. Many coinsurances split the cost of service 80/20, meaning that the insurance will pay 80% of the bill while the patient is responsible for 20% of the bill. The co-pay is the set amount the patient must pay at each visit to the medical office.

93. b. A method of containing hospital costs has been adopted with a system called diagnostically related groups (DRGs). DRGs are used as a scale for reimbursement and are based on the assumption that all patients in the same DRG category will experience the same symptoms and need the same care. An average of the expenses incurred by the patients in a specific DRG is determined, and the inpatient facility is then reimbursed the average expense, not the actual expense of the hospitalization, in an effort to control healthcare spending. ICDs, or International Classification of Diseases, are numbers given to identify each disease or condition and are used on insurance claims. Outpatient prospective payment system (OPPS) is a reimbursement system for outpatients in which procedures and treatments are classified into groups for containing healthcare costs. Allowable amounts are what the insurance carriers pay for provided services.

94. d. Managed care organizations are not federal or state health insurance programs. All of the others listed are federal and state programs. Medicare is mainly for those over 65 years of age; Medicaid is for low-income families; CHAMPUS is for military personnel and families; workers' compensation is for individuals injured or killed while on the job.

95. d. Medicare pays 80% of the amount allowed on a claim. For example, if the physician charged $100 for services provided to a patient, Medicare might allow $80. Of this $80 allowed, Medicare would pay 80%, or $64. The patient is responsible for the remaining 20%, or $16. The physician who participates with Medicare must write off $20, thus equaling out the bill to the $100 charged. The $64 paid by Medicare plus $16 paid by the patient equals $80. This is the total amount allowed by Medicare and the maximum the physician may collect. The remaining $20 plus the $80 collected equals the $100 originally charged.

96. c. Mrs. Lee will have to pay the physician $12. Medicare pays 80% of the amount allowed. Because the amount allowed is $60 and Medicare pays $48, the difference (for which the patient is responsible) equals $12. The physician must write off the difference ($20) between the allowed amount ($60) and the amount charged by the physician's office ($80) in the adjustment column.

97. c. Volumes I and II of the ICD-9-CM books are needed to code diseases and conditions in the medical office. Volume I is a numeric list of the diagnostic codes, and Volume II is a tabular list of all diagnostic codes. Volume III is used for inpatient procedure coding and is not used in the medical office for outpatient coding.

98. d. All the last names are the same, so Unit 2 should be the next consideration when filing in alphabetic order. Frances with an "e" comes before Francis with an "i", so record 2 is the first one alphabetically. Numbers come before letters, making record 3 the next to be filed. The letter "J" comes before "S," placing record 4 come before record 1. The correct order for filing is 2, 3, 4, 1 when the names are alphabetically arranged using the rules of indexing units.

99. c. Codes that cannot stand alone are E codes. External cause codes (E codes) classify external causes of poisoning and injuries and identify medications. E codes are used to provide additional information and cannot be used alone. Modifiers are used with procedure codes. V codes (supplementary health factor codes) are classifications of factors that influence the health status of a patient; they identify reasons for healthcare other than diseases or injuries such as pregnancy. ICD-9-CM codes are the basis for the diagnostic coding system and may be used alone.

100. a. Traditional insurance policies include coverage on a fee-for-service basis. Traditional insurance plans will reimburse the insured for a specific amount of money based on a fee-for-service schedule outlined by the insurance carrier. Medicare is government insurance, usually for individuals age 65 and over. Medicaid is government insurance for low-income individuals. TRICARE is government insurance for retired military personnel and their families.

101. a. The claim will be denied, and the physician will not receive payment. A claims remittance will be sent to the physician's office with details of the error. The patient will not be charged or notified of the error.

102. b. The final step to the aging and collection process for a patient with private insurance is to send an overdue notice with the intent of turning the bill over to a collection agency if not paid promptly. Automatically sending a bill to the collection agency will not help the finances of an office because a collection agency usually keeps between 40% and 50% of whatever it collects. Calling the patient to request payment is not the final step in the aging process, nor is sending an itemized bill because these actions should have been done much sooner. Calling a patient's employer is against the privacy rule.

103. d. Non-duplication of benefits means that benefits will be coordinated between two separate insurance companies and the amount between the two insurance carriers will not exceed 100% of the billed amount. Some insurance carriers have rules that require the subscriber to wait a period of time before the insurance will pay (preexisting conditions). Recurring conditions treated on separate days are paid by insurance carriers.

104. e. Medical expenses for a patient injured at his or her place of employment should be submitted for workers' compensation. Each employer is required by law to carry workers' compensation insurance. The workers' compensation form lists the address to which the form should be sent to receive reimbursement for services provided. No bill should be sent to the patient, the patient's employer, or the patient's private insurance carrier. Unless there is a problem with the workers' compensation process, no information would be sent to the state insurance commissioner.

105. a. The name of the beneficiary and the patient's ID number will be listed on the front portion of a patient's Medicare card. No information is provided about the address of the patient or the expiration date of the Medicare card because the card may last the patient a lifetime unless he or she decides to change insurances. Physician information is also not included on the patient's Medicare card.

106. e. A 15-year-old girl would require the consent of an adult before treatment may be given by a physician. A 15-year-old girl is not considered an adult. An emancipated minor is an individual no longer under the care, supervision, or custody of parents; a 15-year-old girl who is living with her parents does not meet those requirements. The unconscious adult patient would be able to receive emergency care with an implied consent because he or she would not be able to make a decision while unconscious.

107. b. Scheduling a well-baby clinic on Tuesday mornings is an example of the clustering style of scheduling. Clustering is scheduling similar procedures for a specific time slot so that time and staff will be used more efficiently. Other examples of clustering would be school physicals and immunizations.

108. d. Practice-based scheduling can be a mix of any or all of the scheduling styles, to set up a system that works best for the individual office. For example, in a pediatric office, clustering may be used one morning a week for immunizations, and set appointments may be scheduled using the stream scheduling style for the remainder of the day.

109. d. Precertification, also referred to as preauthorization, is the required prior permission or approval from the insurance carrier before the patient may be treated or have a specific procedure performed by the physician. A referral is a request from the primary physician to another physician to have the patient examined and treated. Protocol is the act of following a set of rules. Capitation is a type of insurance that pays the physician per patient, not per visit. Prepayment is paying ahead of time before receiving service.

110. a. Charges for a patient's office visit is an example of an account receivable. Accounts receivable deals with money owed to the medical office for services provided to a patient. Accounts payable deals with money owed by the medical office for services or supplies purchased on credit or for work performed by others, such as the maintenance crew.

111. d. The one-write system is also referred to as the pegboard system. The pegboard system is made up of no carbon required (NCR) forms that allow multiple forms to be layered, so that information has to be written only once yet will be applied to many documents with one writing. The POMR and SOMR are types of patient documentation used in the patient's medical record. The encounter form is used to itemize patient services.

112. d. Allowing three months to pass before billing the patient for the office visit will not help the collection process, because the longer the time from the service, the more difficult it is to collect the payment. Notifying a patient about his or her financial responsibility before an appointment is helpful in collecting the money due at the time of service. Return envelopes make it easier to send in payments and calling about overdue accounts may be helpful if the patient needs to be reminded of the financial obligation or a payment plan needs to be arranged.

113. c. A restrictive endorsement is the safest type of endorsement. It is a stamp marked "Pay to the order of" listing the name of the bank where the deposit will be made and followed by the physician's name. A blank endorsement is a signature only, and if the check is made out to "cash," anyone may sign and cash the check. The other terms listed are not types of check endorsement.

114. c. Payroll documents for employees need to be kept for a minimum of four years.

115. d. Unemployment insurance is not paid through FICA contributions; it is paid by the employer, not the employee. Through FICA deductions, the employee contributes to retirement income, Medicare coverage, disability insurance, and benefits for survivors through the percentage of employee wages withheld by the employer. The employer matches the FICA contribution of the employee—that is, it pays the same amount the employee does.

116. c. Major medical insurance—a type of traditional insurance—is most commonly used to cover serious medical expenses or catastrophic illness and injuries. Medicare is government insurance mainly for the elderly. Medicaid is government insurance, mainly for low-income individuals. CHAMPVA is a health benefit program for veterans with 100% service-related disabilities and the veterans' family members. HMOs are insurance organizations offering a range of healthcare coverage.

117. e. The usual fee is the amount a physician charges for a service or procedure. The customary fee is the average fee charged by a provider in a specific geographical area for a specific service or procedure. The reasonable fee is the fee charged for an exceptionally difficult or complex procedure requiring more time and effort on the part of a provider. The usual, customary, and reasonable charges are not based on regulations of the government.

118. b. The Truth-in-Lending Act is a law designed to protect consumers and requires full disclosure of any additional charges that may apply to a bill, such as interest. The Fair Debt Collection Practices Act was enacted to protect individuals owing money from abusive, unfair collection procedures. The Good Samaritan law protects an individual performing first aid from liability. The Americans with Disabilities Act protects individuals with disabilities from discrimination.

119. e. Some insurance carriers require pre-authorization before a patient can be seen by another physician if reimbursement is expected for the care given, so it is not true that patient referrals may be made without pre-authorization from the insurance carrier.

120. a. Patient advocates are liaisons between the patient and the physician or healthcare provider. A healthcare agent is the person selected to make healthcare decisions for a patient when he or she is no longer able to make healthcare decisions. An advance directive is a type of living will filled out by a patient listing his or her of end-of-life healthcare decisions and naming the healthcare agent. An attorney is used in court cases and may be chosen as the patient's healthcare agent, but is not automatically a patient's healthcare agent or the patient advocate.

121. a. Ergonomics is the science of helping workers reach maximum productivity and reduce fatigue and discomfort through office furniture and equipment design. Kinesiology is the study of body movement. Physiology is the study of how the body functions. Body mechanics is the process of using the correct muscle during movement to prevent injury. Etiology is the study of causes, such as the cause of a specific disease or condition.

122. b. The Centers for Disease Control and Prevention is the organization that developed rules regarding the proper handling of blood products and other infectious material. Universal Precautions is the practice of avoiding contact with body fluids of patients by wearing gloves, goggles, and gowns. The Occupational Safety and Health Administration is the organization involved in ensuring employee safety and health in the working environment. The Food and Drug Administration is the agency that regulates foods and patent medicines. The Controlled Substances Act was established to put a tighter control on the substances being abused by the public.

123. c. Marking exits only in Braille would not help the safety of the medical office, because all exits should be marked for everyone to see clearly. Marking an exit in Braille only would not be sufficient. Working smoke alarms and fire alarms are essential for safety. Training all employees on safety measures is important for safety. Most offices prohibit smoking in buildings, but may provide a sand-filled receptacle outside, allowing people to safely dispose of extinguished cigarettes.

124. e. Perspiration is not considered a biohazardous fluid mainly because it does not contain blood. A biohazardous material is an infectious waste harmful to humans and animals usually including blood and blood products. Synovial fluid from joint cavities, pleural fluid from the lung cavity, and cerebrospinal fluid from the spinal cord cavity all have the potential to have blood mixed in with the fluid, thus making them potentially biohazardous substances. Blood and blood products are considered biohazardous substances.

125. d. Completing bookkeeping once every two weeks is not a bookkeeping guideline because bookkeeping should be done on a daily basis. Using dark blue or black ink makes the work done easier to see over time. Careful checking of numbers and math is essential to accurate bookkeeping.

126. e. An encounter form is not considered the universal insurance claim form; the CMS 1500 is considered the universal claim form. An encounter form is also called a superbill or a charge slip and does provide an itemized account of an office visit made by the patient. Because it comes in a triplicate form, it is convenient to give a copy to the patient, place a copy in the patient's medical record for documentation, and occasionally attach a copy to an insurance claim for paper submission.

Clinical Medical Assistant Knowledge

127. b. Furosemide (Lasix) should be included on a crash cart. Furosemide (Lasix) helps to reduce fluid buildup in people with congestive heart failure. The other choices are drugs that are not considered necessary or useful in an emergency.

128. b. The medical assistant should immediately resume chest compressions and rescue breathing. The only other reasonable choice is to give 30 chest compressions and deliver another shock, but the correct protocol is to continue with chest compressions and rescue breathing until EMS help arrives.

129. d. An automated external defibrillator (AED) is used to treat heart arrhythmias by delivering an external shock to the patient. The other choices will not be helped by the use of an AED. A CVA is a cerebrovascular accident. A diabetic coma occurs when blood sugar gets too high and the body becomes severely dehydrated. Seizures are symptoms of a brain problem that happen because of sudden, abnormal electrical activity in the brain. A stroke is generally considered another term for a CVA.

130. b. The medical assistant is not protected from liability simply because the patient agrees to treatment. Just because the patient agrees to treatment does not mean that the medical assistant will remain blameless if something goes wrong. However, if the medical assistant provided reasonable care, acted in good faith, and did not go beyond the scope of a medical assistant's skills during patient care, then he or she is protected from liability. Once the medical assistant decides to and begins to help, he or she must also stay with the injured person until some with equal or greater skill arrives to take over.

131. d. The medical assistant should apply ice directly to the burn and keep it there until the pain is relieved. Cool water will warm up when placed on the burn and is not as effective as ice. Opening the blister increases the chances of infection. Applying ointment is ineffective on the burn, and covering the burn may cause the covering to stick to the burn. Applying pressure to the area that is burned causes pain, and the absorbent pad may stick to the burn.

132. b. According to basic cardiac life support procedures, one breath every five seconds describes appropriate rescue breathing for an adult patient. Constant and frequent rescue breathing is used to get and keep blood flowing to the brain and to buy time until EMS personnel, or other qualified individuals, arrive.

133. c. To control bleeding or hemorrhaging, the medical assistant should initially apply direct pressure. Applying direct pressure will help slow or stop the blood flow. Applying heat to the wound will increase blood flow. Applying ice over the wound will slow down the swelling, but should not be used until after the bleeding is under control. Applying a tourniquet is the last resort in controlling bleeding, because using a tourniquet on a limb can cause complete cutoff of blood circulation to the limb and lead to amputation. Immobilizing the body part will not control bleeding or hemorrhaging.

134. a. A third-degree burn destroys the epidermis and dermis, including the nerve endings. A first-degree burn involves the epidermal layer only. A second-degree burn involves the epidermis and upper dermis. A minor burn is a first-degree burn. An acid burn could be first-degree, second-degree, or third-degree.

135. d. A strain is a muscle injury. A fracture is a broken bone. A ligament injury is a sprain. A broken blood vessel and a cartilage injury are called different things depending on where the injury is.

136. e. Checking the airway to make sure that the patient can breathe should be one of the first steps when rendering first aid, because if the patient is not breathing, he or she will not live. The pulse must be checked to make sure the heart is pumping, but only after the airway has been checked. Capillary action is a general term relating to how liquid moves along the surface of a solid; it doesn't relate to first aid treatment. Pain or injury to limbs would not be assessed until the medical assistant has made sure that the patient is able to breathe. Checking the patient's emotional state is not as urgent as checking his or her breathing.

137. c. Strains are not a cause of breathing emergencies. Strains are injuries caused by stretching or tearing of muscle or tendons.

138. c. The amount of body surface represented by the head and neck is 9%. According to the rule of nines, each body part is considered 9% of the body surface.

139. b. Shock is caused by lack of blood flow and oxygen to body tissue. A tear in a ligament is a sprain. A heart attack is a myocardial infarction. A stroke, or cerebrovascular accident, happens when blood flow is cut off to part, or parts, of the brain. Epistaxis is a nosebleed.

140. c. A seizure is the involuntary contraction/relaxation of a muscle. There are many causes, including brain injury or high fever. Myocardial infarction is a heart attack. Syncope is fainting. Hemorrhage is excessive bleeding. Abrasion is an open wound resulting in the scraping off of skin layers.

141. b. Insulin shock causes severe hypoglycemia, a drastic drop in blood glucose levels. Hyperkalemia is indicated by high potassium levels in the blood. A diabetic coma causes severe hyperglycemia, an extreme increase in blood glucose levels. Hypokalemia is indicated by low levels of potassium in the blood. Syncope is fainting.

142. d. An autoclave sterilizes items using steam pressure at a temperature of 250°F to 270°F (120°C to 130°C) with 15 lbs. of pressure for a specific amount of time.

143. c. The Environmental Protection Agency is one of the agencies that regulates the disposal of infectious waste outside the workplace. The other agency that sets policies and guidelines for disposing of hazardous materials is the Occupational Safety and Health Administration. The Association for Professionals in Infection Control works to improve health and patient safety by reducing risks of infection through education, research, consulting, collaboration, and public policy. The Centers for Disease Control and Prevention is a federal agency under the Department of Health and Human Services that focuses on disease prevention. The Exposure Control Plan outlines protective measures to be followed in efforts to limit the exposure of employees to blood-borne pathogens and other infectious agents. The Department of Health and Human Services, part of the executive branch of the U.S. government, oversees any activity relating to health and medicine, including food and drug safety, health insurance, and the like; it also oversees activities relating to the human services and welfare, such as Temporary Assistance to Needy Families.

144. e. Sterilization is a method used for the complete destruction of all microorganisms, pathogenic or otherwise. An antiseptic is any substance that limits the development of bacteria. Aseptic refers to the actions practiced to make and maintain an area or object free from infection or pathogens. Disinfection is killing or rendering inert most but not all pathogenic microorganisms. Sanitization is a process used to lower the number of microorganisms on a surface by cleansing the surface with soap, detergent, water, and manual friction.

145. c. When a patient has taken a drug for an extended period of time and the desired effect lessens or does not occur at all, it is called tolerance. When a patient has a tolerance for a drug, the patient's body has become accustomed to it. A toxic effect is a harmful effect, such as those resulting from chemotherapeutic drugs. An idiosyncratic effect is an abnormal response to a drug in a patient with a peculiar defect in body chemistry. A vasoconstrictor controls hemorrhage and relaxes the bronchioles to relieve asthma attacks. Potentiation is an interaction between two drugs that enhances the effect of either drug.

146. b. The Drug Enforcement Administration is responsible for enforcing the Controlled Substance Act. The American Medical Association is the professional association of physicians, which advocates for them and their concerns. The Food and Drug Administration determines the safety and effectiveness of prescription and nonprescription drugs. The Federal Trade Commission works to eliminate unfair or deceptive marketplace practices. The Physician's Desk Reference contains information on most major prescription pharmaceutical products.

147. b. A prophylactic medication is a drug used to lessen or prevent the effects or symptoms of a disease. A curative is a medicine that cures disease or relieves pain. A replacement drug is used to replace a substance that is missing. A therapeutic drug is used to treat a disease or condition. A supplemental drug supplies the body with something that the body lacks.

148. a. Meats and nuts are a source of protein. Raw vegetables are a source of fiber. Citrus fruit is a source of fiber. Butter and oils are fats.

149. d. Dairy products are sources of calcium and vitamin D. Meats and nuts contain vitamin B6 and vitamin E. Raw vegetables contain vitamin C, vitamin E, and vitamin B6. Citrus fruits contain vitamin C. Oils do not contain vitamins.

150. c. Anaerobes survive in the absence of oxygen; they must have an oxygen-free environment in order to grow. The term *spore* refers to a dormant type of bacteria, or a part of a bacteria, that has formed a thick capsule around itself; spores are very resistant to chemicals and heat. Aerobes are microorganisms that need oxygen to live and grow. A vector carries an infective agent from one host to another organism. A fomite is any inanimate object that can carry a microorganism.

151. b. Bleach is an effective disinfecting agent used in the medical office to destroy blood-borne pathogens and is appropriate for instruments, surfaces, furniture, and equipment. A one-to-ten bleach-and-water solution is used (one part bleach, ten parts water). Alcohol is widely used as an antiseptic, but is not as effective as other products in inhibiting the growth and reproduction of microorganisms. Chlorhexidine gluconate is an antibacterial agent used on the skin and mucous membranes. Formaldehyde is a powerful disinfectant gas. Phenol is a very poisonous colorless compound used as an antimicrobial agent.

152. a. Disinfecting the examination table after each patient is one method outlined in standard precautions, used to prevent the transmission of disease to another patient. Emptying the garbage can weekly will not prevent the transmission of disease. The garbage can should be emptied every day or when full. Needles should never be recapped because of the risk of a needle stick injury. Wearing heavy gloves to remove instruments from the autoclave will prevent a burn only; it will not prevent the transmission of disease. Wearing two sets of gloves when cleaning surgical instruments will prevent an injury from a sharp instrument.

153. b. A generic drug is not protected by a trademark but is registered by the Food and Drug Administration; a generic drug has no patent. A controlled drug has abuse potential. A research drug has not been approved by the FDA. An over-the-counter drug can be purchased without a prescription. A trademark drug is officially registered with the FDA and can legally be sold only by the company that owns the trademark.

154. d. If a physician prescribes amoxicillin 500 mg capsules po qid for 10 days, then 40 capsules should be dispensed because qid is four times a day: $4 \times 10 = 40$ capsules.

155. b. An antiarrhythmic is used for a heart condition to prevent or alleviate irregularities in the force or rhythm of the heart. Antacids are used to relieve heartburn, sour stomach, or acid reflux. Anesthetics are medications that are used to reduce pain. Antibiotics are used to prevent, control, or reduce a bacterial infection. Analgesics are used to relieve pain.

156. c. The food pyramid does not suggest eating more carbohydrates. The food pyramid includes less emphasis on carbohydrates.

157. d. Vitamin E is an example of a fat-soluble vitamin. All of the other vitamins listed are water-soluble vitamins.

158. a. Chain of infection means "all of the factors required for infectious disease to spread." The chain of infection is a series of steps that must occur for disease to spread. Droplet transmission is a way for the infectious disease to spread through a cough or a sneeze. Infection control is a method used to reduce the chances of infection by using standard hygienic measures, such as washing hands and wearing gloves. Inflammatory response is a reaction to an infection, chemical, or physical injury that can include redness, swelling, heat, and pain. Nosocomial infection is an infection acquired or occurring in a hospital.

159. d. Washing hands is the most important medical aseptic technique to prevent the transmission of pathogens. Cleaning the examination table, sanitizing the patient's skin, sterilizing instruments, and wearing gloves are also important medical aseptic techniques, but none of those steps is as important as washing hands.

160. d. A mask is used to prevent the air droplets from being transmitted to the medical assistant. Gloves would prevent a contact transmission, and goggles would be a barrier for the medical assistant's eyes, but neither of these items would prevent the medical assistant from breathing in air droplets. Using a gown would prevent spills and splashes from contaminating the medical assistant's clothing, but would not prevent the medical assistant from breathing in the air droplets. A laboratory coat would protect the medical assistant from transmitting microorganisms from his or her work area to the public and would protect his or her clothing, but, again, would not prevent the medical assistant from breathing in the air droplets.

161. d. Substances that prevent or inhibit the growth of a fungus are known as fungicides. Antiseptics inhibit the growth and development of microorganisms. Disinfectants are antimicrobial agents. Germicides are agents that destroys germs. Analgesics are used to relieve pain.

160. b. A drug that is given sublingually is placed under the tongue. A drug that is injected into the deltoid muscle would be an intramuscular injection. A drug that is administered buccally would be put between the lower teeth and the cheek. A drug that is injected into the muscle is an intramuscular drug. An intradermal injection is injected into the dermis, that is, under the epidermis, or outer layer.

163. c. The dose would be two capsules.
1 g = 1,000 mg
0.5 g = 0.5 × 1,000 = 500 mg
(D / H) × Q = 500 / 250 = 50 / 25 = 2 × 1
= 2 capsules

164. a. High-protein diets are often used before surgery to help build and heal body tissues. Protein does not help when there is an infection present. Protein-rich diets are not used to treat hypothermia (low body temperature) or hyperthermia (high body temperature). Protein-rich diets are also not used to treat hypertension, which requires a low-sodium diet.

165. b. The recommended amount of water to ingest daily is eight eight-ounce glasses of water. Water is the body's principal chemical component, and continual daily replenishment is critical.

166. d. Red leakproof bags are used for contaminated supplies such as gloves, gauze, bandages, gowns, and linens. OSHA's Blood-borne Pathogens Standard requires that containers and appliances containing biohazardous materials be labeled with a biohazard warning label. The biohazard warning label must be fluorescent orange or orange-red and contain the biohazard symbol and the word "biohazard" in a contrasting color.

167. d. The waist is considered the lower limit of a sterile surgical field. A sterile field is considered a one-inch border surrounding the tray, and only the area between the shoulders and the waist is sterile. In order to keep your hands sterile, you must keep sterile, gloved hands above the waist.

168. b. Gloves, gowns, and face shields are examples of personal protective equipment. Personal protective equipment is used to decrease or eliminate exposure to potentially infectious materials. Asepsis means "free from pathogens." Engineering controls are methods used to change the way something is made in order to make the item safer for healthcare workers to use. For example, to prevent needle stick injury after phlebotomy, an engineered needle cover is attached to a needle holder to eliminate the need for removal of the needle from the needle holder. Sterilization is a method used for the complete destruction of all microorganisms, pathogenic or otherwise. Decontamination involves the application of a substance to equipment, surfaces, or other items to kill pathogenic microorganisms.

169. b. Acute infection typically has a quick onset and short duration, similar to the common cold. A chronic infection lasts for a long time—sometimes years or a lifetime. An example of a chronic infection is hepatitis C. A latent infection is an infection in which the patient experiences alternating periods of being symptomatic and being symptom-free. A purulent infection is an infection that contains, produces, or consists of pus. A congenital infection is any infection present at birth that was acquired by the infant either in the uterus or during passage through the birth canal.

170. c. Unsaturated fats are liquid at room temperature and may help reduce blood cholesterol. Unsaturated fats are found primarily in vegetables and olive oils. Saturated fats are found in meat, butter, and egg yolks and increase blood cholesterol. Lipids transport fat-soluble vitamins, insulate the body, and provide fatty acids. Fatty acids are either saturated or unsaturated fats. Amino acids are the building blocks of proteins and are not directly linked to cholesterol or its ability to be metabolized.

171. c. The vastus lateralis is the most common intramuscular injection site for infants less than seven months old because it is located away from any major blood vessels and nerves. The deltoid is not used because the muscle is not large enough to absorb the medication. The gluteus maximus is not used because of the lack of muscle in this area. The epidermis is not used because the medication needs to be administered intramuscularly. The dorsogluteal is not used because of the suboptimal immune response.

172. c. The subscription part of a prescription consists of directions for the pharmacist. Directions for the patient are part of the signatura. Refill information includes the number of times the prescription can be refilled. Information that is included on the medication label is part of the signature. The DEA number is included only on the label if the drug is a controlled substance.

173. d. The dose would be 0.8 cc.
5 oz / 16 oz = 0.3125 = 0.3 lbs + 12 lbs = 12.3 lbs.
12.3 lbs. / 2.2 kg = 5.6 kg
3 mg a day × 5.6 kg = 16.8 mg/day
16.8 mg / 4 times/day = 4.2 mg/dose
(4.2 mg / 150 mg) × 3cc = 0.08 cc

174. c. A VIS is a form that explains the safety and efficacy of the vaccine and adverse reactions caused by the vaccine. A DEA number is requested through the Drug Enforcement Agency. A vaccination record is used to document vaccinations. An immunization schedule tells the patient the timetable for immunization shots. A form used to request controlled substances from the pharmacy is a prescription.

175. c. An allergy to a drug that the patient had taken would be noted in past medical history, where the reaction to the drug would also be recorded. The patient's chief complaint is the reason for his or her current visit. Family history refers to the health information of the patient's blood relatives. Present illness refers to the current illnesses and conditions experienced by the patient. The patient's social history relates to the patient's living arrangements, occupation, hobbies, and so on.

176. d. The semi-Fowler position is used to relax tension of the abdominal muscles, allowing for improved breathing. The dorsal recumbent position is when the patient is lying on his or her back. The lithotomy position is when the patient is lying on his or her back with feet in stirrups. The Trendelenburg position is when the patient lies with his or her head approximately 30° lower than his or her outstretched legs and feet. Supine is when the patient is lying on his or her back.

177. c. A newborn's pulse should be taken over the apex, or pointed lower end, of the heart. This is called the apical pulse; at this site, the beat of the heart itself can be felt. It is located to the left of the breastbone and above the bottom of it. All other pulse sites are taken over an artery: the popliteal pulse, behind the knee; the brachial pulse, inside the forearm, on the inner aspect of the elbow; the carotid pulse, in the neck on either side of the trachea (windpipe); the radial pulse, on the inside, or thumb-side, of the wrist at the base of the thumb.

178. e. The dorsalis pedis is the pulse site at the top of the foot. The popliteal pulse is behind the knee; the brachial pulse is inside the forearm, on the inner aspect of the elbow; the carotid pulse is in the neck on either side of the trachea (windpipe); the radial pulse is on the inside, or thumb-side, of the wrist at the base of the thumb.

179. d. Objective symptoms can be observed by an examiner. Constitutional symptoms refer to a group of symptoms that can affect many different systems of the body. Diagnostic refers to a medical condition or disease identified by its signs, symptoms, and the results of various diagnostic procedures. A functional symptom has no identified cause despite extensive diagnostic assessments. Subjective symptoms are felt by the patient but are not observable by an examiner.

180. c. A sitting position would prevent syncope, or fainting, because orthostatic hypotension happens when the blood pressure has momentarily dropped and the person feels dizzy and may have blurred vision. The other choices don't relate to changes in blood pressure. Defecation is the final act of digestion through which waste material (feces) is eliminated from the digestive tract via the anus. Incontinence generally refers to urinary incontinence, or the loss of bladder control. Pyrexia is a term that means fever, and colic refers to apparent abdominal pain in early infancy.

181. a. The general physical examination involves a thorough assessment of all the body systems; the physician uses an organized and systematic approach starting with the head and moving toward the feet.

182. b. An ophthalmoscope is used to examine the interior of the eye. An audiometer is used to measure hearing. An otoscope is used to examine the outer parts of the ear. A stethoscope is used to amplify and, therefore, hear sounds produced by the body. A tympanometer analyzes the status of the middle ear.

183. e. Dyspnea is a term that indicates shortness of breath or difficulty in breathing. The other terms represent conditions relating to respiration or heartbeat. Bradypnea is an abnormal decrease in the respiratory rate of fewer than ten respirations per minute. Tachypnea is an abnormally fast heart rate (greater than 100 beats per minute). Eupnea refers to normal respiratory rate, and apnea refers to the temporary cessation of breathing.

184. c. Palpation is the process of feeling with the hands to detect signs of disease. The other choices are also methods that can be used during a patient examination. Auscultation is the process of listening to the sounds produced within the body to detect signs of disease. Mensuration is the process of measuring the patient. Manipulation is the process of moving a patient's body parts. Observation involves looking at the patient and his or her complexion, movements, reactions, and so forth.

185. b. Demographic information includes the patient's name, address, telephone number, employment information, and insurance information. The chief complaint is the reason for the patient's visit. The family history is a review of the health status of the patient's blood relatives. Medical history is a review of the patient's medical condition, surgeries, hospitalizations, and current medical conditions. The medications part of a patient's record consists of a review of the current medications that the patient is taking.

186. c. The correct order of draw is gold-topped, then lavender-topped tubes. Gold is for chemistry, and lavender for hematology. Gold is drawn first to prevent the anticoagulant from the lavender from contaminating the gold-topped tube.

187. e. A positive result on a human chorionic gonadotropin test in a 23-year-old woman most likely indicates pregnancy. Human chorionic gonadotropin is a hormone that is produced by the developing fertilized egg; small amounts are then secreted into the blood and urine. Anemia is a blood disorder. Appendicitis refers to the inflammation of the appendix. Diabetes mellitus is a chronic disease characterized by the inability of the body to regulate the level of glucose in the blood. Hepatitis is a condition in which the liver is inflamed.

188. c. Quality control refers to a combination of activities designed to ensure reliable and valid test results; it is a method used to evaluate the proper performance of testing procedures, supplies, or equipment in a laboratory. Infection control measures are taken to control nosocomial infections (infections that are a result of treatment in a hospital). Safety education includes measures to prevent injuries. Standard precautions are a set of procedures that aim to reduce the chance of transmitting infectious microorganisms in a healthcare setting. Sensitivity training does not relate to laboratory testing at all; it is a form of training intended to make people more aware of their own prejudices and more sensitive to others.

189. d. Measurement of prothrombin time (PT) is the most effective method to monitor patients who take warfarin (Coumadin), an anticoagulant drug, because it assists in the evaluation of bleeding disorders. The other choices do relate to testing of the blood: Bleeding time measures how fast the small blood vessels close; clotting time measures the time it takes for a sample of blood to clot; partial thromboplastin time (PTT) also measures the time a sample of blood takes to clot, but it is the most common coagulation test for assessment of heparin therapy, not warfarin therapy. A lipid profile does not relate to blood clotting: It is a test that measures cholesterol, high density lipoprotein, and low density lipoprotein.

190. b. Urea nitrogen is produced as a waste product in the process of metabolizing proteins. It forms in the liver and travels via the bloodstream to the kidneys to be excreted. Since the kidneys are involved in the elimination of urea from the body, testing the level of urea nitrogen is one way to understand how well the kidneys are functioning. Blood urea nitrogen can be measured to assess a patient's kidney function; because the kidneys are involved in the elimination of urea, which travels to the kidneys trough the bloodstream, a blood urea nitrogen (BUN) test is one way to understand how well the kidneys are functioning. Amylase is an enzyme instrumental in carbohydrate digestion. Cholesterol is a type of blood lipid, or fat. Glucose is the most common form of sugar in the body. Hemoglobin is a molecule that transports oxygen in the red blood cells.

191. b. *Candida* causes yeast infections. All the other choices, except for *Aspergillosus*, are all microorganisms that can be found and reproduce to pathogenic levels in the human body. Aspergillosis is a condition caused by a fungus found in dead leaves, compost, and other decayed vegetation.

192. e. The Mantoux test is used to test for tuberculosis. Mononucleosis testing looks for the heterophile antibody. A pregnancy test looks for HCG. A strep test looks for Group A streptococcal bacteria. An occult blood test looks for hidden blood in the stool.

193. a. The patient complaining of constipation and abdominal pain will require a stethoscope examination, because a stethoscope is an instrument used to amplify and hear sounds produced by the body. The patient with numbness and tingling in his right hand and fingers would not need a stethoscope examination because numbness and tingling do not produce sound. Rheumatoid arthritis, skin lesions, and sore throats do not produce sound either, so a stethoscope would not be used for these examinations.

194. c. Spirometry measures the amount of air moving into and out of the lungs. Bronchoscopy is the examination or treatment of the bronchi by means of a hollow tube or fiberoptic viewing tube with a light and lens attached. Intubation is the process of passing an endotracheal tube (breathing tube) into the trachea (windpipe). Thoracentesis is a surgical puncture of the chest wall into the parietal cavity for aspiration of fluids. A nebulizer is a breathing treatment administered with a bronchodilator (a medicine used to dilate the bronchi).

195. b. To ensure proper ambulation, a walker should be level with the patient's hips. Specifically, the top of the walker should be at the same height as the top of the hip bone, and the elbows should be bent about 30° while the patient uses the walker. If the top of the walker were level with the patient's elbows, waist, or axilla (underarm), then it would be too high for the patient to maneuver the walker safely. If the top of the walker were level with the patient's wrists, then it would be too low for the patient to maneuver the walker safely.

196. d. The specific purpose of spore test monitoring in an autoclave is to determine whether the autoclave is sterilizing instruments properly. If the autoclave has an air leak, the autoclave would cause incomplete sterilization and the sterilization indicators would not change color. Also, the sterilization indicator would be used to tell whether instruments were wrapped properly. If the autoclave's water reservoir has been overfilled, wet steam would be produced, which would cause too much condensation, preventing the sterilization process from being completed.

197. b. Systolic pressure is a measure of blood pressure while the heart is contracting. Mean arterial pressure is a term used in medicine to describe an average blood pressure in an individual. Diastolic pressure is a measure of blood pressure while the heart is relaxed, between heartbeats. Pulse pressure is the difference between systolic and diastolic blood pressure, or the change in blood pressure seen during a contraction of the heart. High heart tension pressure means high blood pressure.

198. c. Medical assistants should check the expiration dates on supplies stored in examination rooms monthly. Supply expiration dates are marked with the month, day, and year of expiration. Checking the expiration dates before reordering supplies will ensure adequate stock of supplies. Checking the supplies daily or weekly is not necessary. Checking the supplies bimonthly or annually will not prevent the use of expired supplies.

199. e. The stage is a flat surface that holds the slide for viewing. An opening in the solid surface allows illumination of the slide from below. The condenser is a lens system between the light source and the object being viewed. The amount of light focused on the object is controlled by the diaphragm. The eyepiece is the first lens system, or ocular lens, located at the top of the body of the microscope. The objective is the second lens system, which consists of three objective lenses located on the revolving nosepiece, each with a different degree of magnification.

200. d. An infant with a rectal temperature of 103.6° F would have an oral temperature of 102.6° F; the oral temperature is one degree lower than the rectal temperature because the rectum is highly vascular and provides a more closed cavity than the mouth does, so it is warmer.

7 ▶ RMA PRACTICE EXAM

This practice exam is designed to help you practice for the Registered Medical Assistant exam by including questions not only in academic and clinical areas in which you have command of important information, but also in areas in which you need more review. Because the format mimics that of the RMA exam, it will also help you familiarize yourself with the format of the actual exam.

One of the main reasons for taking this practice exam, in addition to getting more practice in answering the kinds of questions on the RMA exam, is to identify your strengths and weaknesses. Make a note of the types of questions you missed and the topics on which you need to concentrate your study time further. Do not neglect any subject area unless you have an almost-perfect score in that area. Remember to refer back to Chapter 2 to design a study plan that fits in with your schedule and lifestyle. Good luck!

RMA Practice Exam

1.	ⓐ	ⓑ	ⓒ	ⓓ	36.	ⓐ	ⓑ	ⓒ	ⓓ	71.	ⓐ	ⓑ	ⓒ	ⓓ
2.	ⓐ	ⓑ	ⓒ	ⓓ	37.	ⓐ	ⓑ	ⓒ	ⓓ	72.	ⓐ	ⓑ	ⓒ	ⓓ
3.	ⓐ	ⓑ	ⓒ	ⓓ	38.	ⓐ	ⓑ	ⓒ	ⓓ	73.	ⓐ	ⓑ	ⓒ	ⓓ
4.	ⓐ	ⓑ	ⓒ	ⓓ	39.	ⓐ	ⓑ	ⓒ	ⓓ	74.	ⓐ	ⓑ	ⓒ	ⓓ
5.	ⓐ	ⓑ	ⓒ	ⓓ	40.	ⓐ	ⓑ	ⓒ	ⓓ	75.	ⓐ	ⓑ	ⓒ	ⓓ
6.	ⓐ	ⓑ	ⓒ	ⓓ	41.	ⓐ	ⓑ	ⓒ	ⓓ	76.	ⓐ	ⓑ	ⓒ	ⓓ
7.	ⓐ	ⓑ	ⓒ	ⓓ	42.	ⓐ	ⓑ	ⓒ	ⓓ	77.	ⓐ	ⓑ	ⓒ	ⓓ
8.	ⓐ	ⓑ	ⓒ	ⓓ	43.	ⓐ	ⓑ	ⓒ	ⓓ	78.	ⓐ	ⓑ	ⓒ	ⓓ
9.	ⓐ	ⓑ	ⓒ	ⓓ	44.	ⓐ	ⓑ	ⓒ	ⓓ	79.	ⓐ	ⓑ	ⓒ	ⓓ
10.	ⓐ	ⓑ	ⓒ	ⓓ	45.	ⓐ	ⓑ	ⓒ	ⓓ	80.	ⓐ	ⓑ	ⓒ	ⓓ
11.	ⓐ	ⓑ	ⓒ	ⓓ	46.	ⓐ	ⓑ	ⓒ	ⓓ	81.	ⓐ	ⓑ	ⓒ	ⓓ
12.	ⓐ	ⓑ	ⓒ	ⓓ	47.	ⓐ	ⓑ	ⓒ	ⓓ	82.	ⓐ	ⓑ	ⓒ	ⓓ
13.	ⓐ	ⓑ	ⓒ	ⓓ	48.	ⓐ	ⓑ	ⓒ	ⓓ	83.	ⓐ	ⓑ	ⓒ	ⓓ
14.	ⓐ	ⓑ	ⓒ	ⓓ	49.	ⓐ	ⓑ	ⓒ	ⓓ	84.	ⓐ	ⓑ	ⓒ	ⓓ
15.	ⓐ	ⓑ	ⓒ	ⓓ	50.	ⓐ	ⓑ	ⓒ	ⓓ	85.	ⓐ	ⓑ	ⓒ	ⓓ
16.	ⓐ	ⓑ	ⓒ	ⓓ	51.	ⓐ	ⓑ	ⓒ	ⓓ	86.	ⓐ	ⓑ	ⓒ	ⓓ
17.	ⓐ	ⓑ	ⓒ	ⓓ	52.	ⓐ	ⓑ	ⓒ	ⓓ	87.	ⓐ	ⓑ	ⓒ	ⓓ
18.	ⓐ	ⓑ	ⓒ	ⓓ	53.	ⓐ	ⓑ	ⓒ	ⓓ	88.	ⓐ	ⓑ	ⓒ	ⓓ
19.	ⓐ	ⓑ	ⓒ	ⓓ	54.	ⓐ	ⓑ	ⓒ	ⓓ	89.	ⓐ	ⓑ	ⓒ	ⓓ
20.	ⓐ	ⓑ	ⓒ	ⓓ	55.	ⓐ	ⓑ	ⓒ	ⓓ	90.	ⓐ	ⓑ	ⓒ	ⓓ
21.	ⓐ	ⓑ	ⓒ	ⓓ	56.	ⓐ	ⓑ	ⓒ	ⓓ	91.	ⓐ	ⓑ	ⓒ	ⓓ
22.	ⓐ	ⓑ	ⓒ	ⓓ	57.	ⓐ	ⓑ	ⓒ	ⓓ	92.	ⓐ	ⓑ	ⓒ	ⓓ
23.	ⓐ	ⓑ	ⓒ	ⓓ	58.	ⓐ	ⓑ	ⓒ	ⓓ	93.	ⓐ	ⓑ	ⓒ	ⓓ
24.	ⓐ	ⓑ	ⓒ	ⓓ	59.	ⓐ	ⓑ	ⓒ	ⓓ	94.	ⓐ	ⓑ	ⓒ	ⓓ
25.	ⓐ	ⓑ	ⓒ	ⓓ	60.	ⓐ	ⓑ	ⓒ	ⓓ	95.	ⓐ	ⓑ	ⓒ	ⓓ
26.	ⓐ	ⓑ	ⓒ	ⓓ	61.	ⓐ	ⓑ	ⓒ	ⓓ	96.	ⓐ	ⓑ	ⓒ	ⓓ
27.	ⓐ	ⓑ	ⓒ	ⓓ	62.	ⓐ	ⓑ	ⓒ	ⓓ	97.	ⓐ	ⓑ	ⓒ	ⓓ
28.	ⓐ	ⓑ	ⓒ	ⓓ	63.	ⓐ	ⓑ	ⓒ	ⓓ	98.	ⓐ	ⓑ	ⓒ	ⓓ
29.	ⓐ	ⓑ	ⓒ	ⓓ	64.	ⓐ	ⓑ	ⓒ	ⓓ	99.	ⓐ	ⓑ	ⓒ	ⓓ
30.	ⓐ	ⓑ	ⓒ	ⓓ	65.	ⓐ	ⓑ	ⓒ	ⓓ	100.	ⓐ	ⓑ	ⓒ	ⓓ
31.	ⓐ	ⓑ	ⓒ	ⓓ	66.	ⓐ	ⓑ	ⓒ	ⓓ					
32.	ⓐ	ⓑ	ⓒ	ⓓ	67.	ⓐ	ⓑ	ⓒ	ⓓ					
33.	ⓐ	ⓑ	ⓒ	ⓓ	68.	ⓐ	ⓑ	ⓒ	ⓓ					
34.	ⓐ	ⓑ	ⓒ	ⓓ	69.	ⓐ	ⓑ	ⓒ	ⓓ					
35.	ⓐ	ⓑ	ⓒ	ⓓ	70.	ⓐ	ⓑ	ⓒ	ⓓ					

RMA Practice Exam

101.	ⓐ	ⓑ	ⓒ	ⓓ
102.	ⓐ	ⓑ	ⓒ	ⓓ
103.	ⓐ	ⓑ	ⓒ	ⓓ
104.	ⓐ	ⓑ	ⓒ	ⓓ
105.	ⓐ	ⓑ	ⓒ	ⓓ
106.	ⓐ	ⓑ	ⓒ	ⓓ
107.	ⓐ	ⓑ	ⓒ	ⓓ
108.	ⓐ	ⓑ	ⓒ	ⓓ
109.	ⓐ	ⓑ	ⓒ	ⓓ
110.	ⓐ	ⓑ	ⓒ	ⓓ
111.	ⓐ	ⓑ	ⓒ	ⓓ
112.	ⓐ	ⓑ	ⓒ	ⓓ
113.	ⓐ	ⓑ	ⓒ	ⓓ
114.	ⓐ	ⓑ	ⓒ	ⓓ
115.	ⓐ	ⓑ	ⓒ	ⓓ
116.	ⓐ	ⓑ	ⓒ	ⓓ
117.	ⓐ	ⓑ	ⓒ	ⓓ
118.	ⓐ	ⓑ	ⓒ	ⓓ
119.	ⓐ	ⓑ	ⓒ	ⓓ
120.	ⓐ	ⓑ	ⓒ	ⓓ
121.	ⓐ	ⓑ	ⓒ	ⓓ
122.	ⓐ	ⓑ	ⓒ	ⓓ
123.	ⓐ	ⓑ	ⓒ	ⓓ
124.	ⓐ	ⓑ	ⓒ	ⓓ
125.	ⓐ	ⓑ	ⓒ	ⓓ
126.	ⓐ	ⓑ	ⓒ	ⓓ
127.	ⓐ	ⓑ	ⓒ	ⓓ
128.	ⓐ	ⓑ	ⓒ	ⓓ
129.	ⓐ	ⓑ	ⓒ	ⓓ
130.	ⓐ	ⓑ	ⓒ	ⓓ
131.	ⓐ	ⓑ	ⓒ	ⓓ
132.	ⓐ	ⓑ	ⓒ	ⓓ
133.	ⓐ	ⓑ	ⓒ	ⓓ
134.	ⓐ	ⓑ	ⓒ	ⓓ
135.	ⓐ	ⓑ	ⓒ	ⓓ

136.	ⓐ	ⓑ	ⓒ	ⓓ
137.	ⓐ	ⓑ	ⓒ	ⓓ
138.	ⓐ	ⓑ	ⓒ	ⓓ
139.	ⓐ	ⓑ	ⓒ	ⓓ
140.	ⓐ	ⓑ	ⓒ	ⓓ
141.	ⓐ	ⓑ	ⓒ	ⓓ
142.	ⓐ	ⓑ	ⓒ	ⓓ
143.	ⓐ	ⓑ	ⓒ	ⓓ
144.	ⓐ	ⓑ	ⓒ	ⓓ
145.	ⓐ	ⓑ	ⓒ	ⓓ
146.	ⓐ	ⓑ	ⓒ	ⓓ
147.	ⓐ	ⓑ	ⓒ	ⓓ
148.	ⓐ	ⓑ	ⓒ	ⓓ
149.	ⓐ	ⓑ	ⓒ	ⓓ
150.	ⓐ	ⓑ	ⓒ	ⓓ
151.	ⓐ	ⓑ	ⓒ	ⓓ
152.	ⓐ	ⓑ	ⓒ	ⓓ
153.	ⓐ	ⓑ	ⓒ	ⓓ
154.	ⓐ	ⓑ	ⓒ	ⓓ
155.	ⓐ	ⓑ	ⓒ	ⓓ
156.	ⓐ	ⓑ	ⓒ	ⓓ
157.	ⓐ	ⓑ	ⓒ	ⓓ
158.	ⓐ	ⓑ	ⓒ	ⓓ
159.	ⓐ	ⓑ	ⓒ	ⓓ
160.	ⓐ	ⓑ	ⓒ	ⓓ
161.	ⓐ	ⓑ	ⓒ	ⓓ
162.	ⓐ	ⓑ	ⓒ	ⓓ
163.	ⓐ	ⓑ	ⓒ	ⓓ
164.	ⓐ	ⓑ	ⓒ	ⓓ
165.	ⓐ	ⓑ	ⓒ	ⓓ
166.	ⓐ	ⓑ	ⓒ	ⓓ
167.	ⓐ	ⓑ	ⓒ	ⓓ
168.	ⓐ	ⓑ	ⓒ	ⓓ
169.	ⓐ	ⓑ	ⓒ	ⓓ
170.	ⓐ	ⓑ	ⓒ	ⓓ

171.	ⓐ	ⓑ	ⓒ	ⓓ
172.	ⓐ	ⓑ	ⓒ	ⓓ
173.	ⓐ	ⓑ	ⓒ	ⓓ
174.	ⓐ	ⓑ	ⓒ	ⓓ
175.	ⓐ	ⓑ	ⓒ	ⓓ
176.	ⓐ	ⓑ	ⓒ	ⓓ
177.	ⓐ	ⓑ	ⓒ	ⓓ
178.	ⓐ	ⓑ	ⓒ	ⓓ
179.	ⓐ	ⓑ	ⓒ	ⓓ
180.	ⓐ	ⓑ	ⓒ	ⓓ
181.	ⓐ	ⓑ	ⓒ	ⓓ
182.	ⓐ	ⓑ	ⓒ	ⓓ
183.	ⓐ	ⓑ	ⓒ	ⓓ
184.	ⓐ	ⓑ	ⓒ	ⓓ
185.	ⓐ	ⓑ	ⓒ	ⓓ
186.	ⓐ	ⓑ	ⓒ	ⓓ
187.	ⓐ	ⓑ	ⓒ	ⓓ
188.	ⓐ	ⓑ	ⓒ	ⓓ
189.	ⓐ	ⓑ	ⓒ	ⓓ
190.	ⓐ	ⓑ	ⓒ	ⓓ
191.	ⓐ	ⓑ	ⓒ	ⓓ
192.	ⓐ	ⓑ	ⓒ	ⓓ
193.	ⓐ	ⓑ	ⓒ	ⓓ
194.	ⓐ	ⓑ	ⓒ	ⓓ
195.	ⓐ	ⓑ	ⓒ	ⓓ
196.	ⓐ	ⓑ	ⓒ	ⓓ
197.	ⓐ	ⓑ	ⓒ	ⓓ
198.	ⓐ	ⓑ	ⓒ	ⓓ
199.	ⓐ	ⓑ	ⓒ	ⓓ
200.	ⓐ	ⓑ	ⓒ	ⓓ

1. In the doctor's office, the patient's blood oxygen saturation is measured with
   a. spirometry.
   b. peak flow meter.
   c. pulse oximeter.
   d. arterial blood gas.

2. Which of the following is a source of vitamin C?
   a. meats and nuts
   b. milk
   c. citrus fruits
   d. oils

3. Principles of professional ethics may include all of the following EXCEPT
   a. objectivity.
   b. financial control.
   c. responsibility.
   d. confidentiality.

4. Which type of drug schedule has no acceptable medical use?
   a. schedule I
   b. schedule II
   c. schedule III
   d. schedule IV

5. A medical assistant scheduled to remove stitches from a patient's arm noticed that the area was red, swollen, and painful upon the slightest touch. The patient requested to see the physician and was reluctant to let the medical assistant remove the sutures. Which of the following attribute is most important in dealing with this situation?
   a. flexibility
   b. dependability
   c. initiative
   d. effective communication

6. Which of the following terms means "incision in the muscle"?
   a. cholecystectomy
   b. myotomy
   c. cholecystotomy
   d. myelography

7. Which of the following is a written description of work experiences, skills, and educational background?
   a. cover letter
   b. resume
   c. transcript
   d. diploma

8. What is the term for the visual examination of the vagina and cervix?
   a. colposcopy
   b. colonoscopy
   c. cholecystectomy
   d. endoscopy

9. Which of the following would be an example of personal accountability?
   a. switching days off with a fellow team member
   b. being courteous to patients
   c. admitting to an error made
   d. smiling at all patients as they enter the office

10. Two rescuers are performing CPR on a nine-year-old child who collapsed and is not breathing. Which of the following actions should the rescuers take?
   a. Attach the AED and follow the voice prompts.
   b. Attach the AED only if it has two child-size pads.
   c. Continue CPR (15:2) for 5 cycles, then attach the AED.
   d. Continue CPR (30:2) for 5 cycles, then attach the AED.

11. The RMA certification is maintained by
    a. applying for a license within the state where you are employed.
    b. earning 45 CEUs within three years or 15 CEUs per year.
    c. maintaining a 40-hour-a-week position within a hospital facility.
    d. becoming a member of the AAMA national organization.

12. Which of the following identifies the components that are central to Sigmund Freud's theories of personality?
    a. id, ego, behaviorism, consciousness
    b. id, ego, superego
    c. loss, grief, denial, ego
    d. behavior, needs, desires

13. Which of the following pulses is auscultated with a stethoscope?
    a. apical
    b. brachial
    c. temporal
    d. radial

14. Demographic information to be included in the patient's record includes
    a. vital signs.
    b. results of tests.
    c. name, address, and telephone number.
    d. discharge summary.

15. Which of the following questions is considered legal when conducting a job interview of a perspective employee?
    a. "Tell me about your family. Any children?"
    b. "What an interesting name. What is your ethnic background?"
    c. "Do you have any problems with your health?"
    d. "Are you authorized to work in the United States?"

16. How often should quality control be performed for laboratory procedures?
    a. daily
    b. weekly
    c. biweekly
    d. monthly

17. In a normal blood cell differential, what is the total number of cells counted?
    a. 50
    b. 100
    c. 150
    d. 200

18. The basic parts of the communication process include
    a. message, sender, receiver, channels, feedback.
    b. message, source, patient, receiver, channels.
    c. sender, receiver, message, source.
    d. channels, source, feedback.

19. A capillary puncture is most likely to be performed on the outer edges of the plantar surface (underside) of the heel in which of the following patients?
    a. a 10-month-old infant
    b. a 4-year-old child
    c. a 16-year-old adolescent
    d. a 38-year-old adult

20. Which of the following attributes refers to the ability to understand someone else's feeling or situations?
    a. sympathy
    b. dependability
    c. empathy
    d. responsibility

21. Which of the following terms describes nearsightedness?
a. diplopia
b. myopia
c. cataract
d. hyperopia

22. The process of cleaning and removing debris from instruments is known as
a. aseptic technique.
b. disinfection.
c. sterilization.
d. sanitization.

23. Which of the following is the best source of fiber?
a. meats and nuts
b. dairy products
c. raw vegetables
d. citrus fruits

24. A clear liquid diet consists of all of the following EXCEPT
a. chicken broth.
b. apple juice.
c. milk.
d. tea.

25. All of the following may interfere with impartiality of the treatment of patients EXCEPT
a. bias.
b. stereotyping.
c. prejudice.
d. diplomacy.

26. Dosages for _____ are most frequently calculated according to body weight.
a. children
b. adults
c. teens
d. elderly individuals

27. The study of body language is called
a. kinesiology.
b. gestures.
c. communications.
d. physiology.

28. Which of the following terms means "inflammation of a vein"?
a. angiitis
b. arteritis
c. phlebitis
d. phlebostenosis

29. A procedure to screen for breast cancer is known as which of the following?
a. cystography
b. mammography
c. myelography
d. pyelography

30. Before transferring a call to another extension, which of the following is the most appropriate for the medical assistant to do?
a. Give the patient the extension number to which he or she is being transferred in case the phone gets disconnected.
b. Record the patient's name and phone number.
c. Place the patient on hold while the medical assistant checks to be sure that the extension number is not busy.
d. Ask the patient to describe in detail the reason he or she is calling.

31. Incoming calls should be answered
a. ideally by the first ring and definitely by the third ring.
b. after the medical assistant completes making an appointment with a waiting patient.
c. ideally by the fourth ring and definitely by the fifth ring.
d. after the medical assistant completes a conversation with another patient on the phone.

32. When a responsive adult agrees to receive first aid care, it is known as
    a. refusal.
    b. implied consent.
    c. expressed consent
    d. obligation.

33. When receiving a call from an angry patient, the medical assistant should
    a. transfer the call to the office manager.
    b. transfer the call to the physician.
    c. stay calm and listen to the patient.
    d. agree with whatever the patient says to help calm him or her down.

34. Screening or triaging incoming calls is
    a. obtaining all needed information for new patient registration.
    b. a scheduling style that is based on the patient's type of insurance.
    c. a method of eliminating patients with financial problems.
    d. a method of prioritizing the urgency of calls.

35. Which of the following is included in a patient's vital signs?
    a. chest circumference
    b. height and weight
    c. reflexes
    d. respiration rate

36. When communicating with a hearing-impaired patient, the medical assistant should do all of the following EXCEPT
    a. face the patient when speaking.
    b. tape all conversations for later review by the patient.
    c. speak a little louder.
    d. jot down instructions for the patient.

37. The medical assistant is performing a venipuncture and has just filled the last specimen tube. Which of the following should the medical assistant do before withdrawing the needle?
    a. Have the patient make a fist.
    b. Label the tubes.
    c. Reassure the patient.
    d. Release the tourniquet.

38. All of the following statements about treating children are true EXCEPT
    a. children should be treated with the same respect that an adult patient would receive.
    b. children should be allowed to handle some simple instruments to help decrease fear of treatment.
    c. children should not be told the truth about a procedure to be done because it may frighten them.
    d. children should be told if a procedure is going to hurt.

39. When communicating with an illiterate patient, the medical assistant may
    a. use oral explanations and directions.
    b. write all directions out in details.
    c. speak more loudly to emphasize directions.
    d. use nonverbal forms of communication such as hand signs.

40. Which of the following best describes the location of hypochondriac region of the body?
    a. below the pelvis
    b. below the ribs
    c. distal to the colon
    d. center of the stomach

41. Which of the following techniques is used to protect the patient from exposure to outside pathogens during minor surgery?
   a. asepsis
   b. standard precautions
   c. isolation
   d. reverse isolation

42. Which of the following organizations developed the guidelines for standard precautions?
   a. Occupational Safety and Health Administration
   b. American Medical Association
   c. Centers for Disease Control and Prevention
   d. Joint Commission on the Accreditation of Healthcare Organizations

43. Which of the following instruments is used to look into the ears?
   a. audiometer
   b. otoscope
   c. percussion hammer
   d. ophthalmoscope

44. Which of the following vitamins aids in blood clotting?
   a. vitamin B2
   b. vitamin K
   c. vitamin C
   d. vitamin E

45. Evaluating the effectiveness of communication may be done by
   a. using channels.
   b. using feedback.
   c. asking closed questions.
   d. waiting to see if the patient questions what the medical assistant is saying.

46. Which of the following is the section of a prescription with instructions to the patient on how to take the prescribed medication?
   a. inscription
   b. signature
   c. subscription
   d. superscription

47. Which form, when signed by a patient, allows a representative to act as a healthcare agent for a patient?
   a. implied consent
   b. durable power of attorney
   c. a patient's will
   d. living will

48. Which term means "vomiting blood"?
   a. epistaxis
   b. hemaarthrosis
   c. hematemesis
   d. hyperemesis

49. All of the following events are reportable by the physician EXCEPT
   a. births and deaths.
   b. stab wounds.
   c. child abuse.
   d. hypertension.

50. Which of the following combining forms is matched correctly with the meaning?
   a. *latero* = "below"
   b. *peri* = "around"
   c. *hypo* = "above"
   d. *antero* = "back"

51. Which of the following is the term used to describe the improper release of confidential information?
a. libel
b. slander
c. invasion of privacy
d. misdemeanor

52. A medical assistant who continually asks to leave work early for personal reasons is lacking the quality of
a. foresight.
b. initiative.
c. dependability.
d. efficiency.

53. Triage involves all of the following EXCEPT
a. screening phone calls.
b. diagnosing the patient's condition.
c. determining how serious the illness is.
d. determining if the patient has an emergency.

54. An AED delivers a(n)
a. electrocardiogram.
b. hypovolemic shock.
c. electric shock.
d. cardiopulmonary resuscitation.

55. Which of the following describes a lawful act performed improperly by a physician?
a. malfeasance
b. misfeasance
c. nonfeasance
d. feasance

56. Which of the following terms describes untrue oral statements made to damage an individual's reputation?
a. libel
b. negligence
c. bias
d. slander

57. Which of the following instruments is used by the physician to determine the presence or absence of bowel sounds?
a. audiometer
b. colonoscope
c. dosimeter
d. stethoscope

58. The Occupational Safety and Health Act (OSHA) was legislation passed to ensure all of the following EXCEPT
a. free workplace consultations for help in identifying and correcting workplace hazards.
b. safer and healthier working environments for employees.
c. training in the care of biohazardous waste.
d. legal assistance to employers being sued.

59. All of the following accommodations may be made to comply with the regulations recommended in the Americans with Disabilities Act EXCEPT
a. providing wider, uncluttered hallways for easy maneuvering of wheelchairs.
b. providing Braille signs.
c. roomier examination rooms offering easier access of wheelchairs.
d. inquiring about the mobility devices a patient uses to see whether the office can accommodate them.

60. All of the following statements are true about the Medical Practice Acts EXCEPT
a. each state regulates the licensure of physicians.
b. a medical assistant is under the direct supervision of a physician.
c. a medical assistant may have his or her license revoked for performing certain tasks.
d. a medical assistant may be held responsible for acts done improperly.

61. Which of the following contains the genetic material of the cell?
   a. nuclear membrane
   b. gene
   c. cytoplasm
   d. nucleus

62. The three types of muscle tissue are
   a. respiratory, rough, and skeletal.
   b. cardiac, nervous, and skeletal.
   c. skeletal, smooth, and cardiac.
   d. integumentary, vascular, and skeletal.

63. Which of the following describes the purpose of monitoring autoclaves with spore tests?
   a. to determine whether an autoclave has a leak
   b. to determine whether instruments have been cleaned properly before sterilizing
   c. to ensure that an autoclave is sterilizing instruments properly
   d. to ensure that instruments have been wrapped correctly

64. The process by which nutrients leave the gastrointestinal system and enter the bloodstream is called
   a. ingestion.
   b. digestion.
   c. metabolism.
   d. absorption.

65. When a blood pressure cuff is deflated, the first tapping sound is the
   a. mean arterial pressure.
   b. systolic pressure.
   c. diastolic pressure.
   d. pulse pressure.

66. The Good Samaritan Law protects an individual
   a. who performs first aid voluntarily on an injured person.
   b. who performs first aid as part of his or her job.
   c. no matter what type of help the individual tries to provide an injured person.
   d. who performs first aid without financial compensation.

67. Which of the following classes of drugs is administered as a cleansing preparation before performing a radiologic study of the intestinal tract?
   a. anticholinergics
   b. antiemetics
   c. antispasmodics
   d. cathartics

68. An advance directive
   a. is the same thing as a living will.
   b. allows an individual to describe in detail wishes for end-of-life care and allows a durable power of attorney for healthcare to be selected.
   c. specifically prevents anatomical gifts to be made and specifies which attorney will be used to settle an estate.
   d. is a consent form for surgical intervention when complications arise during medical treatment.

69. Which suffix means "pain"?
   a. *algia*
   b. *iasis*
   c. *rrhea*
   d. *rrhexis*

70. Which term is used to mean ordering an individual to appear in court and to bring any papers, books, or information necessary to explain an issue?
   a. *res ipsa loquitur*
   b. *respondeat superior*
   c. *guardian ad litem*
   d. *subpoena duces tecum*

71. Which of the following is the study and treatment of the colon, rectum, and anus?
   a. urology
   b. colonoscopy
   c. proctology
   d. endoscopy

72. All of the following information about the W-4 form used by the Internal Revenue Service is true EXCEPT
   a. it includes the marital status of an employee.
   b. the employee is responsible for completing the W-4 form.
   c. it is used to calculate the payroll deductions for an employee.
   d. it may be changed only once a year.

73. Which is not an approved right in the Patient's Bill of Rights?
   a. right to patient confidentiality
   b. right to informed consent
   c. right to be treated with dignity
   d. right to refunds for complications that arise during hospital stays

74. The medical assistant is attending to a responsive child injured in a bicycle accident. He has a sharp pain and swelling in the right leg, which looks strangely bent. EMS has been alerted. The medical assistant should
   a. tap the leg and shout, "Are you okay?"
   b. manually stabilize the injured leg.
   c. firmly snap the dislocated bone ends back into place.
   d. apply ice.

75. Which term describes legal techniques used to resolve disputes between parties, such as a physician and a patient, without going to court?
   a. affirmative defense
   b. arbitration
   c. implied consent
   d. jurisprudence

76. Contributory negligence
   a. tries to show that the plaintiff (patient) is totally at fault.
   b. tries to show that the defendant (physician) is totally innocent.
   c. tries to show that the plaintiff (patient) is partially responsible for the injury or complication.
   d. is a type of arbitration.

77. A patient comes to the office and says, "I have pain in the right lower side of my abdomen." This is an example of which component of the patient's history?
   a. chief complaint
   b. family history
   c. past medical history
   d. review of systems

78. During a spirometery, how many good efforts at inhaling deeply and exhaling must a patient make to ensure an accurate measurement?
a. one
b. two
c. three
d. four

79. Which of the following is a screening test for tuberculosis?
a. Schick
b. Schilling
c. radioallergosorbent test (RAST)
d. Mantoux

80. An example of an emancipated minor is
a. a 17-year-old married female.
b. a 26-year-old single male.
c. a 22-year-old army private.
d. a 16-year-old severely mentally challenged female living at home.

81. All of the following are techniques for active listening EXCEPT
a. giving the patient 100% of one's attention.
b. spending more time listening than talking.
c. stating opinions and interjecting questions to ensure clear understanding of the message.
d. nodding appropriately as the patient talks.

82. Which of the following terms means "nosebleed"?
a. emphysema
b. epistaxis
c. syncope
d. pleurisy

83. Dysmenorrhea means
a. absence of menstruation.
b. excessive menstruation.
c. painful intercourse.
d. pain during menstruation.

84. A healthcare professional should wear a face shield for protection when performing which of the following tasks?
a. administering an injection
b. inoculating a culture plate
c. removing staples from an incision
d. transporting sharps containers

85. Eating contaminated food is an example of which of the following links in the chain of infection?
a. means of transmission
b. portal of entry
c. portal of exit
d. reservoir

86. A patient with high cholesterol should be instructed to avoid intake of which of the following?
a. caffeine
b. all dairy products
c. raw vegetables
d. red meat

87. Which of the following thermometers would be used when taking a temperature via the ear canal?
a. temporal
b. axillary
c. tympanic
d. disposable

88. Workers' compensation is a law that covers all of the following EXCEPT
   a. an employee who has been injured on the job.
   b. an employee who suffers from lung damage because of prolonged exposure to hazardous chemicals while remodeling his or her home.
   c. an employee who has been injured while working with the provided safety glasses.
   d. an employee with a known history of asthma who has developed complications after inhaling a toxic chemical while working.

89. The most appropriate step immediately after administering a subcutaneous injection is to
   a. apply antiseptic to the injection site.
   b. cover the puncture site with a sterile bandage.
   c. check the drug label.
   d. massage the injection site.

90. Which type of letter formatting aligns all lines with the left margin of the paper except for the date line, complimentary closing line, and signature line?
   a. simplified
   b. full block
   c. modified block
   d. indented

91. Which suffix means "fixation"?
   a. *rrhage*
   b. *ptosis*
   c. *pexy*
   d. *rrhexis*

92. Which of the following items would NOT be included when preparing minutes of a meeting?
   a. name of the meeting and the date, time, and place of the meeting
   b. names of members present and absent
   c. schedule of all past and future meetings
   d. name of the person presiding over the meeting

93. The root word *enter* refers to which of the following?
   a. head
   b. intestines
   c. liver
   d. neck

94. Data processing involves all of the following EXCEPT
   a. entering data.
   b. repairing computer equipment.
   c. maintaining data.
   d. updating data.

95. Which part of the computer is responsible for allowing the computer to perform all operations?
   a. modem
   b. monitor
   c. flash drive
   d. central processing unit

96. Which of the following is the universal sign that a person is choking?
   a. clutching the neck
   b. placing hands on the abdomen
   c. placing hands on the chest
   d. raising arms in the air

97. Which of the following is the abbreviation for the medical term for a stroke?
a. CVD
b. CVA
c. CHF
d. CAD

98. Data storage devices include all of the following EXCEPT
a. flash drive.
b. CPU.
c. CDs.
d. CD-R.

99. All of the following statements about computer software are true EXCEPT
a. computer software helps the user perform specific tasks.
b. computer software consists of a modem and a printer.
c. computer software is used to control computer hardware.
d. computer software performs specific data-processing functions.

100. The circumference of the head should be measured during regular checkups until a pediatric patient reaches which of the following ages?
a. 12 months
b. 18 months
c. 24 months
d. 36 months

101. Which of the following is an advantage of the electronic medical record (EMR)?
a. easy for all medical personnel to use
b. inexpensive to maintain
c. available quickly in emergency situations
d. passwords do not need to be changed

102. Before drawing blood for a lipid profile, the patient must be instructed to fast for how many hours before the test?
a. 1 to 2
b. 3 to 4
c. 6 to 8
d. 12 to 14

103. A paper medical record should be corrected by which of the following methods?
a. Neatly cover the error with correction fluid so that the correct information can be entered.
b. Draw a double line through the error in red ink.
c. Write "error" on the red line, completely covering the incorrect entry.
d. Draw a single line through the error with red ink, write "corr," write the correction, initial, and date.

104. One concept that is central in cognitive theory is
a. irrational beliefs.
b. hierarchy of needs.
c. stages of grief.
d. antisocial behavior.

105. In a filing system, the release mark
a. determines the indexing units of the item to be filed.
b. indicates, usually by the physician's initials or signature, that the item has been seen and read by the physician and is ready to file.
c. is the process of inspecting all items before they can be filed.
d. indicates the cross-reference information placed on an item to be filed.

106. The endocrine system is responsible for
   a. excretion of wastes.
   b. breakdown of food.
   c. gas exchange.
   d. regulating the body's metabolic activities.

107. Which of the following is the abnormal outward curvature of the spine?
   a. lordosis
   b. scoliosis
   c. kyphosis
   d. osteoporosis

108. Which of the following words or phrases means "all of the factors required for infectious disease to spread"?
   a. chain of infection
   b. droplet transmission
   c. inflammation response
   d. portal of entry

109. Which of the following is NOT considered appropriate barrier protection?
   a. face shield
   b. gloves
   c. gown
   d. prescription eyeglasses

110. The primary source of energy in food comes from which of the following?
   a. vitamins
   b. carbohydrates
   c. fats
   d. triglycerides

111. Knowing how to index, or order, names is necessary in deciding where to place a file in an alphabetical filing system. Which of the following names is indexed correctly?
   a. Ellen Frances St. James:
      St. James Ellen Frances
   b. John Thomas Walters-Higgins, Sr.:
      Walters-Higgins John Thomas Sr
   c. Arnold J. Smith-Jones:
      Smithjones Arnold J.
   d. Dr. George Arthur Waters:
      Dr. Waters George Arthur

112. Lidocaine and procaine are examples of
   a. analgesics.
   b. anesthetics.
   c. hypnotics.
   d. sedatives.

113. Which term refers to a record of picture of a blood vessel?
   a. endoscope
   b. otoscope
   c. angiogram
   d. angioplasty

114. The advantages of postage meters include all of the following EXCEPT that they
   a. are disposable.
   b. provide faster delivery of mail.
   c. eliminate the need for letters to be canceled or postmarked at the post office.
   d. are economical to use.

115. Which of the following terms refers to the cessation of menstruation?
   a. menarche
   b. menopause
   c. menorrhagia
   d. menorrhea

116. Notations on envelopes such as "Special Delivery" or "Certified" would be typed
   a. directly below the return address.
   b. directly below the stamp.
   c. in the lower right-hand corner of the envelope.
   d. in the lower left-hand corner of the envelope.

117. Characteristics of a first-degree burn include
   a. blistered skin.
   b. charred skin.
   c. reddened skin.
   d. edema of the skin.

118. All of the statements about special delivery mail are true EXCEPT
   a. it is charged at a special delivery rate.
   b. it ensures that the mail will be delivered as soon as it reaches the destination post office.
   c. it does not speed up delivery between cities.
   d. it offers proof of delivery.

119. Which of the following procedures should be used when a letter addressed to another medical office is opened in error?
   a. Reseal the envelope, write "opened in error," and then mail it again.
   b. Place the letter in a new envelope, address the envelope, and then mail it again.
   c. Read the letter and then fax it to the correct office.
   d. Discard the letter if it does not contain important information.

120. The lithotomy position is used for patients in which circumstance?
   a. needing a breast exam
   b. needing sigmoid exam
   c. experiencing an asthma attack
   d. needing a cervical exam

121. The approved USPS state abbreviation for Minnesota is
   a. MI.
   b. MN.
   c. MA.
   d. MS.

122. Tests for occult blood in the stool should be performed after a patient has been on a three-day diet that is free from which of the following?
   a. alcohol
   b. fresh fruit
   c. raw vegetables
   d. red meat

123. In which manner is a letter to be handled when it will be mailed in a window envelope?
   a. The letter is folded in thirds by fan folding the letter with the name and address fitting into the window.
   b. The name and address need to be typed on a separate cover sheet to place in the window of the envelope.
   c. The letter is taped to the inside of the envelope to be sure that the name and address stays centered in the window.
   d. The letter should be typed in extra large font so that the name and address are clearly visible.

124. Which of the following situations should be recorded in the patient's medical record?
   a. an established patient reschedules an appointment
   b. an established patient makes an appointment
   c. an established patient cancels an appointment
   d. an established patient is late for his or her appointment

125. Which of the following is the largest organ in the body?
a. heart
b. stomach
c. skin
d. kidney

126. Anatomy is the study of the
a. functions of the body.
b. blood.
c. structures of the body.
d. diseases of the body.

127. Each of the following is a method of sterilization to achieve surgical asepsis EXCEPT
a. dry heat.
b. gas processing.
c. microwaving.
d. steam under pressure.

128. Patients that need to follow a low-sodium diet include all of the following EXCEPT
a. a patient with kidney disease.
b. a patient with high blood pressure.
c. a patient with edema.
d. a patient with diabetes.

129. Which of the following would be appropriate when setting up the matrix in an appointment book?
a. entering patient names in appointment slots
b. placing an "X" through the vacation days in red ink
c. marking in blue the times the physician will be seeing patients
d. placing an "X" through vacation days in pencil

130. The physician orders a buccal medication. The medical assistant should instruct the patient to
a. swallow the medication.
b. chew the medication.
c. place the medication between the lower teeth and cheek.
d. place the medication under the tongue.

131. The type of scheduling style that assigns a specific time for each patient throughout the day is called
a. modified wave.
b. stream.
c. clustering.
d. open hours.

132. Which of the following suffixes means "swallowing"?
a. *emesis*
b. *phagia*
c. *lysis*
d. *pepsia*

133. Which of the following is NOT a government-sponsored healthcare insurance plan?
a. Medicare
b. TRICARE
c. Blue Cross/Blue Shield
d. CHAMPVA

134. If a provider accepts assignment on a Medicare claim, this means that
a. the insurance payment will be sent to the patient.
b. the insurance payment will be sent to the medical office.
c. the patient does not have to pay a deductible.
d. insurance covered 100% of the bill.

135. Coordination of benefits (COB) is used by insurance carriers
   a. to avoid duplication of payments for the same service or procedure.
   b. as a method of scheduling appointments for patient services.
   c. to organize medical records.
   d. to separate multiple insurance claims with similar services.

136. When rendering first aid to a choking infant, all of the following may be performed EXCEPT
   a. back blows.
   b. chest thrusts.
   c. abdominal thrusts.
   d. finger sweep.

137. Which of the following checks has a stub attached to the check for recording information about the transaction?
   a. voucher check
   b. traveler's check
   c. cashier's check
   d. personal check

138. Which of the following checks is the patient's personal check?
   a. money order
   b. cashier's check
   c. traveler's check
   d. certified check

139. What piece of equipment is helpful during a physical exam to determine hearing?
   a. stethoscope
   b. watch with a second hand
   c. otoscope
   d. tuning fork

140. If the patient has a history of returned checks for non-sufficient funds, the medical assistant may accept all of the following types of checks EXCEPT
   a. personal check.
   b. money order.
   c. traveler's check.
   d. cashier's check.

141. Which of the following is the most appropriate method to obtain a sputum specimen?
   a. Aspirate the posterior pharynx with a bulb syringe.
   b. Have the patient cough deeply and expel the material into a sterile container.
   c. Have the patient gargle with saline and expel the liquid onto an agar plate.
   d. Lift the tongue and swab with a culturette.

142. Insurance policies that require policy holders to seek medical care from preferred providers only are called
   a. traditional policies.
   b. group policies.
   c. managed care policies.
   d. indemnity policies.

143. All of the following are stages in Elizabeth Kübler-Ross's theory of five stages of grief EXCEPT
   a. denial.
   b. anger.
   c. bargaining.
   d. confusion.

144. Policies that are supplementary to Medicare insurance are known as
   a. interim policies.
   b. Medicaid policies.
   c. Medicare assignment policies.
   d. Medigap policies.

145. Epithelial tissue covers all of the following EXCEPT
   a. cavities.
   b. cartilage.
   c. vessels.
   d. canals.

146. What term indicates a hole in the lining of the stomach?
   a. gastroenteritis
   b. ulcerative colitis
   c. hemothorax
   d. peptic ulcer

147. Standard precautions apply to each of the following EXCEPT
   a. amniotic fluid.
   b. saliva.
   c. sweat.
   d. urine.

148. Medicare claims are handled in the state or region by
   a. health maintenance organizations.
   b. CMS 1500.
   c. a fiscal intermediary.
   d. senior citizens' organizations.

149. An idiosyncratic effect is
   a. normal.
   b. a drug effect that is characteristic of a specific person.
   c. caused when two drugs with opposing actions interact.
   d. the study of what the body does to a drug.

150. Why is it important for the medical assistant to understand medical insurance coding?
   a. Insurance coding is needed to transfer all patient-related information.
   b. Insurance coding may be used to explain office expenses to the patient.
   c. Insurance coding is needed to file patient claims in order to receive reimbursement from insurance carriers.
   d. Insurance coding is the basis of medical office success.

151. The medical specialty study of and treatment of diseases and disorders of the urinary tract is
   a. urology.
   b. dermatology.
   c. cardiology.
   d. otolaryngology.

152. The ICD-9-CM coding book was compiled by
   a. the AMA.
   b. Medicare.
   c. WHO.
   d. CPT.

153. Which of the following is the required insurance form for government-run programs such as Medicare and Medicaid?
   a. ICD-9-CM
   b. CMS 1500
   c. CPT
   d. ICD-10

154. Which prefix means "inside"?
   a. *para*
   b. *intra*
   c. *endo*
   d. *epi*

155. All of the following are reasons that an insurance carrier may reject a claim EXCEPT
   a. the CPT code is not appropriate for the diagnosis listed.
   b. the procedure is not documented in the patient's medical record.
   c. the procedure does not include a required modifier.
   d. the five-digit CPT code matches the appropriate diagnosis.

156. The first aid priority for an injured victim is to
   a. make sure a patent, or cleared, airway exists.
   b. initiate breathing.
   c. stop bleeding.
   d. immobilize injuries.

157. The most common insurance form used in the medical office is
   a. CMS 1490.
   b. the universal insurance form.
   c. UB04.
   d. CMS 1500.

158. Of the following choices, which is the most important point to remember when completing an insurance claim form?
   a. to use the UB-04, the standard form for outpatient visits in the physician's office
   b. to check each carrier's regulations
   c. to complete the form manually before entering it on the computer
   d. to print copies to place in the patient's chart and to send to the patient

159. Measuring the circumference of an infant's head is an example of
   a. percussion.
   b. manipulation.
   c. mensuration.
   d. inspection.

160. Which item may be used to check a patient's insurance eligibility?
   a. a POS device
   b. a claims register
   c. a claim form
   d. an EOB

161. The life of an RBC is
   a. 80 days.
   b. 100 days.
   c. 120 days.
   d. 150 days.

162. Collection of fees when a patient has died may be directed to
   a. the executor of the estate.
   b. small claims court.
   c. probate court.
   d. collection agency.

163. Which of the following body fats is protective against cardiovascular disease?
   a. chylomicron
   b. high-density lipoprotein (HDL)
   c. low-density lipoprotein (LDL)
   d. triglycerides

164. A statement for an overdue bill should no longer be sent to a patient when the patient
   a. changes address or moves out of state.
   b. declares bankruptcy.
   c. leaves town.
   d. loses in small claims court.

165. The inguinal region is the
   a. region above the navel.
   b. middle lateral regions.
   c. lower lateral groin region.
   d. upper lateral region below the ribs.

166. Which of the following will result if a physician fails to assign a diagnostic code for an insurance claim?
- **a.** The physician will write off the bill.
- **b.** The insurance claim will be rejected.
- **c.** The information will be released illegally.
- **d.** The insurance payments will be lower than expected.

167. Calculate the following drug dosage:
The physician orders 750 milligrams of ciprofloxacin (Cipro). The label of the bottle in the office says 250 milligrams per tablet.
- **a.** one-half tablet
- **b.** one tablet
- **c.** two tablets
- **d.** three tablets

168. The combining form *pulmon/o* refers to the
- **a.** diaphragm.
- **b.** ear.
- **c.** kidney.
- **d.** lungs.

169. An assignment of benefits signature by the patient gives the insurance company authorization to do which of the following?
- **a.** pay benefits directly to the physician
- **b.** pay benefits directly to the patient
- **c.** pay benefits to a third party
- **d.** withhold benefits entirely

170. A parenteral drug is
- **a.** taken orally.
- **b.** dissolved in water and swallowed.
- **c.** a drug that is in capsule form.
- **d.** injected.

171. When a new patient claims coverage under Medicare, the medical assistant in a medical office should check the patient's Medicare card to be sure that it includes
- **a.** Part A.
- **b.** Part B.
- **c.** Part C.
- **d.** Part D.

172. Which of the following terms means "abnormal inflammation of the liver"?
- **a.** hepatitis
- **b.** hepatomalacia
- **c.** hepatomegaly
- **d.** nephritis

173. All of the following statements are true for the Uniform Anatomical Gift Law EXCEPT
- **a.** the law applies for organ donation before and after death.
- **b.** all organs—regardless of their condition—may be donated.
- **c.** there is no charge to the patient or his or her family for removing organs for donation.
- **d.** an individual has the right to decide how many organs and which organs he or she wishes to donate.

174. In human behavior, defense mechanisms include all of the following EXCEPT
- **a.** rationalization.
- **b.** projection.
- **c.** denial.
- **d.** substitution.

175. Which of the following is a proper technique for disposing of biohazardous waste?
   a. placing contaminated gloves in a plastic biohazard bag
   b. placing full sharps containers on a countertop in an examination room until pickup
   c. placing microscope slides in a biohazardous waste basket
   d. placing soiled surgical gowns in an open hamper

176. The yearly amount a patient must pay before an insurance carrier reimburses medical expenses is called a
   a. premium.
   b. coinsurance.
   c. deductible.
   d. co-pay.

177. Which of the following should be done first when a patient is suffering from insulin shock?
   a. administer sugar
   b. administer fluids
   c. treat for shock
   d. lay the victim down

178. The term used to describe the sharing of medical expenses between the patient and the insurance carrier with the patient paying a percentage of the bill (usually a split of 80% insurance and 20% patient) is called
   a. coinsurance.
   b. a co-pay.
   c. a premium.
   d. a deductible.

179. In which of the following positions should the patient be placed for an abdominal examination?
   a. knee-chest
   b. prone
   c. semi-Fowler
   d. supine

180. Which of the following is the medical term for bruise?
   a. concussion
   b. fracture
   c. contusion
   d. strain

181. All of the following are ways for a medical assistant to protect confidential information on a computer from unauthorized personnel EXCEPT
   a. lock the computer at night.
   b. provide an individual password for each user.
   c. change passwords frequently.
   d. share password only with medical personnel.

182. Why would a medical assistant use the z-track method to administer a drug?
   a. The drug needs to be absorbed by the gastrointestinal tract.
   b. The drug needs to be deep intramuscular (IM) and can stain or irritate the subcutaneous tissue.
   c. The drug is given to a patient with no large muscle mass.
   d. The patient is under two years of age.

183. The pegboard system is also referred to as the
   a. POMR system.
   b. SOMR system.
   c. balance statement system.
   d. write-it-once, or one-write, system.

184. A minor wound includes all of the following EXCEPT
    a. abrasion.
    b. laceration.
    c. puncture.
    d. open fracture.

185. Aging of accounts should be done for which of the following reasons?
    a. to keep track of accounts payable
    b. to determine the amount a patient owes on a bill and for how long
    c. to locate the oldest patient in the practice
    d. to determine when it is time to purge old material

186. The prefix *tachy* means which of the following?
    a. fast
    b. fixed
    c. thick
    d. thin

187. Which of the following describes the antagonism effect?
    a. two drugs that have a greater effect when taken together
    b. two drugs taken together that have no effect on each other
    c. two drugs working in opposition to each other
    d. drugs that have an interaction

188. The amount of air remaining in the lungs after normal expiration is called the
    a. forced vital capacity.
    b. functional residual capacity.
    c. inspiratory capacity.
    d. total lung capacity.

189. How often should equipment and instruments be checked to ensure that they are working properly?
    a. daily
    b. weekly
    c. biweekly
    d. monthly

190. When a physician orders a nebulizer treatment, the administration of the drug is through which process or route?
    a. injection
    b. inhalation
    c. sublingual
    d. oral

191. One of the primary functions of vitamin D is to
    a. support the metabolism.
    b. support bone development.
    c. function as an antioxidant.
    d. aid weight loss.

192. If an ECG recording appears as a series of small uniform spikes in the baseline, the medical assistant should
    a. check for nearby electric appliances.
    b. ask the patient to lie still.
    c. help the patient to relax and stay warm.
    d. check the cable connection to the electrodes.

193. Which of the following practices ensures the most effective restocking of supplies?
    a. immediately opening supplies and placing them on a storage shelf
    b. keeping a list of inventory and noting diminishing supplies
    c. ordering large quantities of supplies that are on sale
    d. qualifying for introductory offers by using a new vendor

194. Lead I of the electrocardigraph transmits and records electrical activity between which of the following limbs?
   a. left arm and left leg
   b. left arm and right leg
   c. right arm and left arm
   d. right arm and left leg

195. How much water is recommended to be consumed in a 24-hour period?
   a. three eight-ounce glasses
   b. ten eight-ounce glasses
   c. six eight-ounce glasses
   d. eight eight-ounce glasses

196. Which of the following is used in the autoclave for sterilization of packaged instruments?
   a. sterile water
   b. tap water
   c. distilled water
   d. mineral water

197. In approximately how many hours will a plaster cast be completely dry?
   a. 10
   b. 12
   c. 24
   d. 72

198. Which of the following is a device used when full weight cannot be placed on an injured area?
   a. crutches
   b. cane
   c. walker
   d. cast

199. Which of the following is an instrument that measures a person's ability to hear variations in sound intensity and pitch?
   a. audiometer
   b. glucometer
   c. otoscope
   d. sphygmomanometer

200. A patient states that he has had no digestive problems. This statement should be recorded in which of the following parts of the patient's medical record?
   a. chief complaint
   b. physical examination
   c. present illness
   d. review of systems

Answers and Explanations

1. c. In the doctor's office, the pulse oximeter is used to measure the oxygen saturation of arterial blood. Spirometry measures air taken into and expelled from the lungs. The peak flow meter assesses the ability of the patient to move air into and out of the lungs. Arterial blood gas is a test to determine the acidity or alkalinity of the blood and the concentrations of oxygen, carbon dioxide, and bicarbonate in the blood.

2. c. Citrus fruits are a source of vitamin C. Meats and nuts contain vitamin B6 and vitamin E. Milk is a source of vitamin D. No vitamins are found in oils.

3. b. Financial control has nothing to do with ethics. Ethics is a set of values, or knowing the difference between right and wrong and acting accordingly. An ethical professional is responsible for his or her own behavior, treating each patient with fairness (objectivity) and never revealing any private information about a patient (confidentiality).

4. a. The drugs in schedule I, such as heroin, have no acceptable medical use. Drugs in schedule II have medical use with precautions and limitations and have a high potential for abuse. Drugs in schedule III have medical use with precautions and limitations and have a moderate potential for abuse. Drugs in schedule IV have medical use with precautions and limitations and have low potential for abuse.

5. a. Flexibility is the ability to change or adapt plans or schedules because of an emergency. Instead of removing the sutures as instructed, a flexible medical assistant might notify the physician of the inflamed wound and have the physician discuss the situation with the concerned patient. The goal of treatment is to provide quality care and meet the needs of the patient. The other attributes listed—dependability, initiative, and effective communication—are also important, but are not necessarily the most important attribute needed in this situation. A less flexible medical assistant may insist that the sutures be removed because this was the procedure requested to be done.

6. b. Myotomy. *My* = "muscle" + *otomy* = "surgical incision."

7. b. A resume is a written description of work experiences, skills, and educational background. A cover letter is usually sent with a resume providing additional information explaining why the applicant feels he or she is the right person for the position being offered. A diploma is issued by an educational facility such as a school or college, showing that an individual has successfully completed a course or degree. A transcript is a document listing courses taken and grades received.

8. a. Colposcopy. *Colp/o* = "vagina" + *scopy* = "visual examination."

9. c. Accountability means being responsible for one's own actions and admitting to an error made. No matter how difficult it is to admit one's errors, it is the right thing to do. Although they are good behavioral traits, smiling and being courteous have nothing to do with acting accountable for one's actions. Switching days off with a fellow worker may be a responsible thing to do, as long as it is cleared by the office manager or other supervisor.

10. a. The rescuers should attach the AED and follow the voice prompts. Adult-size pads can be used in place of the child-size pads. A ventricular fibrillation victim who gets his or her heart pattern restored immediately following a sudden cardiac arrest has about a two-thirds chance of recovery. The AED automatically analyzes the patient's heart rhythm when the electrodes are fully attached. It should be used only when the patient is unresponsive and not breathing adequately.

11. b. The medical assistant must earn 45 CEUs within three years or 15 CEUs per year in order to maintain the RMA credential. Medical assistants are not licensed, nor do they have to work 40 hours per week in order to maintain the RMA credential. The AAMA is the national association for the CMA, not the RMA, although an RMA may voluntarily join the AAMA organization.

12. b. The id, ego, and superego are how Freud viewed the human personality. The id is the collection of basic drives and impulses that arise from our concerns about survival, preservation, and procreation of life; the ego is the part of individual's personality that operates in the realm of awareness, and comprises perception, cognition, and action; the superego is concerned with elements outside the individual, such as family, societal values, social mores, and the like.

13. a. The apical pulse—found at the apex of the heart—is measured by placing a stethoscope at that location and counting the pulse. All other choices can be palpated, or felt.

14. c. Name, address, and telephone number are all examples of the demographic information that should be taken from the patient and included in his or her record. The other choices should also be included in the record as well.

15. d. "Are you authorized to work in the United States?" is a legal question. It is illegal to ask about an individual's ethnic background, which may lead to discrimination. An employer has the responsibility to be sure employees are legally able to be employed in the United States. Asking about disabilities, marital status, children, or ethnic background during a job interview is illegal.

16. a. Quality control should be performed daily for laboratory procedures. Daily quality controls are performed to ensure the accuracy and reliability of test results. If controls were performed only weekly, biweekly, or monthly, the medical office could not ensure accurate results.

17. b. In a normal blood cell differential, the total number of cells counted is 100. Using this number, the percentage of each type of cell can be readily calculated.

18. a. The message, sender, receiver, channels, and feedback are the basic parts of the communication process. The source describes with whom the message originated such as the patient or the medical assistant, and the patient may be either the sender or the receiver. Channels are the various types of verbal and nonverbal methods that may be used to convey the messages.

19. a. A capillary puncture is most likely performed on the outer edges of the plantar surface (underside) of the heel of an infant (newborn to one year old). Once a child is walking, the finger is used for a capillary puncture. For all of the other patients listed, the finger can be used for a capillary puncture because the feet have become too callused, and the finger will have more tissue than the finger of an infant does.

20. c. Empathy is being able to understand another person's situation or being sensitive to the needs of another person by putting oneself in someone else's position. Sympathy is sharing the same feelings with an individual or feeling sorry for someone. A sympathetic medical assistant often lacks the ability to be helpful to a patient or to be able to make objective decisions in order to meet the needs of a patient, because he or she may not have enough objectivity.

21. b. Myopia describes nearsightedness. Diplopia means double vision. A cataract is an opaque formation or cloudiness of the lens and surrounding tissue of the eye. Hyperopia means farsightedness.

22. d. The process of cleaning and removing debris from instruments is known as sanitization. Sanitization reduces the number of microorganisms on an inanimate object to a relatively safe level. Aseptic technique refers to actions performed to make and maintain an area or object free from infection or pathogens. Disinfection is killing or rendering inert most but not all pathogenic microorganisms. Sterilization is a method used to kill all microorganisms from an item.

23. c. Raw vegetables are the best source of fiber. Meats and nuts contain protein and vitamins. Dairy products contain vitamin D, vitamin A, and B vitamins. Citrus fruits contain vitamin C.

24. c. Milk is not part of a clear liquid diet. A clear liquid is a liquid that one can see through. A clear liquid diet is recommended for patients recovering from diarrhea or surgery.

25. d. Diplomacy is the ability to speak without offending or insulting an individual or being sensitive and considerate when choosing words to use when discussing issues with patients or coworkers. Diplomacy would not interfere with impartiality of the treatment of patients. Stereotyping, bias, and prejudice are all terms that refer to having a predetermined attitude or making assumptions about an individual without getting all the facts; these traits may interfere with the impartial treatment of patients.

26. a. Dosages for children are frequently calculated according to body weight.

27. a. Kinesiology is the study of body language and how it is used in communication. Gestures are movements that are made to express emotions or feelings that an individual may have; smiling, for example, may show happiness. Communication is the exchange of information between two or more individuals. Physiology is the study of living systems.

28. c. Phlebitis. *Phleb/o* = "blood" + *itis* = "inflammation."

29. b. Mammography. *Mammo* = "breast" + *graphy* = "recording process."

30. a. The medical assistant should record the patient's name and phone number in case the line is disconnected during the transfer of the call. Giving the patient the extension of the person he or she is trying to reach would be helpful if the patient got disconnected or needed to call that person back, but having the name and phone number so that the medical assistant can call the patient back is the most helpful and courteous thing to do if the call is disconnected.

31. a. Incoming calls should be answered ideally by the first ring and definitely by the third ring because the call may be an emergency. It is respectful and courteous to answer calls promptly, because this demonstrates the medical assistant's willingness to be helpful to the patient. If the medical assistant is busy making an appointment with a patient in person, the medical assistant should ask the patient with whom he or she is speaking to please excuse the interruption, and then the medical assistant should answer the incoming call, questioning to see if it is an emergency. If the incoming call is not an emergency, the medical assistant should ask the permission of the patient on the phone to be put on hold.

32. c. When a responsive adult agrees to receive first aid care, he or she is giving "expressed consent." Implied consent means that it is assumed that the patient consents, based on his or her actions.

33. c. The medical assistant should stay calm and listen to the patient; this approach gives the patient the opportunity to vent his or her emotions. By listening carefully, the medical assistant will be able to identify the problem and then offer help. Transferring the call to either the physician or the office manager will probably anger the patient even more because the patient will be put on hold or get voicemail if the person to whom the call was transferred is not immediately available. The solution may be for the physician to make a return call to the patient, but only after it is determined that the physician is the best person to handle the call and that he or she has time to review the patient's medical record. The patient does not want to hear arguments or any defense from the medical assistant. A calm approach by the medical assistant will do more to calm the patient than any other action.

34. d. Screening or triaging incoming calls is a method of prioritizing the urgency of calls. When incoming calls are screened, urgent problems can be identified and patient needs can be met more quickly. By triaging incoming calls, the medical assistant can handle emergency situations immediately. This allows the proper time allotment to be given for needed appointments, and patients can be scheduled according to the urgency of the problem.

35. d. The act of taking vital signs normally entails measuring and recording the respiratory rate (breathing), as well as temperature, pulse rate, and blood pressure. The other choices may offer useful information about a patient's health condition, but they are not vital signs.

36. b. The medical assistant should not tape all conversations for later review by the patient because the hearing-impaired person may have trouble hearing the tape. In addition, often a patient will feel uncomfortable discussing private information if a tape recorder is running. There are much better ways to communicate with a hearing-impaired patient, such as speaking a little bit more slowly, speaking a little bit louder, and jotting down instructions for the patient. Facing the patient directly may also be helpful if the individual reads lips.

37. d. Before withdrawing the needle, the medical assistant should release the tourniquet because the pressure on the vein from the tourniquet could cause internal and external bleeding around the puncture site. The tourniquet should not be left on the patient for more than one minute because it may alter test results (it is also uncomfortable for the patient), so the medical assistant should remove the tourniquet before labeling the tubes or reassuring the patient. The medical assistant should not have the patient make a fist, because this would cause more bleeding from the puncture site.

38. c. Children should be told the truth about a procedure to be done, even if it may frighten them. A child will lose trust in an adult if he or she is lied to. It is better to state the truth in basic simple terms, giving just the information needed. An informed child will be more cooperative, and communication and trust will create a better patient-healthcare provider relationship for future procedures and care. Allowing a child to handle instruments that are simple and safe will help familiarize him or her with the environment, thereby reducing fear of the medical office.

39. a. When communicating with an illiterate patient, the medical assistant may use oral explanations and directions. Being illiterate simply means that the individual is lacking the ability to read, not the ability to hear and understand. Speaking louder or making gestures will not help if there is nothing wrong with the patient's hearing, and drawing pictures will probably be more confusing to the patient if he or she needs to guess what the picture is supposed to represent.

40. b. Below the ribs best describes the location of the hypochondriac region, which is the upper side section of the body. Below the pelvis is the iliac region. Distal to the colon is the hypogastric region. The center of the stomach is called the umbilical region.

41. a. Asepsis is used to protect the patient from exposure to outside pathogens during minor surgery; it is a condition that means free from pathogens. Standard precautions is a set of principles and practices used to prevent the transmission of infectious materials and reduce the occurrence of nosocomial infections, that is, infections that develop in hospitals or healthcare settings. Isolation refers to the practice of separating infected patients from individuals who are not infected, while reverse isolation refers to keeping a patient away from potentially infected individuals.

42. c. Centers for Disease Control and Prevention (CDC) developed guidelines called standard precautions to advise healthcare providers about the proper handling of any blood or body fluids that may contain blood or infectious organisms.

43. b. An otoscope is an instrument used to look into the ears in order to examine the external ear canal and tympanic membrane. An audiometer is an instrument used to measure hearing. A percussion hammer is an instrument with a rubber head that is used for testing reflexes. An ophthalmoscope is an instrument used to examine the interior of the eye.

44. b. Vitamin K aids in blood clotting. Vitamin B2 helps to metabolize energy, releasing energy from nutrients in body cells. Vitamin C is an antioxidant and plays a vital role in the immune system. Vitamin E is an antioxidant that protects cellular structure.

45. b. Evaluating the effectiveness of communication may be done by using feedback. Feedback, the final part of the communication process, is the response made back to the sender of the message. Feedback gives the sender the opportunity to evaluate whether the message sent was understood correctly by the receiver and to correct any misunderstandings in the message. Feedback can be accomplished by restating or paraphrasing the words of the sender and should not be just repeating the exact words of the message. Channels are the various types of verbal and nonverbal methods that may be used to convey messages, such as written messages, spoken messages, or body gestures. Closed questions require a yes-or-no answer and do not give the medical assistant the opportunity to gather information as to the understanding of the message, because even though the patient may respond with a yes, that does not mean that the message was correctly understood.

46. b. The signature is the section of a prescription that indicates the directions to the patient for taking the medication. The inscription states the name of the drug and dose. The subscription gives the directions to the pharmacist. The superscription consists of the symbol Rx and means "take."

47. b. A durable power of attorney for healthcare is a document that names the person chosen to represent an individual (a healthcare agent) and be the person to make the final decisions about an individual's end-of-life healthcare. A living will is a type of advance directive and often does not list the name of the individual who was chosen as the healthcare agent for the patient. A patient's will is the legal distribution of his or her estate.

48. c. Hematemesis. *Hemat/o* = "blood" + *emesis* = "vomiting."

49. d. Hypertension, or high blood pressure, is a health issue that is not reportable to the state or federal agencies. Because hypertension is not a contagious condition, it does not need to be reported. Stab wounds and child abuse are violent crimes and thus reportable incidences. Births and deaths are reported for statistical information about infant mortality which may be helpful in identifying those at risk and in offering prevention education.

50. b. *Peri* = "around."

51. c. Invasion of privacy is the unauthorized intrusion into or release of an individual's personal private information without cause. Libel is false written statements about an individual, and slander is speaking falsely about an individual, both of which may cause harm to an individual or damage the individual's reputation.

52. c. Dependability means trustworthiness or the quality of being able to be counted on to carry out a request. A medical assistant who is always asking to leave early is not someone a coworker can count on to do the required job properly. Foresight is the ability to see ahead and plan for the future. Initiative means that the individual does a task without being asked or reminded.

53. b. Triage does not involve diagnosing the patient's condition. Diagnosing patient conditions is beyond the medical assistant's scope of practice. Triage does involve screening phone calls, determining how serious the patient's illness is, and determining whether or not the patient has an emergency.

54. c. An AED provides an electric shock. An electrocardiogram records the electrical activity of the heart. Hypovolemic shock is a condition in which there is insufficient blood volume. Cardiopulmonary resuscitation provides ventilation and blood circulation when a person has none.

55. b. Misfeasance is improperly performing a legal act, such as a medical assistant measuring a patient's blood pressure but getting the incorrect reading. Malfeasance is performing a wrong or unlawful act, such as selling signed prescription forms to a patient. Non-feasance is failure to perform a required duty or obligation, such as a physician not ordering a test for a patient that a reasonable physician would order (e.g., an ECG for a patient complaining of chest pain). Feasance is a generic term for the performance of an act and does not specify if the act was performed correctly or incorrectly.

56. d. Slander is *speaking* falsely about someone in a way that may harm or damage the person's reputation. Libel is *writing* false statements about an individual, which may harm or damage the individual's reputation. Bias is a predetermined attitude about a person or situation, usually one that can interfere with impartial judgment. Negligence is failing to use a reasonable amount of care, resulting in harm or damage to an individual.

57. d. The stethoscope amplifies sounds produced by the body and is therefore useful in analyzing bowel sounds. An audiometer is an instrument used to measure hearing. A colonoscope is an instrument used to examine the colon. A dosimeter is a device used for measuring exposure to radiation.

58. d. OSHA does not provide legal assistance to employers being sued. OSHA regulations provide assistance to employees and employers to help make the work environment a safer and healthier place.

59. d. Inquiring about the mobility devices a patient uses to see whether the office can accommodate them is not part of the ADA, because the ADA was enacted to provide access to all types of facilities for individuals with disabilities.

60. c. Medical assistants are not licensed, but rather are certified or registered, so they cannot have a license revoked. However, medical assistant may be held accountable for acts done improperly. Medical assistants work under the supervision of a physician but they may be held responsible for performing any tasks not within the scope of training (tasks not learned) or if tasks are performed improperly. A medical assistant is responsible for knowing the federal and state regulations in the state where he or she works and for following them.

61. d. The nucleus contains deoxyribonucleic acid (DNA), which is the genetic material that contains the instructions for building proteins and other structures. The nuclear membrane is a flexible membrane that serves as a barrier by enclosing the cell contents. A gene is the basic unit of heredity in a living organism. The cytoplasm consists of cellular material outside the nucleus and inside the cell membrane.

62. c. The three types of muscle tissue are skeletal, smooth, and cardiac.

63. c. Monitoring autoclaves with spore tests is a quality control for the autoclave, to ensure that an autoclave is sterilizing instruments properly. A sealed pack with spores is placed in an autoclave during operation and then sent to a lab, which performs a culture test to see if spores grow.

64. d. Absorption is the process by which nutrients leave the gastrointestinal system and enter the bloodstream. Ingestion is the process of taking in nutrients. Digestion is the process of breaking down the nutrients for absorption into the bloodstream. Metabolism is the synthesizing of nutrients.

65. b. When a blood pressure cuff is deflated, the first tapping sound is the systolic pressure. The systolic pressure is the point at which the blood first begins to spurt through the artery as the cuff pressure begins to decrease. The mean arterial pressure is an average blood pressure during a cardiac cycle. The diastolic pressure represents the pressure that occurs on the walls of the arteries during diastole, that is, when the blood is flowing freely through the brachial artery. The pulse pressure is the difference between the systolic pressure and the diastolic pressure.

66. a. The Good Samaritan law protects an individual performing first aid voluntarily on an injured person and providing reasonable care. Although performing first aid is voluntary, an individual may be sued if he or she did not at least summon help by calling 911. A medical healthcare worker is not covered by the Good Samaritan law while at work and therefore may be liable for improperly performed procedures.

67. d. Cathartics are administered as a cleansing preparation before performing a radiologic study of the intestinal tract; they are used to empty the bowels. Anticholinergics are used to reduce muscle spasms. Antiemetics are used to reduce vomiting and nausea. Antispasmodics are used to reduce spasms.

68. b. An advance directive allows an individual to describe in detail wishes for end-of-life care and allows a durable power of attorney for healthcare to be selected. A living will is a type of advance directive that takes effect when a patient is terminally ill and usually does not name a healthcare agent. An advance directive is not a consent form for surgical intervention when complications arise during medical treatment. An advance directive does not specifically prevent anatomical gifts to be made, nor does it specify which attorney will be used to settle an estate because it is designed to specify wishes about healthcare for an individual who is incapacitated.

69. a. *Algia* means "pain."

70. d. A *subpoena duces tecum* is an order to appear in court and to bring any papers, books, or information necessary to explain in detail the issue in question. *Res ipsa loquitur* is the Latin term meaning "the thing speaks for itself" when explaining negligent actions, and *respondeat superior* is the Latin term for the law that states that physicians are liable for the negligent actions of any employee working under the physician's supervision. A *guardian ad litem* is a representative of the court used on behalf of a minor injured through negligent medical care.

71. c. Proctology. *Proct/o* = "anus" or "rectum" + *logy* = "study of."

72. d. The W-4 form should be amended or changed every time there is a change in status of the employee's information. Marriage, divorce, or a change in the number of dependents should be updated throughout the year. It is the responsibility of the employee to keep the W-4 form current.

73. d. The right to receive refunds for complications is not listed in the Patient's Bill of Rights. The patient does have the right to be treated with dignity and respect; to have his or her private personal information kept confidential; and to be informed about the details of the procedure to be done, the risks involved, and alternate treatments available.

74. b. The medical assistant should manually stabilize the injured leg. Because the medical assistant can observe the leg that is strangely bent, there is no need to ask the child if he or she is okay. Snapping the bone back in place may cause internal damage. Applying ice, while often used to reduce swelling, will not stabilize the wound.

75. b. Arbitration is a legal technique used to resolve disputes between parties, such as a physician and a patient, without going to court. A panel of neutral parties who are knowledgeable about the subject will listen to both sides of the dispute and will make an impartial judgment that both sides agree to obey. Arbitration may be selected over trying the case in court because the resolution to the dispute is more confidential, less expensive, and more convenient, and usually a decision is accomplished within a much shorter period of time compared to a court case, which may last years. Arbitration statutes apply the same measure of damages as a decision in a court case. Affirmative defense is when the defendant tries to share the blame with the plaintiff in hopes of winning the case.

76. c. Contributory negligence tries to show that the plaintiff (patient) is partially responsible for the injury or complication. For example, if the patient was informed about the risks of an elective surgery but chose to have the surgery anyway, the defense may be able to prove that the patient was partially responsible for any complications that occurred because of the surgery.

77. a. The chief complaint identifies the patient's reason for seeking care. The other choices are important to include in a patient's record also. Family history is a review of the health status of the patient's blood relatives. Past medical history is a review of the patient's past medical status. Review of systems information is the result of a systematic review of each body system.

78. c. During a spirometry, the patient must make three good efforts at inhaling deeply and exhaling to ensure an accurate measurement. The maneuver is highly dependent on patient cooperation and effort; it is normally repeated at least three times to ensure reproducibility. After three attempts, fatigue may prevent the patient from giving accurate results.

79. d. The Mantoux test is a skin test used to screen for tuberculosis. The other terms refer to tests for other diseases or disorders: The Schick tests screens for diphtheria, the Schilling test screens for pernicious anemia, and the RAST test screens for allergies.

80. a. A 17-year-old married female is considered an emancipated minor. She is under the legal age for an adult, which is age 18 in most states, but she is married and not under the care of her parents. The 26-year-old male and the 22-year-old army private are too old to be considered minors. The 16-year-old severely mentally challenged female is not self sufficient, is living at home under her parents' care, and does not meet the definition of an emancipated minor. An emancipated minor is no longer under the care, supervision, or custody of parents.

81. c. Stating opinions and interjecting questions to ensure clear understanding of the message are not techniques for active listening. The patient should be allowed to finish what he or she is saying before the medical assistant asks any questions to clarify what the patient has said. Interrupting the patient may interfere with his or her concentration and the content of the message the patient is trying to convey. Nodding appropriately is a nonverbal communication method that shows the patient that the medical assistant is listening and paying attention to what the patient is saying.

82. b. Epistaxis is a nosebleed. Emphysema is the enlargement and loss of elasticity of the alveoli because of partial blockage of alveolar spaces. Syncope means fainting. Pleurisy is inflammation of the pleural membranes.

83. d. Dysmenorrhea means pain during menstruation. The absence of menstruation is amenorrhea. Excessive menstruation is menorrhagia. Painful intercourse is dyspareunia.

84. b. A healthcare professional should wear a face shield when inoculating a culture plate, because a face shield is used to minimize the entry of infectious material into the body. When administering an injection, removing staples from an incision, or transporting sharps containers, the medical assistant does not need to wear a face shield because the risk of exposure to air droplets containing a microorganism is minimal.

85. b. All the answer choices are parts of the chain of infection, but eating contaminated food is an example of portal of entry; it is a way for an infectious organism to enter the body.

86. d. A patient with high cholesterol should be instructed to avoid intake of red meat. Cholesterol is found in meat and animal products. Some, but not all, dairy products are high in cholesterol.

87. c. The tympanic thermometer is a type of thermometer that is put in the ear. The temporal thermometer is used across the forehead. The axillary thermometer is an oral thermometer, which can also be used to take a temperature in the axilla (underarm). A disposable thermometer is a single-use thermometer designed to prevent cross-contamination that is used either orally or on the forehead.

88. b. Workers' compensation will not cover an employee who suffered illness resulting from work done at a person's home, even though it may have been caused by exposure to hazardous material. An employee will be covered under workers' compensation laws only if safety glasses, a requirement, are worn. An injury does not have to occur immediately for insurance coverage, but the injury will be covered if the employee can prove that the condition resulted from prolonged or repetitious behavior. For example, inhaling toxic fumes over time may cause lung damage, and repetitive motions of the wrist may cause carpal tunnel syndrome.

89. d. The most appropriate step immediately after administering a subcutaneous injection is massaging the injection site. Applying antiseptic to the injection site immediately after administering a subcutaneous injection would cause a burning sensation. A sterile bandage is not necessary after an injection. Checking the drug label should be done before the injection.

90. c. In the modified-block formatting style, all lines are aligned with the left margin of the paper, except for the date line, complimentary closing line, and signature line, which are centered on the page. Indented modified-block follows the directions for modified-block use, but allows the paragraphs to be indented five spaces. All lines are aligned with the left margin of the paper when using full-block formatting. The simplified formatting style aligns all lines with the left margin of the paper and omits the salutation and the complimentary closing.

91. c. *Pexy* means "fixation."

92. c. The schedule of all past and future meetings is not part of the information included in the minutes of a meeting. The minutes of the meeting include the date, place, and time of the next meeting. The name of the meeting, members present and absent, and the person presiding over the meeting are all items included in the minutes of a meeting.

93. b. *Enter* refers to the intestines.

94. b. Repairing computer equipment is not part of data processing, although it may be necessary in order to accomplish data processing. Data processing, also called data entry, is the conversion of data into a form that can be used by a computer. Data processing includes entering, updating, and maintaining data, or information, on a computer system, including data contained in archives.

95. d. The central processing unit (CPU) allows the computer to perform all functions. The monitor is the computer screen. The modem is used to transmit signals across telephone or cable lines. A flash drive is an external drive that is used to store information.

96. a. Clutching the neck is the universal sign that a person is choking. This is a signal that this person cannot breathe.

97. b. The abbreviation for stroke is CVA; it stands for "cardiovascular accident." CVD stands for "cardiovascular disease." CHF stands for "congestive heart failure." CAD stands for "coronary artery disease."

98. b. The CPU, or central processing unit, allows the computer to perform all functions. A flash drive, CD, and CD-R are all storage devices.

99. b. Computer hardware consists of devices that are connected to the computer, such as a printer, monitor, keyboard, and central processing unit. Computer software describes the programs that allow users to perform various tasks on the computer, including tasks that control the hardware.

100. d. The head circumference of children younger than three years (36 months) should be routinely measured and plotted on a head circumference growth chart.

101. c. EMRs can be accessed quickly in cases of emergencies, even when the patient's physician is not available or the medical office is closed. If an emergency arises when the patient is away traveling, his or her records will be available for use by facilities with EMR systems. EMRs are expensive to establish and maintain, and it can take staff members weeks and even months to feel comfortable using this type of system. Security issues are a problem for EMRs; maintaining security requires passwords to be changed frequently.

102. d. Before drawing blood for a lipid profile, the patient must be instructed to fast for 12 to 14 hours. Eating food within 12 to 14 hours before a lipid profile will not affect the HDL or total cholesterol test results, but it may affect the test results for triglycerides and LDL. If the patient needs to take medications within 12 to 14 hours before the exam, he or she may take the medications with a small amount of water.

103. d. A paper medical record should be corrected by drawing a single line through the error with red ink, writing "corr," and the correction needed, initialing it, and writing the date. The medical record is a legal document, and correction fluid is never used to correct errors in the medical record. Errors in the medical record should not be scribbled out because they must remain readable.

104. a. Through cognitive theory, psychologists have developed approaches to help their patients identify irrational beliefs, which are parts of individuals' understanding of themselves and the world that does not match reality or possibility—such as "I must be the prettiest girl in the world." Hierarchy of needs is a concept from theorist Abraham Maslow, who established a pyramid-type model of most basic needs, such as for food, up to more advanced needs, such as self-esteem. The stages of grief are the central theory in Elizabeth Kübler-Ross's model of how individuals handle trauma, loss, and death. Antisocial behavior may be exhibited in people undergoing cognitive therapy, but it is not a central concept in cognitive theory.

105. b. The release mark, usually the initials placed on the item by the physician, indicates that the item has been seen, read, and approved for filing. The physician's initials serve as a safety check, preventing any unread items, such as test results, from being filed.

106. d. The endocrine system is responsible for regulating the body's metabolic activities. Excretion of wastes and breakdown of food are done by the digestive system. Gas exchange is done by the respiratory system.

107. c. Kyphosis is an abnormal outward curvature of the spine. Lordosis is an abnormal inward curvature of the spine. Scoliosis is an abnormal sideward curvature of the spine. Osteoporosis is the condition of having brittle, porous bones that are susceptible to fractures.

108. a. Chain of infection means "all of the factors required for infectious disease to spread." In order for a pathogen to survive and produce disease, a cycle called chain of infection must be followed. If the cycle is broken at any point, then the pathogen dies. Droplet transmission is how a pathogen is transmitted from one person to another when a person coughs or sneezes. Inflammation response is a reaction to an infection, a chemical, or a physical injury can include redness, swelling, heat, and pain. Portal of entry is how the pathogen gains entry into the body.

109. d. Prescription eyeglasses are not considered an appropriate barrier protection because they do not allow enough coverage of the eyes to be considered an adequate barrier. The other choices—face shields, gloves, and gowns—are all considered adequate barrier protection.

110. b. Carbohydrates in food are the primary source of energy. Vitamins are needed for metabolism and prevention of certain diseases. Fats transport fat-soluble vitamins, insulate the body from the cold, and provide fatty acids. Triglyceride is a component molecule of fat found in fatty foods.

111. c. Smithjones is indexed correctly. With a hyphenated name, the hyphen is removed and only the first letter of the name is capitalized. St. James needs the period removed and a lowercase "j"; and Walter-Higgins needs the hyphen removed and the "H" entered in lowercase (Walterhiggins). Last names should be included first, and titles and other identifying information (Sr. or Jr., Dr., Prof., etc.) should be the last information to be indexed.

112. b. Lidocaine and procaine are examples of anesthetics, which are medications are used to reduce pain. (The name of many anesthetics ends in "caine.") Analgesics are medications used to relieve pain. Hypnotics are medications that induce sleep. Sedatives are medications that have a tranquilizing effect.

113. c. Angiogram. *Angi/o* = "blood vessel" + *gram* = "picture, record."

114. a. Postage meters are not disposable. They can be leased or purchased and refilled as needed for whatever amount the office selects. Once the letter has been canceled by attaching the adhesive sticker containing the postage, the item does not have to be canceled or postmarked at the post office, which speeds up the delivery time. Using exact postage based on the weight of the letter saves money because the amount of postage needed is calculated for each individual letter.

115. b. Menopause. *Men/o* = "menstruation" + *pause* = "stop."

116. b. Notations on letters such as "Special Delivery" or "Certified" would be typed directly below the stamp and typed in all uppercase letters. Nothing is entered in the lower corners of the letter since that space is left available for bar codes when the letter is read by an OCR scanner.

117. c. Characteristics of a first-degree burn include reddened skin. A first-degree burn involves the epidermis layer only. Blistered skin would appear with a second-degree burn. Charred skin would appear with a third-degree burn. Edema of the skin would appear with a second-degree burn.

118. d. Special delivery mail does not offer proof of delivery. Using special delivery does not speed up the travel time between cities. First-class mail, registered mail, or insured mail can be sent using special delivery and the mail is charged a special delivery rate. The advantage of special delivery is the immediate delivery of the mailed item as soon as it reaches the post office of the final destination.

119. a. The correct procedure for how to handle a letter opened in error would be to reseal it, write "opened in error" across the envelope, and either put it back in the mail or hand it to the mail carrier. Mail addressed to other offices should not be read once it is discovered the envelope was opened in error and should not be faxed to the other party. Discarding the letter is an unacceptable choice. The best procedure when opening mail is to be careful and to check all addresses before opening the envelope.

120. d. Lithotomy—when the patient is lying on his or her back with feet in stirrups—is used for a cervical exam. For a breast exam, the patient would be in the supine position. For a sigmoid exam, the patient would be in the knee-chest or Sims position. For an asthma attack, the patient would be in the Fowler's position.

121. b. MN is the approved two-letter USPS abbreviation for Minnesota.

122. d. Tests for occult blood in the stool should be performed after a patient has been on a three-day diet that is free from red meat because the meat contains animal blood.

123. a. Letters intended for window envelopes are fan folded by folding the bottom edge up one third of the length of the paper. The letter is then turned over, and the top of the letter is folded down to the crease. The letter is placed in the envelope with the address showing in the window. A cover sheet is not needed for window envelope use. The font size remains the same as the font size of the letter.

124. c. Canceled appointments and no-show appointments need to be marked, preferably in red, in the paper appointment book, and in a special section of the computer software system. They should also be recorded in the patient record. It is up to the individual office whether or not this entry in the medical record is done in red ink, but it is essential that the date of the missed appointment is recorded. Because the medical record is a legal document, entries made can be used to document that a patient has been noncompliant to the physician's request when he or she canceled the appointment without rescheduling or that the patient failed to show up for recommended medical care. If the patient decides to sue the physician because his or her medical condition did not improve, the physician can show the court that the patient did not carry out his or her responsibility by keeping the recommended appointment. If a patient cancels an appointment but makes another appointment for a few days later, there is no need to record this information in the medical record. Rescheduling an appointment is not a necessary piece of information needed in the medical record.

125. c. The skin is the largest organ in the body. The heart is about the size of a fist. The stomach in an adult has capacity of 1 liter to 1.5 liters. The kidney is a bean-shaped organ of the urinary system. The average weight of a kidney is 120 g to 150 g.

126. c. Anatomy is the study of the structures of the body. Physiology is the study of the functions of the body. Hematology is the study of blood. Pathology is the study of diseases of the body.

127. c. Microwaving is not a method of sterilization used to achieve surgical asepsis because it does not have adequate pressure, time, and temperature to kill the microorganisms. The other choices—dry heat, gas processing, and steam under pressure—are all methods of sterilization used to achieve surgical asepsis. Dry heat is used to sterilize articles that cannot be penetrated by steam or may be damaged by it, such as oil, petroleum jelly, and powder. Gas processing is used to sterilize heat-sensitive items such as syringes, sutures, and catheters. Steam under pressure helps maintain a high temperature to kill all microorganisms.

128. d. The most important dietary concern for a patient with diabetes is his or her sugar intake. A patient with kidney disease, a patient with high blood pressure, and a patient with edema all need to follow a low-sodium diet.

129. d. Setting up the matrix of an appointment book is the process of marking off, in pencil, the times the physician will not be available to see patients, the times the office will be closed, vacation days, medical meetings, or any other times when no appointments should be scheduled. Ink is not used because the times marked off could change and it would be difficult to remove the crossed-out sections, thus creating a messy, hard-to-read appointment book. Computerized software allows the appointment book to set up the matrix in a similar fashion, including a place to list the reason for the office closing. Entering patient names in appointment slots comes after the matrix has been set up.

130. c. If the physician orders a buccal medication, then the medical assistant should instruct the patient to place the medication between the lower teeth and cheek. A medication that is swallowed or chewed is an oral medication. A medication that is placed under the tongue is a sublingual medication.

131. b. The stream style of scheduling allows a specific number of minutes for each visit. Clustering groups together similar procedures or problems, such as a block of time reserved for flu shots or physical exams. Modified-wave schedules two patients at the beginning of each hour and one patient at half past the hour with the goal of starting and finishing the hour on time and treating three patients within each hour. Open hours scheduling does not give any appointment times to patients. Patients are free to walk in during any time that the facility is open.

132. b. *Phagia* means "swallowing."

133. c. Blue Cross/Blue Shield is a private insurance company. Medicare is a government sponsored healthcare programs. TRICARE and CHAMPVA are military healthcare programs.

134. b. Assignment of benefits means that the patient has signed a consent form releasing the insurance payment to the healthcare provider, therefore allowing the payment to be sent to the provider. Nonassignment of benefits means that the patient did not give permission for the insurance carrier to send the payment to the provider, so the payment will be sent to the patient. The medical office will then bill the patient for the services provided.

135. a. Coordination of benefits (COB) is used by insurance carriers to avoid duplication of payments for the same service or procedure. It is sometimes referred to as non-duplication of benefits. When both spouses have insurance through their places of employment, the claim is first sent to the patient's insurance, the primary insurance. After payment has been received, the claim is then sent to the secondary insurance, the insurance of the spouse. The maximum payment for the service can be only 100% divided between the two insurances.

136. c. Abdominal thrusts can damage the internal organs of infants and should not be performed on a choking infant.

137. a. A voucher check has a stub attached to the check for recording information about the transaction. None of the other types of checks has attachments to be used for recording information.

138. d. A certified check is the patient's personal check that the bank has cleared or "certified." A certified check guarantees that sufficient funds are available and on reserve in the patient's account and cannot be withdrawn for any other use. The money order and traveler's checks are from banks, companies, or the post office, and the patient purchases them for cash.

139. d. The tuning fork—a stainless steel instrument with a handle at one end and two prongs at the other end—is used to test for hearing. The other choices are instruments that can also be used during a patient examination. A stethoscope amplifies sounds produced by the body. A watch with a second hand is used to measure pulse and respirations. An otoscope is used to examine the outer ear.

140. a. If the patient has a history of returned checks for non-sufficient funds, the medical assistant should avoid taking a personal check from this patient. A personal check from the patient offers no guarantees that the money will be available when the check is cashed. The money order, traveler's check, and cashier's check were either purchased with cash or guaranteed by the bank that sufficient funds will be available when the check is cashed.

141. b. Having the patient cough deeply and expel the material into a sterile container is the most appropriate method to obtain a sputum specimen.

142. c. Insurance policies that require policyholders to seek medical care from preferred providers only are called managed care policies. Most patients seek medical attention from physicians who accept the insurance that they have, but the patients are not required to select a physician from a specific list. Group policies are policies that are offered to a group usually offering a lower price for the patient. Indemnity healthcare insurance, also known as fee-for-service, is a plan where the insured pays for the medical service and then seeks reimbursement from the insurance carrier, so the patient is not limited to a specific list of physicians.

143. d. Although a person who is undergoing trauma and loss may experience confusion, it is not one of the stages described by Kübler-Ross in her theory of the five stages of grief. The five stages, in order, are denial, anger, bargaining, depression, and acceptance.

144. d. Policies that are supplementary to Medicare insurance are known as Medigap policies because they pay the parts of the medical bill that Medicare does not cover. Depending on the type of Medigap policy, the yearly deductible and the 20% not covered by Medicare may be covered by a patient's Medigap insurance.

145. b. Epithelial tissue does not cover cartilage. Cartilage is connective tissue.

146. d. Peptic ulcer is a hole in the lining of the stomach or duodenum. Gastroenteritis is an inflammation of the stomach and intestines. Ulcerative colitis is an inflammation and ulcers of the lining of the colon. Hemothorax is blood in the chest cavity.

147. c. Standard precautions do not apply to sweat. Sweat is not considered an infectious material by the CDC. Amniotic fluid, saliva, and urine are all considered by the CDC to be contaminated with infectious microorganisms.

148. c. Medicare claims are handled in the state or region by a fiscal intermediary. A fiscal intermediary is a private company that contracts with Medicare to manage and pay Medicare Part A expenses and some of Medicare Part B expenses. A senior citizens' organization has nothing to do with paying medical expenses for patients. CMS 1500 is the form used to complete insurance claims. A health maintenance organization is a type of company that is similar to an insurance company and has the goal of employing physicians to give good care at a lower price.

149. b. An idiosyncratic effect is a drug effect that is characteristic of a specific person. It is not a normal reaction; a normal reaction would be therapeutic. Antagonism is caused when two drugs with opposing actions interact. Pharmacodynamics is the study of what the body does to a drug.

150. c. Insurance coding is needed to file patient claims in order to receive reimbursement from insurance carriers. CPT codes, used for procedures and services rendered to a patient, and ICD-9 codes, used for diagnosis of conditions, are required by insurance carriers for reimbursement of patient claims. Coding is not needed to transfer all patient-related information or to explain office expenses. Coding is not responsible for the success of a medical office either. A medical office succeeds because of the service and care provided and the proper management of all areas of the medical practice.

151. a. Urology. *Ur/o* = "urinary tract" + *logy* = "study of."

152. c. The World Health Organization (WHO) is responsible for publishing and updating the International Classification of Diseases 9 Revision Clinical Modification (ICD-9-CM) volumes used to translate diagnoses and conditions into numbers. The data collected by the ICD system is used for reimbursement purposes and to collect morbidity and mortality statistics. The American Medical Association (AMA) is the national association for physicians. Medicare is government-sponsored insurance, mainly for the elderly. Current Procedural Terminology (CPT) codes are used to translate procedures and services into numbers.

153. b. The CMS 1500 is the required insurance form for government-run programs such as Medicare and Medicaid, although it may be used for most types of insurance claims. ICD-9-CM is used to code diseases and conditions, and ICD-10 is the newer edition of ICD-9. CPT is used to code procedures and services.

154. c. *Endo* means "inside."

155. d. If the five-digit CPT code matches the patient's diagnosis, then the insurance carrier must pay the claim. If a procedure was done to test urine for glucose (sugar), a diagnosis is needed to justify the procedure (such as diabetes). If the claim listed the CPT code for a urine test but entered a diagnosis that the patient had trouble sleeping, then the CPT code would not match the diagnosis because there would be no reason to test the urine for a patient who had trouble sleeping. The claim would be rejected.

156. a. The first aid priority for an injured victim is to make sure a patent (open or cleared) airway exists. Without a cleared airway, the patient will not be able to breathe, so the patent airway must be the priority. The medical assistant should first create an airway and get the patient breathing, and then tend to injuries.

157. d. The Centers for Medicare and Medicaid (CMS) 1500 is the most common insurance form used in a medical office. The UB-04 form is used for completing claims covering services such as inpatient admissions, outpatient procedures, and care in facilities such as psychiatric and alcohol clinics and nursing facilities.

158. b. It is most important to check each carrier's regulations to be sure the claim will be completed properly. There is no need to complete the form manually before entering it into the computer. Copies do not need to be placed in the patient's medical record.

159. c. Mensuration is the process of measuring the patient. The other choices are also methods that can be used during a patient examination. Percussion involves tapping the patient with fingers and listening to the sounds produced to determine the size, density, and location of an organ. Manipulation is the process of moving a patient's body parts. Inspection involves observation of the patient for any signs of disease.

160. a. A point-of-service device (POS) allows direct communication between the physician's office and the insurance carrier to verify membership of a patient with a particular insurance. The claims register keeps track of insurance claims sent in to the insurance carrier. The claim form is the form sent to the insurance carrier either by paper or electronically. An EOB is an explanation of benefits that is sent to a patient by the insurance carrier, describing the charges and payment made on a claim.

161. c. The life of an RBC, or red blood cell, is 120 days.

162. a. Collection of fees when a patient has died may be directed to the executor of the patient's estate. The executor of the patient's estate is the person responsible for handling financial matters for the deceased patient's bills. Going to small claims court or to a collection agency is not the proper way to handle collection for a deceased patient.

163. b. High-density lipoprotein (HDL) is the one form of fat in the body that protects against cardiovascular disease. Known as the "good cholesterol," HDL removes excess cholesterol from the cells and carries it to the liver to be excreted. The other choices are types of fat molecules in the body, but they do not actively remove cholesterol from the body.

164. b. When a patient declares bankruptcy, bills should no longer be sent to the patient. The medical office is notified that the patient has declared bankruptcy by the court. Many times the court will request that any patient bills be submitted for payment consideration. Medical offices should pursue payment of bills from patients who have changed addresses or moved out of state. Detailed patient registration records may provide clues—such as a driver's license, place of employment, next of kin, or the person who referred the patient to the office—that may be helpful in contacting an individual to collect overdue bills.

165. c. Inguinal region is the lower lateral groin region. The region above the navel is the umbilical region. The middle lateral region is the lumbar region. The upper lateral region below the ribs is the iliac region.

166. b. The insurance claim will be rejected because the insurance carrier will consider the claim incomplete. No one will be paid until the claim is resubmitted with all areas completed.

167. d. The dose would be three tablets: $750 \div 250 = 3$ tablets.

168. d. The root word *pulmon* refers to the lungs.

169. a. An assignment of benefits signature by the patient gives the insurance company authorization to pay benefits directly to the physician. Non-assignment would give permission for the insurance carrier to send the payment to the patient.

170. d. Parenteral drugs are those taken through any route other than the mouth—for example, a drug that is given by injection.

171. b. Medicare Part B covers outpatient services, which include physician's offices. Part A covers inpatient services; Part C is coverage for alternate insurances, but the Medicare card would not list this information because the patient would have a different type of insurance card. Part D is prescription coverage, which does not affect coverage for medical office visits.

172. a. Hepatitis. *Hepata/o* = "liver" + *itis* = "inflammation."

173. b. The Uniform Anatomical Gift Law does not state that all organs—regardless of their condition—may be donated. The physician responsible for harvesting the donated organs may make the decision to reject an organ if the patient had certain infectious diseases or some types of cancer.

174. d. Substitution is not a defense mechanism. The other choices are all common defense mechanisms. Rationalization is when a person makes excuses to justify inappropriate behavior. Projection is when a person experiencing difficult or negative feelings or thoughts may accuse others of thinking or feeling the way they do. Denial is a complete rejection of a difficult fact or feeling.

175. a. Placing contaminated gloves in a plastic biohazard bag to prevent exposure is a proper technique to dispose of biohazardous waste. Placing a full sharps container on a countertop in an examination room until pickup is not a proper technique for disposal. The full sharps container must be placed in a biohazard cardboard box lined with a biohazard bag. Placing a microscope slide in a biohazard waste basket is not a proper technique for disposal because the slide is sharp and it can penetrate the bag, leading to an exposure risk.

176. c. A deductible is the amount of money a patient must pay each year before the insurance carrier will start to reimburse a patient's medical expenses. A co-pay is a specific amount paid at the time of medical treatment to offset a portion of the medical costs. Coinsurance is a percentage of the medical bill owed by the patient. A premium is a yearly amount of money paid in order to keep the insurance active.

177. a. When a patient is suffering from insulin shock, the medical assistant should immediately administer sugar. If the person is conscious, give sugar in any form. If a person is suffering from a diabetic coma, the sugar is not required, but it will not cause the person further harm. Insulin shock is severe hypoglycemia and a diabetic coma is severe hyperglycemia. Administering fluids, treating for shock, or laying the victim down will address the hyperglycemia or hypoglycemia problem, but the first thing that should be done is to administer sugar.

178. a. Coinsurance is the sharing of the medical expenses between the patient and the insurance carrier, with the patient paying a percentage of the bill (for instance, 20%) and the insurance carrier paying the remaining percentage. A co-pay is the set amount of money the patient pays at each visit. The deductible is the amount the patient must pay yearly before the insurance carrier will start to reimburse medical expenses. The premium is the yearly charge to keep the insurance active.

179. d. Supine position is used for examination of the head, chest, abdomen and extremities. The knee-chest position is for examination of the rectal area. The prone position is used to examine the back and assess the extension of hip joint. The semi-Fowler position is used to examine the upper body of patients with cardiovascular and respiratory problems.

180. c. The medical term for bruise is contusion. A bruise, or contusion, is caused when blood vessels under the skin are damaged or broken as the result of a blow. A concussion is an injury to the brain. A fracture is a broken bone. A strain is stretching or tearing of muscle tissue.

181. d. A medical assistant should not share his or her password with medical personnel because each computer user should have his or her own password. Passwords should be changed frequently. Locking the computer at night will help protect the information stored in the computer.

182. b. A medical assistant would use the z-track method to administer a drug if the drug needs to be deep intramuscular (IM) because the drug can stain or irritate the subcutaneous tissue. A drug that needs to be absorbed by the gastrointestinal tract is an oral drug. The z-track is given intramuscularly, so it would not be appropriate for the drug to be given to a patient with no large muscle mass. The z-track method can be used regardless of age.

183. d. The pegboard system is also referred to as the write-it-once, or one-write, system. The pegboard system is made up of no carbon required (NCR) forms that allow multiple forms to be layered, so that information has to be written only once, yet will be applied to many documents with one writing. The POMR and SOMR are types of patient documentation used in the patient's medical record.

184. d. An open fracture is a major injury in which the bone has broken through the skin. Abrasion, laceration, and puncture are all minor wounds.

185. b. The aging of accounts should be done to determine the amount a patient owes on a bill and for how long it has been owed. Aging accounts is important because the longer the time from the service, the more difficult it is to collect the money from the patient. Insurance carriers also have a time limit on how long claims may be submitted for reimbursement. A claim sent after the time limit will not be paid, and the patient is not responsible for the bill, causing the physician to lose money. Aging accounts has nothing to do with accounts payable or purging material no longer needed. It is not a way to locate the oldest patient in the practice.

186. a. *Tachy* means "fast."

187. c. An antagonism effect occurs when two drugs work in opposition to each other. Synergism occurs when two drugs taken together have a greater effect. Drug interaction is a general term that includes antagonism, synergism, and the like.

188. b. The amount of air remaining in the lungs after normal expiration is called the functional residual capacity (FRC). The forced vital capacity (FVC) is the maximum volume of air that can be expired when one exhales as forcefully and as rapidly as possible. The inspiratory capacity is the volume of gas that can be taken into the lungs in a full inhalation. Total lung capacity is the amount of gas contained in the lung at the end of a maximal inhalation.

189. a. Equipment and instruments should be checked daily in order to ensure that they are in working order when needed for treatment of patients. Checking equipment weekly, biweekly, or monthly is not often enough to ensure that the equipment and instruments will be ready when needed.

190. b. When a physician orders a nebulizer treatment, the route of drug administration is through inhalation of a mist. Injection would be in the subcutaneous tissue or muscle. Sublingual is under the tongue. Oral is by mouth.

191. b. Vitamin D supports bone development. Other vitamins, including some of the B vitamins, support metabolism. Vitamin E functions as an antioxidant. Vitamin D does not help in weight loss.

192. a. The medical assistant should check for nearby electrical appliances, because the electrical appliances will cause the small uniform spikes in the baseline of the ECG. Patient movement will cause a wandering baseline. Muscle movement will cause unwanted jagged peaks of irregular heights and spacing.

193. b. The most effective method of restocking supplies consists of keeping a list of inventory, noting diminishing supplies, and reordering when necessary. Keeping a list of inventory will help the medical assistant know when it is time to restock a particular item. Immediately opening supplies and placing them on storage shelf will help replenish supplies, but it will not help to keep track of the diminished supplies that need restocking. Ordering large quantities of supplies that are on sale will help save money but will not help keep track of inventory. Qualifying for introductory offers by using a new vendor may help save money on supplies during the introductory phase, but it will not help in keeping track of inventory.

194. c. Lead I of the electrocardigraph transmits and records electrical activity between the right arm and the left arm. Lead III of the electrocardigraph records the electrical activity between the left arm and left leg. Lead II records the electrical activity between the right arm and left leg. The right leg is a ground and is not used in the ECG recording.

195. d. In a 24-hour period, eight eight-ounce glasses of water are recommended for consumption.

196. c. Distilled water is used in the autoclave for sterilization of packaged instruments because it contains no chlorine or minerals to damage or block the air exhaust of the autoclave. The types of water included in the other choices contain minerals and/or chlorine, either of which can corrode and block the air exhaust of the autoclave or cause corrosion of the stainless-steel chamber of the autoclave.

197. d. A plaster cast will dry completely in approximately 72 hours.

198. a. Crutches are used when full weight cannot be placed on an injured area. A cane is used by patients who have weakness on one side of the body, such as hemiparesis or a joint disability. A walker is used by patients who have weakness or balance problems. A cast is used to stabilize a broken bone.

199. a. An audiometer is an instrument that measures a person's ability to hear variations in sound intensity and pitch; it therefore helps to measure hearing loss. The other choices are instruments used to test different bodily functions or examine parts of the body. The glucometer is a machine used to measure glucose levels. The otoscope is an instrument used to look into the ears. A sphygmomanometer is used—with a stethoscope—to measure blood pressure.

200. d. A review of systems is when each body system is reviewed by the physician during the physical exam. The patient's chief complaint is the reason for his or her visit. Physical examination includes a range of activities: measuring vital signs, reviewing of the body's systems, and diagnostic screening tests. Present illness is the current condition or illness the patient is showing symptoms of.

ABBREVIATIONS AND GLOSSARY

Commonly Used Medical Abbreviations

ABBREVIATION	DEFINITION	ABBREVIATION	DEFINITION
ABG	arterial blood gas	HTN	hypertension
a.c.	before meals	Hx	history
AD	right ear	ID	intradermal
a.m.a.	against medical advice	IM	intramuscular
AP	anteroposterior	IV	intravenous
AS	left ear	IVP	intravenous pyelogram
b.i.d.	twice a day	NKA	no known allergies
BP	blood pressure	NSAID	nonsteroidal anti-inflammatory drug
bpm	beats per minute	OD	right eye
BUN	blood urea nitrogen	OS	left eye
Bx	biopsy	OTC	over the counter
CBC	complete blood count	PE	physical exam
CC	chief complaint	PERRLA	pupils equal, round, reactive to light and accommodation
cc	cubic centimeter	PI	present illness
cm	centimeter	po	orally
CNS	central nervous system	qid	four times a day
D/C	discharge	QNS	quantity not sufficient
DNI	do not intubate	R/O	rule out
DNR	do not resuscitate	ROM	range of motion
Dx	diagnosis	SOB	shortness of breath
GI	gastrointestinal	TIA	transient ischemic attack
GTT	glucose tolerance test	TPN	total parenteral nutrition
HCT	hematocrit	TPR	temperature, pulse, respiration
HGB	hemoglobin	UA	urinalysis
HPI	history of present illness	WNL	within normal limits

Glossary

ABCs airway, breathing, circulation; the primary aspects of assessment in an emergency

absorption the method the body uses to transfer nutrients from the gastrointestinal, or digestive, tract into the bloodstream

accession record preassigned numbers given to medical records in a numeric filing system

active files medical records of patients currently under the care of the physician

active listening listening with a purpose or reason, paying close attention to the words used in the conversation as well as to the tone of the words spoken; restating what a patient has said to be sure it was correctly understood

acute infection an infection with a quick onset and short duration

advance directives a set of instructions created by an individual about his or her future medical care, should he or she become incapacitated and unable to make his or her own healthcare decisions. A healthcare agent is appointed by the individual to make healthcare decisions for him or her.

aerobic growing, living, or occurring in the presence of oxygen

afebrile without fever

affirmative defense a type of legal defense commonly used in malpractice cases whereby the patient and the physician share the blame for the injury received by the patient

aging of accounts the length of time an account has been overdue, beginning from the time the first billing statement is sent to the patient

alternating current interference in an ECG readout, a type of artifact that appears as a series of spikes on the paper; could be caused by nearby equipment

Americans with Disabilities Act (ADA) a law enacted in 1991 that is designed to protect the rights of people with physical and mental disabilities

ampule a small sealed glass or plastic container designed to preserve its sterile contents

anaerobic growing, living, or occurring in the absence of oxygen

anemia a condition marked by deficiency of red blood cells

antagonism the reduced effectiveness of one or both drugs with opposing actions when they are taken at the same time and cancel each other out

antecubital the space located at the front of the elbow

antibody a substance produced by the body in response to it being invaded by an antigen

antigen a substance capable of stimulating the formation of antibodies in an individual

apnea the temporary cessation of breathing

arbitration a legal technique used to resolve disputes between parties, such as a physician and a patient, without going to court

arteriovenous fistula an abnormal linkage or passageway from an artery to a vein

assignment of benefits a method used by the insurance carrier to determine to whom the payment will be sent. If a patient accepts assignment, the payment will be sent to the physician's office.

asymptomatic having no noticeable signs of disease

auscultatory gap in sphygmomanometry, a period of abnormal silence or diminished intensity during one of the Korotkoff sound phases

auscultation the method of listening to the sounds produced by and emanating from within the body for diagnostic purposes

autoclave a piece of equipment used to sterilize materials and instruments, using steam under pressure

axilla the armpits

bacillus a rod-shaped bacterial cell that causes tuberculosis and tetanus, among other diseases

bacteria a group of single-cell microorganisms, some of which cause disease

bias a predetermined attitude about a person or situation, usually one that can interfere with impartial judgment

bilirubinuria bilirubin in urine

bioavailability the amount of a drug that reaches the bloodstream and the length of time needed for it to do so

biohazardous waste contaminated waste that is potentially infectious to humans or animals

biologic indicator a preparation of living bacterial spores

birthday rule the guideline that states that the parent whose birthday falls first in the year is the primary insurance carrier for the child

blind copy used when a letter or an e-mail will be sent to individuals other than the person to whom the letter was written without the knowledge of the person to whom the letter was written

body mechanics a method of movement and coordination to preserve and promote good posture, balance, and body alignment

bradypnea abnormally slow breathing

buccal pertaining to the cheek

calorie a unit that measures the amount of heat produced by energy

cannula a tube that can be inserted into a body cavity or duct

capillaries small blood vessels that carry blood to and from the small arterioles to the tissues and return blood to the small venules

capitated plan a form of managed care designed to provide healthcare to members for a fixed monthly cost

cardiac arrhythmia an irregular heartbeat

cardiopulmonary resuscitation (CPR) a standard approach to providing first aid—rescue breathing and heart massage—in a situation in which the victim is not breathing and the heart may have stopped beating

cardiovascular system a system that circulates blood, via the heart, arteries, veins, and capillaries, throughout the body to transport oxygen and nutrients to cells and to carry waste products to the kidneys, where waste is removed by filtration

catalyst a substance that helps move a chemical reaction forward

cell the structural and functional unit of life

Centers for Medicare and Medicaid Services (CMS) 1500 a standardized form used in the medical office to submit insurance claims

channel a type of verbal or nonverbal method that may be used to convey a message

Chlamydiae a type of bacteria that multiply only within a host cell and have a unique growing cycle

chromatin the long, slender, filamentous threads that are the genetic material (i.e., deoxyribonucleic acid or DNA) in a nondividing cell

chromosomes rodlike structures that condense from chromatin in a cell's nucleus during mitosis

chronic infection an infection that lasts for a long time—sometimes for years or a lifetime

chronological filing a method in which patient information is filed with the most recent material of the medical record on top

civil law regulations concerning the rights of private citizens and the relationships between individuals

claims register also called an insurance log; a method of keeping track of claims submitted to an insurance carrier

clean claims insurance claims containing no errors, which are readily accepted and paid by the insurance carrier

closed files medical records that no longer needed (for example, those of deceased patients)

closed question an inquiry that requires only a one-word answer—yes or no

cocci spherical bacteria, including staphylococci, streptococci, and diplococci

coinsurance the percentage that an insured person pays once the insurance policy's deductible is exceeded, up to the policy's stop-loss

Commission on Accreditation of Allied Health Education Programs (CAAHEP) an agency that accredits medical assistants and other allied health programs offered by private and public postsecondary educational facilities

communication the exchange of information using verbal and nonverbal means

connective tissue a basic type of tissue that consists of cells within an extracellular matrix; includes bone, cartilage, and blood

consent agreeing to or giving approval

contract law a body of law established to govern agreements, either oral or written, between individuals

contributory negligence a type of affirmative defense that is one of the most common and effective types of defenses used in malpractice cases. The defense tries to show that the patient's behavior or negligence was partially responsible for the injury or complication that occurred, although the physician will admit to performing the procedure that led to the patient's injury.

coordination of benefits (COB) a system used by insurance carriers to avoid duplication of payments for the same service or procedure

co-pay a fixed fee paid by a patient for a visit to a medical office, for a medical procedure, or to have a prescription filled

cover letter a memo, usually sent with a resume, providing additional information explaining why the applicant feels he or she is the right person for the position being offered

criminal law a body of law that deals with crimes against society, such as murder or burglary

cross-reference a notation placed in one file area listing other areas within the file system where a specific piece of information may be found

customary fee the average fee charged by a provider in a specific geographical area for a specific service or procedure

cycle billing a once-a-month billing system that allows the office to divide the accounts into sections and then bill each section every so many days, which allows patients to receive bills on a monthly basis, but spreads the work out over a longer time period

cyst stage the dormant stage in the life cycle

cytoplasm gel-like fluid inside the cell

database (data bank) specific data collected and arranged for easy and fast searching and retrieval of information

day sheet the basic form that is placed on the pegboard and is used to record all transactions that are posted each day

decibels (dB) a unit used to measure sound level; also widely used in electronics, signals, and communication

deductible the portion of an insurance claim that is not covered by an insurance company

defendant the person being sued (as opposed to *plaintiff*)

defibrillator a specialized device used to deliver an electrical shock to a patient suffering from a life-threatening cardiac arrhythmia; an automated external defibrillator (AED) uses automated instructions and actions to help the individual perform defibrillation on the patient

deltoid the muscle over the shoulder joint

deoxyribonucleic acid (DNA) genetic material; a double-stranded polymer of nucleotides, each containing a phosphate group, a nitrogenous base, and the sugar deoxyribose

diabetic coma severe hyperglycemia in diabetics characterized by rapid respirations, warm, dry skin, thirst, and confusion

diagnostically related groups (DRGs) categories of diagnoses used in a hospital inpatient prospective payment system (IPPS); divided into 467 illness categories, with each illness attributed an ICD code; insurance reimbursement for medical care is based on the assumption that all patients in the same DRG category will experience the same symptoms and need the same care

digestion the breaking down of food into smaller components that the body can absorb

digestive system a system responsible for digestion of food via the mouth, esophagus, stomach, small intestine, large intestine, liver, and pancreas, so that nutrients from the food can be absorbed into the bloodstream and waste can be eliminated

diplomacy the skill of handling affairs without offending or insulting an individual; being sensitive and considerate when choosing the appropriate words to use in discussing issues with patients or coworkers

dirty claims insurance claims containing errors, which are rejected and will not be paid by the insurance carrier

disinfection the application of a cleaning substance to equipment, surfaces, or other items to kill pathogenic microorganisms

dislocation a separation of two bones where they meet at a joint

distal remote; farther from any point of reference; opposed to *proximal*

dosage the amount of a drug to be taken at one time

durable power of attorney for healthcare a document that names the person chosen to represent an individual (a healthcare agent) who will be the person to make the final decisions about the individual's end-of-life healthcare

dysphagia difficulty swallowing

electrodes sensors that are placed on the patient's arms, legs, and chest to pick up the electrical activity of the heart in an ECG

electronic claims transmission (ECT) an insurance claim submitted via the Internet

electronic health record (EHR) a record of the total care provided to a patient from all sources

electronic medical record (EMR) a computer-generated record of a patient's care from one source, such as a medical office, a hospital, or a pharmacy

elimination the method through which the body removes, or excretes, waste

emancipated minor an individual who has not yet reached the age of majority—in most states, 18 years old—but who is no longer under the care, supervision, or custody of his or her parents

empathy an understanding of another's situation; sensitivity to the needs of another person by putting oneself in someone else's position

enclosure notation a note added to a letter to indicate that other documents are being sent with the letter

encounter form also called a charge slip or superbill; an itemized account of the patient's visit, listing the procedures, diagnosis, and charges for the visit

encryption a software program designed to protect information from being read by unauthorized individuals

endocrine system a system responsible for integrating all body functions via the adrenal glands, gonads, pancreas, parathyroids, pineal, pituitary, thymus, and thyroid

endorsement a signature used to transfer a check legally to the bank in exchange for cash. In a medical office, a stamp marked "pay to the order of" listing the name of the bank where the deposit will be made, followed by the physician's name, is often used as endorsement.

enzyme a substance, usually made of protein, that catalyzes a chemical reaction—that is, helps to move the reaction forward

epilepsy a brain disorder that causes seizures

epithelial tissue tissue that covers all external and lines all internal body surfaces

Epstein-Barr virus the infection that causes mononucleosis

erythema a redness of the skin caused by congestion of the capillaries in the lower layers of the skin

ethics a set of values; the difference between right and wrong

excretion the elimination of waste products from the body

explanation of benefits (EOB) a report sent to the patient from his or her insurance carrier itemizing the benefits paid for services provided on a specific date

expressed consent a spoken or written agreement that provides consent; many times, a handshake is considered an expressed consent

external cause codes (E codes) codes classifying external causes of poisoning and injuries, and identifying medications; used to provide additional information and cannot be used alone

feedback the response given to the sender of the message

felony a serious crime that is usually punishable by prison time; may include actions such as murder, selling illegal drugs, or practicing medicine without a license

forced vital capacity (FVC) the maximum volume of air (measured in liters) that can be expired when the patient exhales as forcefully and rapidly as possible and for as long as possible

formaldehyde a powerful disinfectant gas

fornix arches or folds in parts of the anatomy, including the vault of the pharynx or the upper part of the vagina

fraud an intentional deception usually made for personal gain

fundus the interior surface of the eye, opposite the lens; includes the retina, optic disc, macula and fovea, and posterior pole

fungus a simple, single-celled organism, such as yeast, or multicellular colonies, such as mold and mushrooms

gait manner or style of walking

gamma glutamyl transpeptidase a liver enzyme

glycosuria glucose in urine

government insurance plan a government-run plan that is supported financially by tax revenues, and, in some cases, individual premiums; includes Medicare, Medicaid, TRICARE, and CHAMPVA

guarantor the person responsible for paying a medical bill

guardian ad litem a representative of the court used on behalf of a minor injured through negligence of medical care

glycemic index a scale that indicates the amount of time it takes a food to raise blood glucose levels

Health Insurance Portability and Accountability Act of 1996 (HIPAA) a law administered by the U.S. Department of Health and Human Services and enforced by the Office for Civil Rights that governs the rules and procedures that provide for the privacy and security of a patient's protected health information (PHI)

health maintenance organization (HMO) a type of managed care system that offers comprehensive healthcare to an enrolled group for a fixed amount of money

helminthes parasitic worms

hematuria blood in urine

heterophile antibodies the antibody found in individuals suffering from infectious mononucleosis

high density lipoprotein (HDL) a type of fat in the body known as "good cholesterol" because HDL removes excess cholesterol form the cells and carries it to the liver to be excreted

human chorionic gonadotropin (HCG) a hormone secreted by a fertilized egg; used in pregnancy testing

hypercholesterolemia high levels of cholesterol in the blood

hyperopia farsightedness

hypertriglyeridemia high levels of triglycerides in the blood

idiosyncratic effect an effect that is characteristic of a specific person

implied consent indirect acceptance, such as when an individual extends an arm to have his or her blood pressure measured

inactive file a medical record of a patient who has not been recently treated

incontinence the inability to control excretory functions, such as defecation or urination

independent practice association (IPA) a group of physicians in private practice who join together to treat members at a discounted fee or on a capitation basis

induration an abnormally hard, inflamed area

infant mortality rates the death rate of infants categorized by the infant's birth weight, mother's age, prenatal care, smoking and alcohol use during pregnancy, and mother's education

informed consent a written statement signed by the patient agreeing to the procedure or treatment recommended by the physician only after receiving a detailed explanation of the procedure to be done, the reasons for the procedure, the risks involved, complications that may occur, and any alternate methods of treatment that may be used instead of the procedure being discussed

ingestion the consumption of nutrients; eating and drinking

inguinal hernia a hernia in the groin

inpatient prospective payment system (IPPS) reimbursement system for hospital inpatients designed to contain healthcare costs; based on DRGs

insulin shock severe hypoglycemia in diabetics characterized by rapid heart rate, cold clammy skin, and confusion

integumentary system the skin and its accessory structures

intermittent occasional; not continuous

interrupted baseline a type of artifact that occurs when the electrical connection has been interrupted on an ECG

intradermal injection a shot of medication into the dermis, or deep layer of the skin

intramuscular injection a shot of medication into the muscle tissue

invoice a record of the charges for items or services delivered, which implies a request for payment; also called a bill

Joint Commission on Accreditation of Healthcare Organizations (JCAHO) an organization designed to improve healthcare in medical facilities

jurisprudence a department of law that deals with legal issues and decisions

ketonuria ketones in urine

ketosis a condition in which large amounts of ketones, the normal products of fat metabolism, accumulate in the tissues and body fluids

kinesics the study of body language

lancet a short, wide surgical knife

latent infection an infection with alternating periods of being symptomatic and periods of being symptom free

lead any of the conductors connected to the electrocardiograph; also, any of the records made by the electro-cardiograph

ledger cards cards (one per patient) that are used to record patient transactions, such as charges and payments, and to keep track of the balance a patient owes

leukocyturia an excess of white blood cells in urine

libel false written statements about an individual which may harm or damage his or her reputation

lipodystrophy a disorder in which the body's fatty tissue degenerates or otherwise becomes abnormal

living will a limited type of advance directive that takes effect when the individual is terminally ill

low density lipoprotein (LDL) a type of fat in the body known as "bad cholesterol" because an excess amount of LDL in the blood can cause plaque to build up on the arterial walls

lymphadenopathy any disorder of the lymph nodes or lymph vessels

macula an oval-shaped, yellow pigmented part of the human eye that absorbs excess blue and ultraviolet light

major medical insurance coverage for the most serious medical expenses or catastrophic illnesses

malfeasance a wrong or unlawful act

managed care a general term used to indicate lower-cost healthcare coverage

manipulation skillful use of the hands in diagnostic procedures

Material Safety Data Sheet (MSDS) a data sheet that contains basic information about a specific chemical or product

Mayo stand a wide metal tray used to hold sterile instruments and supplies

Medicaid a government-run insurance program providing healthcare to individuals regardless of age whose income is insufficient to meet medical expenses; also known as Title XVIX

medical asepsis the removal of pathogens and the reduction of the transfer of microorganisms through cleaning any body part or surface

Medicare a government-run health insurance program under Social Security, Title XVIII, that was started in 1965 for individuals who are either age 65 and over or under age 65 but disabled and unable to work

meniscus the curved surface on a column of liquid in a tube

mensuration the process of measuring the patient

message in the communication cycle, the content or information being transferred

metabolism (of a drug) the chemical breakdown of a drug to inactivate and eliminate it after the body has used it

metabolism the total of all biochemical reactions that take place in the body; includes anabolism and catabolism

microorganism a tiny plant or animal that cannot be seen with the naked eye; a "microscopic" organism

microscope an optical instrument consisting of one or more lenses that is used to magnify objects

minerals inorganic elements vital to a range of bodily functions, for example, structural components of tissue and cellular compounds, and as catalysts for enzyme activity

misdemeanor a crime that is less serious than a felony; examples include fraud or falsifying medical records

misfeasance improperly performing a legal act

modalities treatment methods

modifiers two-digit numbers used in coding to indicate specific circumstances about the procedure or service

monitor a screen used to view activity on the computer

morbidity the relative incidence of ill health or disease in a population

morphology codes (M codes) five-digit codes used mainly for cancer registries. The first four digits indicate the specific histological term, and the last digit indicates if the tumor is benign or malignant.

mortality the incidence of death in a population

motherboard a circuit board in a computer that allows all other parts in the computer to communicate with one another

mouse a handheld pointing device that controls the cursor of a computer

musculoskeletal system a system of the body consisting of bones, joints, muscles, ligaments, and tendons. Its function is to provide support and protection for the body's structures, as well as to allow for physical movement.

myocardial ischemia a decrease in blood flow to the heart, caused by constriction or plugging of the arteries supplying blood to the heart

myopia nearsightedness

nares nostrils

National Uniform Claims Committee (NUCC) a voluntary organization that was developed to institute changes in the claim forms used in the reimbursement process

nebulizer a breathing treatment with a bronchodilator (a medication to dilate the bronchi), such as albuterol, which is used for patients who have asthma symptoms

negligence the failure to use a reasonable amount of care, resulting in harm or damage to an individual

nervous system a system of the body consisting of the nerves, brain, and spinal cord, responsible for coordinating the reception of stimuli

networking the cultivation of relationships for business or for job searching

nonfeasance the failure to perform a required duty or obligation

nonpathogen a microorganism that does not cause disease

nonverbal communication the exchange of information without speaking words, but rather using gestures

normal flora microorganisms, including bacteria and fungi, normally occurring in or on an organ; also known as resident flora

nosocomial an infection acquired or occurring in a hospital among patients

nucleus the control center of the cell that directs all the cell's activities

Occupational Safety and Health Administration (OSHA) a federal agency involved with safety issues in the workplace

open-ended question an inquiry that requires the patient to give more than a one-word answer

ophthalmoscope a lighted instrument used to examine the interior of the eye

optic nerve a nerve that transmits visual information from the eye to the brain

optical character reader (OCR) a type of scanner that electronically transforms the address information on a letter into a bar code, which is placed at the bottom edge of the letter

otoscope a device that is used to look into the ears to investigate symptoms

oximeter a device that measures the oxygen saturation level in the patient's blood as well as the patient's pulse rate

palliative care medical care that aims to reduce the negative effects of the symptoms of a disease, but that does not aim to cure it

palpation the method of feeling with the hands to detect signs of disease

parasite an organism that must live inside another living organism in order to survive

parenteral in pharmacology, the introduction of medication into the body through routes other than oral, primarily injection

pathogen a microorganism that causes disease

patient advocates liaisons between the patient and the physician or healthcare provider

perception the method in which an individual sees a situation or another individual

percussion the method of tapping the body to detect signs of disease

pharmacodynamics the study of the body's biochemical and physiological response to a drug

pharmacokinetics the study of the action of drugs as they move through the body

pharmacotherapeutics the study of the use and effect of drugs in the treatment and prevention of disease

pinna the projecting part of the ear lying outside of the head

plaintiff a person initiating the lawsuit (as opposed to *defendant*)

pneumothorax a collapsed lung

point-of-service (POS) device a device that allows direct communication with the insurance carrier to verify the status of a patient's insurance coverage

point-of-service (POS) plan an HMO plan that allows the member to choose a physician from a list of physicians who have previously agreed to the discounted payment schedule

potentiation an interaction between two drugs that enhances the effect of either drug, producing a heightened response similar to an overdose

precordial leads chest leads

preferred provider organization (PPO) a managed care plan consisting of a group of physicians who agree to a predetermined pay scale for provided services

prejudice a predetermined conclusion or judgment without knowledge, thought, or reason, many times in a negative manner

presbyopia deterioration of near vision, commonly associated with aging

prescription an order to a pharmacist to dispense a supply of medication

private insurance (also called commercial insurance) healthcare coverage provided to individuals or groups (usually companies or associations) by private insurance companies

prophylactic drug medication taken to maintain health and prevent the spread of disease

protected health information (PHI) any information about the provision of healthcare, healthcare status, or payment for healthcare that can be linked to a particular person

proteins amino acids linked together in chains and branching arrangements, that are essential to the structural components of body tissues

proteinuria protein in urine

protozoan a single-celled parasite, worm, or insect

purging the process of appropriately disposing of information or files no longer needed in a medical office

radioimmunoassay a technique used to determine antibody levels

radiopaque dye a dye injected into patients to aid in the visualization of body parts; also known as a contrast medium

range of motion range in degrees of an angle through which a joint can be extended and flexed

reasonable fee the charge for an exceptionally difficult or complex procedure requiring more time and effort on the part of a provider

reference initials the abbreviated signature of the person who typed or keyed a letter

relative value studies a method created to develop a unit value for every medical procedure in order to develop a fair and accurate fee schedule

remittance advice a notification sent to the physician's offices that summarizes all the benefits paid to the provider for the claims submitted

reproductive system a system of the body consisting of the penis and testicles in men, and the ovaries, uterus, and vagina in women, that produces new life

res ipsa loquitur a Latin term meaning "the thing speaks for itself" when explaining negligent actions

resident flora nonpathogenic microorganisms that normally live on and in the human body; also known as normal flora

resource-based relative value scale (RBRVS) a formula used to calculate reimbursement amounts for various procedures, based on resources involved in providing services rather than on fees charged by providers in the past

respiratory system a system of the body consisting of the nose, pharynx, trachea, larynx, and lungs that brings oxygen into the body for transportation to the cells

respondeat superior a Latin term for the law that states that physicians are liable for the negligent actions of any employee working under the physician's supervision

resume, chronological a document that summarizes an applicant's background in reverse chronological order, meaning that the most recent information is listed first

resume, functional a document that emphasizes the most valuable experiences and skills that the applicant can bring to the job

resume, targeted a document written specifically for the advertised position, emphasizing the education and experiences that are directly related to fulfilling the expectations of this particular job

salutation the greeting of a letter; for example, *Dear Dr. Smith*

sanitization the removal of microorganisms using chemicals, heat, or ionizing radiation

screen saver an image that appears on a computer monitor when no activity has been detected for a time; used to protect the computer screen from burn-in

sensory system a system of the body consisting of the organs of sight, hearing, smell, taste, and touch that is responsible for sight, hearing, taste, and sensations

sequela a morbid secondary condition that occurs as a result of a less serious primary infection—for instance, a *sequela* of a streptococcal infection is rheumatic fever

shock a life-threatening condition related to inadequate oxygen supply

slander false, spoken statements about someone that may harm or damage the person's reputation

software a term that describes the programs that perform various tasks on the hardware

somatic tremor a muscle movement most often caused by patient discomfort, apprehension, talking, or uncontrollable body movement.

source-oriented medical record (SOMR) a method of record organization that files patient information according to the type of source, or subject matter, generating the information

speculum an instrument for opening a body orifice or cavity for viewing

sphygmomanometer an instrument used to measure blood pressure

spirometer a device that provides numerous measurements that help the physician assess lung functioning and help to determine the extent of pulmonary disease

splenomegaly the enlargement of the spleen

spores a hard, thick-walled capsule formed by some bacteria that contains only the essential parts of the protoplasm of the bacterial cell

sprain a stretching or tearing of ligaments within a joint

spreadsheets software programs used for organizing and computing numerical data and arranging the data in charts, graphs, and models for displaying statistical information for businesses

spriochetes long, spiral, flexible bacteria, which cause diseases such as syphilis and Lyme disease

staphylococci a type of cocci—that is, a spherically-shaped bacteria—that live in clusters on the skin and mucous membranes

statute of limitation the time period after an event in which a legal proceeding may be filed in a court of law

stereotype a generalized assumption of a group of individuals that can be either positive or negative

sterile field an area free of all microorganisms, pathogenic and nonpathogenic

sterilization the complete elimination of all microorganisms from a surface or instrument through exposure to chemicals, ionizing radiation, dry heat, gas, or steam

sterol any of a group of predominantly unsaturated solid alcohols of the steroid group, such as cholesterol and ergosterol, present in the fatty tissues of plants and animals

stethoscope an instrument used to study sounds in the body

strain a stretching or tearing of muscle or tendons

subcutaneous a shot of medication into the layer of tissue beneath the skin into the body's fatty layer

subjective symptom a symptom that is felt by a patient but is not observed by an examiner

sublingual the administration of medication under the tongue, where it will dissolve and be absorbed into the body

subpoena duces tecum an order to appear in court and bring any papers, books, or information necessary to explain in detail the issue in question

supplementary health factor codes (V codes) codes found in Volume II that include classification of factors that influence the health status of a patient

surgical asepsis the practice of destroying all pathogenic organisms so that none is able to enter the body

surgical scrub a type of hand washing that is designed to reduce the number of pathogenic microorganisms on the hands and forearms

sympathy the sharing of the same feelings with an individual; feeling sorry for someone

symptom any change in the body or its functioning that indicates a disease may be present

symptomatic having noticeable signs of disease

syncope a sudden drop in blood pressure or oxygen levels in the brain resulting in loss of consciousness; fainting

synergism a pharmacological property relating to how two drugs have a greater therapeutic effect when administered together than the expected effects of each drug alone

tachypnea abnormally fast breathing

teamwork a group effort to reach a common goal

telephone personality the tone, pitch, volume, and speed of speaking, as well as the warmth and friendliness that the medical assistant expresses when answering the phone and carrying on a conversation with a caller

third party someone other than the patient who is responsible for paying the patient's medical expenses or a portion of the expenses

tickler file a reminder system used to indicate that some type of action is needed on a particular file in the medical office

tissues groups of similar cells that perform a specialized function

tolerance the lessening of the desired effect of a drug the longer a patient uses it

topical medicine that is applied to the skin, through which the drug will be absorbed

tort law rules and regulations that deal with wrongful acts other than a breach of contract against another person, such as injury, libel, or slander

toxic effect the damaging cumulative effect of a drug that is not metabolized or properly excreted

traditional insurance plan health coverage that will reimburse the insured for a specific amount of money based on a fee-for-service schedule outlined in the insurance

transcription the preparation of accurate, formatted reports by converting dictated physician notes into written documents

transdermal the application of a drug through the skin

transient ischemic attack a brief and sudden decrease in the functioning of the brain, caused by a disturbance of blood supply to it

triage the screening of patients at medical facilities in order to treat the most seriously injured or the sickest patient first

TRICARE formally known as the Civilian Health and Medical Program of the Uniformed Services (CHAMPUS); a healthcare program designed and managed by the Department of Defense that provides civilian healthcare to military personnel and their families

triglyceride a component molecule of fat found in fatty foods

UB-04 form a document used for completing claims covering services such as inpatient admissions, outpatient procedures, and care in facilities such as psychiatric and alcohol clinics and nursing facilities

Uniform Bill 92 (UB92) the standard insurance claim form used by institutions

urinary system a system of the body that filters blood via the kidneys, ureters, urinary bladder, and urethra to remove waste and maintains the electrolyte and fluid balance within the body

urochrome the pigment in urine responsible for its yellow color; produced by the breakdown of hemoglobin

usual fee the average price a physician charges for a service or procedure

V codes (supplementary health factor codes) classification of factors that influence the health status of a patient; identify reasons for healthcare other than diseases or injuries

vasoconstrictor an agent that causes a contraction of the wall of the blood vessel

vasodilator an agent that causes an expansion in the diameter of a blood vessel

vector a carrier that transfers an infective agent from one host to another

ventricular fibrillation extremely abnormal heart rhythm

ventricular tachycardia (V-tach or VT) a rapid heartbeat, originating in one of the heart's ventricles of the heart

verbal communication the spoken word and the tone and inflections of the voice

virus a pathogen that can grow and reproduce only after infecting a host cell

vitamins organic substances found naturally in foods and needed in small amounts for metabolism and prevention of certain diseases

voucher a form filled out when minor expenses are paid using the petty cash fund, listing the date, the amount and reason for the expenditure, and the initials of the person taking the money

W-4 a tax form that new employees must complete, listing the number of withholding allowances claimed; more formally known as Employee's Withholding Allowance Certificate

waiting period a specified amount of time that must pass before a person's insurance coverage may begin

wandering baseline a type of artifact where the stylus gradually shifts away from the center of the paper on an ECG

warranty a guarantee by the manufacturer of a product or piece of equipment that the equipment purchased is free of any known defects

workers' compensation a type of insurance that provides an employee who has been injured or disabled in a job-related incident with coverage for medical expenses

z-track injection a modified intramuscular injection technique, in which the skin is pulled to one side and held while the needle is inserted at a 90° angle, leaving a zigzag needle track from the surface of the skin to the muscular layer

ADDITIONAL ONLINE PRACTICE ▶

Whether you need help building basic skills or preparing for an exam, visit the LearningExpress Practice Center! On this site, you can access additional practice materials. Using the code below, you'll be able to log in and take an additional practice test. This online practice will also provide you with:

- **Immediate scoring**
- **Detailed answer explanations**

- **Personalized recommendations for further practice and study**

Log in to the LearningExpress Practice Center by using this URL: **www.learnatest.com/practice**

This is your Access Code: **9247**

Follow the steps online to redeem your access code. After you've used your access code to register with the site, you will be prompted to create a username and password. For easy reference, record them here:

Username: _____   **Password:** _____

With your username and password, you can log in and access your additional practice materials. If you have any questions or problems, please contact LearningExpress customer service at 1-800-295-9556 ext. 2, or e-mail us at **customerservice@learningexpressllc.com**.

NOTES

NOTES

NOTES

NOTES

NOTES